Nurses in practice

A perspective on work environments

Nurses in practice
A perspective on work environments

Edited by

MARCELLA Z. DAVIS, RN, DNSc

Associate Professor-in-Residence, School of Nursing,
University of California, San Francisco

MARLENE KRAMER, RN, PhD

Professor of Nursing, Department of Social
and Behavioral Sciences, School of Nursing,
University of California, San Francisco

ANSELM L. STRAUSS, PhD

Professor of Sociology, Department of Social and
Behavioral Sciences, School of Nursing,
University of California, San Francisco

THE C. V. MOSBY COMPANY
SAINT LOUIS 1975

Printed in the United States of America

Distributed in Great Britain by Henry Kimpton, London

Library of Congress Cataloging in Publication Data

Davis, Marcella Zaleski.
    Nurses in practice.

    1. Nurses and nursing. 2. Nurse and patient.
3. Nurses and nursing—Study and teaching.
I. Kramer, Marlene, 1931-   joint author.
II. Strauss, Anselm L., joint author. III. Title.
[DNLM: 1. Nursing care. WY100 D263n]
RT42.D38   610.73   74-13232
ISBN 0-8016-1208-X

E/VH/VH 9 8 7 6 5 4 3 2 1

Contributors

CHARLOTTE F. BAMBINO, RN, PhD

Chief Clinical Nursing Researcher, Veteran's Administration Hospital,
San Francisco

PATRICIA BENNER, RN, MS

Associate Specialist on Anticipatory Socialization Grant, School of Nursing,
University of California, San Francisco

JEANNE QUINT BENOLIEL, RN, DNSc

Professor of Nursing, School of Nursing, University of Washington, Seattle

MARCELLA Z. DAVIS, RN, DNSc

Associate Professor-in-Residence, School of Nursing,
University of California, San Francisco

SHIZUKO YOSHIMURA FAGERHAUGH, RN, DNSc

Research Assistant, School of Nursing, University of California, San Francisco

RUTH FLESHMAN, RN, MS

Assistant Professor, School of Nursing, University of California, San Francisco

BARNEY GLASER, PhD

Professor-in-Residence of Sociology, Department of Social and Behavioral Sciences,
School of Nursing, University of California, San Francisco

HELEN GLASS, RN, EdD

Professor and Director of School of Nursing, University of Manitoba, Winnipeg, Manitoba

MARLENE KRAMER, RN, PhD

Professor of Nursing, Department of Social and Behavioral Sciences, School of Nursing, University of California, San Francisco

EVELYN T. PETERSON, RN, MA

Associate Professor, School of Nursing, University of Minnesota, Minneapolis

CATHERINE POPELL, RN, MS

President of Catherine Popell & Associates: Nurse Consulting Firm, Los Altos, California

LAURA REIF, RN, MA, MS

Doctoral Student in Sociology, Department of Social and Behavioral Sciences, School of Nursing, University of California, San Francisco

KAREN SCHOLER, RN, BS

Senior Nursing Student in Baccalaureate Nursing Program, University of California, San Francisco

ANSELM L. STRAUSS, PhD

Professor of Sociology, Department of Social and Behavioral Sciences, School of Nursing, University of California, San Francisco

Preface

This book, for students and teachers of nursing, is about the work of nurses in a variety of settings. A recurrent theme throughout is that work behavior—professional ideology notwithstanding—is greatly influenced by organizational and structural elements in each place of work, as well as by social and cultural features in the society at large. On the whole, the performance of all professionals is influenced by elements in the work environment and by developments in society in general. However, because of a variety of structural features characteristic of the profession of nursing itself, the work performance of the nurse would seem to be highly vulnerable to the influence of external elements.

One feature to consider is the relative lack of autonomy in some spheres of practice within the profession. Nowhere is this more evident than in the situation of the practitioner of nursing. Whatever autonomy the practitioner of nursing has is delegated through informal arrangements made among those with whom she works (for example, the physician) and not by way of any formal institutional fiat. A second feature is that the profession is comprised mainly of women; consequently, whatever attitudes about the role of women exist in society at large apply to nurses as well. A third feature is that a key value of the profession is the care of the whole patient rather than one segment. Today the practice of nursing, however, reflects less the care component of that value and more the coordination of the care components offered by a wide variety of other health professionals. The material throughout the book illustrates these and other features as they influence and in turn are influenced by a wide range of elements in the work environments of nurses.

The reader should be cautioned here that this material is not intended as a moral lesson on how nursing ought to be done or *not* to be done. Rather, since nurses occupy a primary position as providers of health care and the education of nurses is seen as a significant route to the improvement of that care, this material provides a point of departure for examining both. Thus, by looking at the performance of the nurse in work environments, we can begin to extract realistic guidelines for alterations in the education of nurses that would redound to the improvement in health care for patients.

Major portions of the material presented here are observations of nurses at work in such places as the intensive care unit, the pediatric ward, the emergency room, and the patient's home and neighborhood. These observations were made in the main by nurses who, while in the roles of participant-observer and nurse-researcher, observed other nurses at work. The observations appear in two forms: (1) as raw data; that is, they are presented here just as they were originally written up as field notes; and (2) as analyzed data; that is, the observations (raw data) have been analyzed and organized according to some conceptual scheme and written into a completed piece, as we see in the chapters on public health nursing and on chronic illness. Most of the field observations were part of larger ongoing research studies, such as research grants or doctoral dissertation, and only those parts relevant to this book were used.

Short of being in the actual environment, field notes provide a vivid picture of the situation under study. Therefore, we have purposely used raw data, first for their rich context and second to give the reader some idea of how fieldwork itself is carried out. Fieldwork involves not only observing and recording what people do and say; equally important, it is discovering who the people in the situation are, how they fit into the ongoing action and setting, and what meanings the observed persons themselves give to their behavior.

The field notes of the pediatric unit offer a good example of how the observer notes to himself what he sees, how he identifies who the observed persons are, and how he comes to learn what meanings to attach to what he observed. These pediatric unit field notes tell us that the researcher observed two nurses in "deep conversation." The identity of one nurse is easily established by the tag on her uniform reading "Head Nurse." The researcher inferred the identity of the second nurse from a variety of cues: for example, about her appearance, "She looked very tired, harried, and harassed"; the time of day, "It was 8:15 AM." Since this observer already knew that the night nurse was supposed to be off duty at 7:30 AM, she assumed (and checked out later) not only that this was the night nurse but that her late departure signaled that something was amiss. Further in the field notes we learn that during the night a child had died. The emergence of that piece of information begins to explain the observed tense interaction between the two nurses and the night nurse's late departure.

This vignette, as commonplace as it may appear, contains those elements that distinguish fieldwork as a research method from other methods of investigation. The fieldworker makes observations of behavior in its natural settings as opposed to observing behavior in artificially established settings. Since the fieldwork situation provides many more cues to what the observed action means, the opportunities for correction and refinement of observations are maximized. This method is in contrast to other research methods where meaning must be inferred from a single item of behavior, such as the answer to a questionnaire item or the response to an interviewer's questions.

Both the natural and social sciences—anthropology, zoology, geology, and so on—use the fieldwork method of research. These sciences take as their basic premise the idea that since there are constant transactions between the object and its setting, making each comprehensible only in the context of the other, the study must be conducted in the subject's natural surroundings. The tools used in the act of fieldwork are observation, participation, and written (field notes) and spoken (tapes) recordings. Through the use of these tools, the researcher attempts to provide as representative, comprehensive, and accurate a rendition of the situation under study as possible.

The aspect of fieldwork that requires observations to be made in the environment where the action normally occurs makes it most suitable for the study of nursing practice wherever it is performed. If one accepts the premise that behavior is influenced by environmental and cultural factors, it is obvious that to study the performance of a worker, one would need to observe him where the work is done. For example, the clinical situation as a locale of work is a highly complex environment, the study of which cannot be reduced to simple question and answer items on a questionnaire or interview form. Nor for that matter would setting up small group laboratory experiments get at the complexities of the ongoing transactions. A brief look at one aspect of this environment might illustrate the point. In the clinical situation multiple relationships are formed among persons of differing levels of authority, expertise, and status that constantly influence and play back on each other. For instance, the relationship between nurse and patient can easily affect the one between nurse and doctor; in turn, the doctor-family interaction is bound to play back on the nurse-patient relationship, and so on.

These relationships, complex as they may be, are but one dimension in the work context. Other factors, some widely discrepant, influence the interactions and in turn the work performance. The field notes on the intensive care unit vividly illustrate how the nurse's work is influenced by widely variant factors. At the one end may be the physician's order for minimal care of patients for whom the medical staff no longer hold any hope. At the other end—and having nothing in common other than their mutual influence on the work of the nurse—may be the inconveniently timed rotational schedules of residents and interns.

The nature of the patient's illness is an important dimension whose impact cuts across all work environments. Its significance for nurses derives less from a specific diagnosis but more from problems that confront patients, their families, and significant others when illness is prolonged indefinitely as opposed to when illness is successfully treated and of short duration. The material in the "outside" section is about these issues. They reflect in particular the low priority that the social and psychological problems of the chronically ill and other groups marginal to the mainstream of medical care have been assigned, not only by the nurses but by health professionals in general. Given the devalued status of this patient population,

ix

it should not be surprising to see in the material evidence of gaps in care and the socially isolating and psychologically demoralizing effects of no care.

Through the use of a variety of materials, this book provides a perspective for looking at and talking about the practice of nursing in the context of work environments. So that students might critically examine this material, questions are provided at the end of each entry; some are addressed to them and others to teachers. At the beginning of each chapter, an introductory passage discusses the material to follow and provides the reader with some immediate anchoring foci.

In the book's concern for the actual work of the nurse is the implicit conviction that the concepts of nursing practice must be empirically based. Only in this way can the realities and ideals of nursing be brought into a continuing and fruitful dialogue with each other. We sincerely trust that the book (but more so, what the students shall bring from it) will further this end.

Marcella Z. Davis
Marlene Kramer
Anselm L. Strauss

Contents

Nurses in practice

A perspective on work environments

part I

Inside the hospital

Many factors impinge upon what work is done and how work can be done—in fact, they determine the very nature of the work. In nursing, one of these primary factors is whether the patient or client is an inpatient or an outpatient. An inpatient necessitates and sets into motion a whole array of tasks that at worst become a substitute for the work of nursing and that at best often prevent or vie with nursing work for dominance. It is useful to think of the tasks required when a patient is housed within an institutional setting for protracted periods of time as hotel maintenance tasks. The patient not only must be "doctored" or "nursed," but because he must also be housed while undergoing these ministrations, he must have certain kinds of hotel functions available to him around the clock, such as restaurant, maid, telephone, newspaper, laundry, and mail service.

To accomplish these hotel-type functions as efficiently as possible, departments are created to fulfill specific tasks. For example, in a given patient area the maintenance department is responsible for seeing that the building is heated properly, the plumbing is working, and so on; the housekeeping department is responsible for keeping the unit clean; messenger service might be responsible for the delivery of supplies and pickup of outgoing mail. While each department has its specific tasks and functions, someone must coordinate these various services and functions and maintain the system in operation. This person must notify the housekeeping department, for example that a patient's bathroom needs to be cleaned, since maintenance was there to fix the plumbing.

To summarize, there are two sets of tasks that have implications for the nurses' work in an inpatient setting—in addition to the activities that are called "nursing." There are hotel-like functions, and there are system maintenance functions. Historically, these have all been included in the work of the nurse, due in large measure to what Hans Mauksch refers to as "continuity of time and space." The nurse is the only person who is there around the clock—24 hours a day, 7 days a

1

week. To her quite naturally falls the additional tasks of providing hotel-type functions and keeping the organization running. In many instances, these tasks have been so numerous and overwhelming that they have completely replaced or obliterated the work of nursing.

Currently there is much discussion about these two sets of tasks. It is generally recognized that both of them interfere with nursing. Ward manager systems, unit clerks, and stewardship programs represent but a few of the attempts being made to provide the hotel functions and to maintain the organization without the nurse having to do these tasks. The extent to which they are effective is still to be determined.

In the series of papers presented in this part, the reader will note that some of these hotel and system maintenance tasks are still being done by nurses. In some instances, the work appears to be willingly done and perceived as an inherent part of the nurse's function; in other instances, such as shown in Strauss's description of the nurses at PPI, a private hospital in Chicago, the managerial functions are a major source of role conflict for the nurse. Kramer's field notes on the head nurse at work on a medical unit of a large city hospital, and Fleshman's field notes on emergency ward nurses at work provide an opportunity to compare and contrast the nature of the nurse's work resulting from the patient's constant need for hotel-type services (medical unit setting) or intermittent need for these tasks (emergency room setting).

Closely related to this theme of the type of tasks demanded by the hospital organization is the opposite side of the coin—the primary function of the nurse as perceived by herself and others and as exemplified in her behavior. Is the nurse's primary function the coordination of hotel, maintenance, and care functions, or is her primary function that of "care-giver"? The first paper in this section, describing the head nurse at work, and the series of papers detailing the operation and functioning of nurses in the emergency ward provide an opportunity for the reader to assess the coordinative aspects of the nurse's work. Particularly revealing, and a provocative contrast study with respect to the care and cure functions of the nurse's role as perceived by nurses, are the papers describing the nurses at PPI and the nurses in intensive care unit and pediatric settings.

Another major determinant in understanding and analyzing the nature of the nurse's work stems from variables due to types of patient illnesses and the corresponding expectations of health professionals toward patients with these kinds of illnesses or health problems. There are at least three dimensions of importance in the type of patient illness. One has to do with the expected outcome of the illness—recovery or death or some state in-between. A second is concerned with the expected rapidity of change in the patient's state of health and the potential for controlling these changes, such as the degree to which the nurse can prevent the death of a patient who is in a highly labile state. The third dimension is concerned with the degree of social loss that the death or long-term disability of the patient represents to the health professional and to society at large. (A child, for example, generally represents a much greater social loss than an aged individual.) These dimensions in the type of patient illness and their effect in determining the nature of the nurse's work can be clearly seen by comparing and contrasting the descriptions of the nurse's work in settings such as the intensive care unit (ICU), pediatrics, and the emergency room; it can be seen most particularly in Quint's essay on the dying patient, Glaser and Strauss's excerpt on the perennial problem of caring for patients in pain, and in Fagerhaugh's description of potentially conflicting illnesses (tuberculosis and mental illness).

The type of illness and problem presented leads to a corresponding expectation of patient behavior. Previous experiences with patients having certain kinds of illnesses and presenting certain kinds of problems lead health professionals to expect specific kinds of behavior from the patient and to anticipate predictable kinds of patterns or trajectories of events. These subcultural expectations in large measure provide coping mechanisms for the nurse and other health professionals in dealing with the impact of high-stress situations. When patients, such as Mrs. Abel, the patient described in Strauss's analysis of the problem of pain, do not conform to these expectations, a series of subtle accommodating mechanisms can be perceived as nurses and doctors attempt to alter work or attitudinal patterns in order to bring about a greater degree of consonance. In addition to the Strauss excerpt on pain, this same kind of interplay can be noted in Fagerhaugh's description of the conflict in the care and treatment of phychiatric and tuberculosis patients.

Cultural differences between health care personnel and patients are evident in numerous instances in the articles in this section, particularly in the field notes on the head nurse on the medical unit and in the field notes on the nurses in the emergency ward. A difference in the way in which nurses handle these cultural differences is also noted. Is this because of differences in the backgrounds, training, personalities and life experiences of the nurses? Or is it possible that cultural differences are handled on a more individual basis in a more resident population than in a transient one? Is this a possible variable influencing the nature of the nurse's work in respect to this very important area of individual patient differences?

Values and attitudes associated with cultural and subcultural differences are learned—both prior to professional education and within the professional socialization process itself. If nurses and doctors behave as described by Fleshman, where do they learn this behavior? The conference notes of Benner seem to indicate that these are not the attitudes and values being taught to nurses in school. Benner describes an incident occurring with two students who were having clinical laboratory experience in the same emergency ward described in Fleshman's field notes. The students apparently were blocking the acquisition of the dominant values of the work setting—but at what price? And for how long would they be able to continue doing this after graduation, without the support of an empathic instructor?

3

One last theme that is prevalent throughout many of the papers presented in this section is the aspect of degree of professional autonomy and interprofessional control and collaboration. As previously noted, there are many structural deterrents to nurse autonomy. Other factors, such as intern-resident rotation schedules and rapidity of crises situations, appear to foster opportunity for nurse autonomy. The articles and field observations on the premature infant, the head nurse, and the ICU nurses particularly illustrate these points. Closely coupled with autonomy is the degree of interprofessional control and collaboration and the factors that inhibit or promote this aspect of the nurse's work. That this is one of the major deficits for nurse faculty when nurses are perceived and perceive themselves as "guests in the house" is clearly seen in Glass's description. The interaction between professional groups and the potential affect of these interactions on patient care is also demonstrated in the articles describing the work of psychiatric nurses in PPI, the care of patients with both tuberculosis and psychiatric problems, and the care of patients in pain.

The head nurse at work

The field notes presented in Chapter 1 are abstracted from a series of observations done over a 3-year period. The head nurse, Kelly Bye, was a participant in a 6-year longitudinal research study at the time these observations were done. The total set of observations consists of two formal interviews with Kelly—one in 1968 and one in 1970; 1 week of daily field observations in March of 1970; formal interviews with both Kelly's immediate supervisor and the Director of Nursing in June of 1968 and 1971; and 1 week of daily field observations in June of 1971. Throughout the field observations, informal field interviews were done as needed to clarify observations, obtain additional information, and so on. The same person did all the interviews and made all of the observations.

In this chapter, only 2 days in the work experience of nurse Kelly Bye are presented, but these notes should be sufficient for the reader to elicit patterns of behavior in her work as a nurse. It might be well to identify some of the structural and cultural restraints to Kelly's enactment of the nurse's role. These field notes provide opportunity and enlightenment into two particular organizational and social complexities: (1) nurse role autonomy—how it is exercised and what strategies the nurse uses to augment her autonomy, and (2) doctor (male) and nurse (female) role relationships and the effect of these relationships on medical and nursing care.

1. Field notes on the head nurse

Marlene Kramer, RN, PhD

Marlene Kramer, RN, PhD

Day 1–1970

I remembered Kelly Bye from my initial contact with her during the interview in 1969. She was about 25 years old, very attractive in a pixyish sort of way. She has short, curly, sandy-colored hair and is very lively. I walk fast, but I had to run to keep up with her! Kelly is vivacious, pleasant, talks easily, and gives one the impression of being well educated—she has a good command of English, expresses herself well, and speaks knowledgeably about things other than nursing. She is small in stature and almost wiry, moves quickly and with authority when she walks.

I checked in at the nursing office and called Kelly's floor from there—mainly because I wasn't sure I could find my way up to Ward B. As I walked into the nurse's station, Kelly looked up, saw me, and sort of smiled a bit. She was standing, literally, in the midst of four physicians. Two of them were housemen (I assumed this because they had on whites); the other two were visiting men. All were in the process of discussing the transfer of Mr. J. from Ward B to a nursing home. I quickly picked up that Kelly did not agree that the patient was ready to be transferred. She felt that it was too soon. The visiting physician, Dr. C., addressed Kelly in a somewhat jocular tone. "Oh, come now, Kelly, you know you are all just babying him around here." But also there was some respect in his voice and manner, because after a while he said, "Well, what makes you think he isn't ready?" Kelly answered that the patient's bowels were still impacted, that he was still having difficulty voiding, and that these things would not be corrected in the nursing home, because nursing homes were primarily for maintenance care, rather than for corrective care. Dr. C. raised his eyebrows and responded, "Well, what have you [meaning Kelly] been doing about these things?" Kelly told him about the enema and diet regimen being tried and the particular bladder schedule they had developed

6

for Mr. J. Dr. C. nodded approvingly, and after more discussion he said, "Well, maybe we should delay his transfer for a while and see what the nurses can do for him." That seemed to end it. Mrs. Bye gave him a few prescription blanks and said they needed more SSKI for Mr. J. and more of this and that drug for him. Dr. C. wrote out the prescription blanks. Then Kelly reminded him to cancel the order for the transfer to the nursing home, and to reinstitute previous orders. He did this, then smiled at her and said, "You really like that old man, don't you?" They exchanged a few pleasantries, and this particular conference broke up.

Throughout this dialogue I noticed that Dr. C. addressed Kelly by her first name, and my general impression was that this was a warm, friendly, collaborative conference that had some mutual trust and respect underneath it. I also had the impression that this was not the first time this had occurred.

As the group disbanded, Kelly turned to me and said, "Good morning," and smiled broadly. Dr. C. was about to leave the nurse's station; Kelly detained him by putting her hand on his arm and said, "Dr. C., I would like you to meet Dr. Marlene Kramer," and proceeded to introduce me. She said, "Dr. Kramer is conducting some research, and I am one of her subjects; she will be here all week observing me and the rest of the staff on Ward B." She said this without any kind of embarrassment. Dr. C. immediately responded and said, "Well, Kelly is a good one to study." He smiled, shook my hand, and wished me luck. Kelly then showed me where to put my purse and papers and asked me if there was anything in particular that I wanted to do. I explained that she should just go on about her regular work. She did not seem particularly ill at ease in any way. She introduced me to the nurses in the nurse's station in pretty much the same way as she had introduced me to Dr. C. She particularly introduced me to her ward secretary, whose name is Jo. She did this very warmly, with her arm around Jo's shoulder, and said, "This gal is my right-hand man. Without her I could not exist." Kelly then sat down and began to look at some charts on which the physicians had written orders. The ward secretary was posting the orders, but I noted very quickly that Kelly rechecked all the orders that the ward secretary posted. In one incident, apparently the ward secretary had omitted posting a particular blood test on one of the patients, and Kelly caught this. She asked Jo, "Did you think you had posted this or did you post this on a different chart?" There seemed to be no embarrassment or ill feeling between the two. The ward secretary said she thought she had posted it and proceeded to check all the other charts and found out she hadn't, so the error was remedied.

After a little while one of the physicians came up and requested the blood pressure record. It wasn't there, so the nurse who was pouring medications at the medication counter said, "Well, uh, it is not on the sheet yet." Kelly left the nurse's station, went down the hall to the right, located the nurse who was team leader, and apparently asked her for the blood pressure sheet. She walked so rapidly I couldn't keep up with her.

I should pause for a moment and describe a little bit more of the ward. This

7

medical-isolation ward had 23 patients. It was roughly divided at the nurse's station into two teams. Team One was on the left as you left the nursing station and consisted of 11 patient beds; Team Two was on the right and consisted of 12 patient beds. As I walked down the hall after Kelly, I noted very quickly that all of the patients appeared to be very ill. My basis for this inference was that as I passed the rooms and glanced right and left, there was a great deal of equipment in use—oxygen; it seemed almost every patient had an IV running; there was a circOlectric bed in one room; and a number of patients were on isolation (signs at the door and isolation cards outside). As I looked at the patients when I walked down the hall it seemed that at least half of them were comatose.

The physicians who had requested the blood pressure record were now in Mrs. M.'s room. Kelly had already gotten the blood pressure record and was in Mrs. M.'s room before I caught up with her. I stood at the door of Mrs. M.'s room. In the room there were a visiting man (I judged this by his suit), two interns or residents, Kelly, and the patient lying in bed. I didn't go in; I felt uncomfortable. I thought at first the reason I didn't go in was that the patient was on isolation, but it didn't take me any time at all to realize there was no sign on the door. I don't know why I didn't go in; I just stood at the door. After a few minutes, Kelly came out and said to me, "This is a very interesting patient; she has had a cardiac battery implant. Would you like to meet her?" I said, "Yes," and so I went in with her. When there was a break in the conversation between the patient and the physician, Kelly introduced me to both in almost identically the same way as before. The physician welcomed me, and the patient smiled broadly. I didn't catch anything on the faces of the intern and resident, because I was looking at the other two. Then they went on to discuss how the patient was feeling. There was an informal interchange between the visiting man and the patient; the dialogue was very pleasant, informal, and friendly. Kelly participated freely in the conversation, commenting on observations she had made or reminding the patient of questions she had said she wanted to ask the doctor. I was somewhat surprised at the amount of data being discussed directly in front of the patient, but including the patient. Different kinds of blood reports and the patient's results were presented. Kelly was the one who interpreted to the patient's what they meant, and the interesting thing (in fact, to me, it was startling!) was that the doctor would pause and wait for Kelly to do this interpreting. For example, the physician had asked Kelly what the patient's blood pressure was. She told him that Mrs. M. was slightly hypotensive and that her blood pressure was 90 over something, and then Kelly turned to the patient and explained to her that her blood pressure was a little bit low, that it is expected to be after this type of surgery, and that generally the blood pressure is a bit lower the first couple of days, particularly as you get out of bed. Mrs. M. nodded and said that her other doctor had been in earlier and had said that she could get out of bed if it were all right with this present physician, the one who was in the room now. The physician said, "Think it's okay, Mrs. Bye?" Kelly nodded and said to the patient, "Now you must remember that since your blood pressure is somewhat low you best not get

out of bed without calling us and having one of us here when you get out of bed."
Then she went on and explained how sometimes with low blood pressure you could
feel faint and dizzy and weak. The physician said, "Yes, it is very important that
you call the nurses," and reinforced what it was that Kelly had said. (I was rather
amazed at their collaborative interchange; it's frequently what nurses desire, but I
haven't seen it happen that much! I didn't have any feeling that any of this was put
on. I had a feeling that this kind of interaction was fairly routine.)

The patient and the physician discussed a few other things—bowels, and
stitches, and things of this type—and then the doctor walked out, followed by the
intern and resident. Kelly and I stayed. Kelly had been standing at the foot of the
bed, and as the physician left she moved in and stood directly next to Mrs. M. She
put her hand on Mrs. M's arm and repeated her instructions that Mrs. M. was not to
get up without help. Then she said to Mrs. M., "You look as though you are feeling
kind of blue this morning." Tears welled up in Mrs. M's eyes almost at once, and
she said, "Yes, I thought I would be feeling better by now." At this Kelly
responded, "You're still a little dizzy?" Mrs. M said, "Yes." Kelly said, "You aren't
having any more pain are you?" The patient said, "Oh no, not at all like it was
before the surgery," and then she just repeated, "I thought I would be feeling
better by now." Kelly said, "Do you mean anything other than the fact that you're
still dizzy and weak?" The patient said, "No, that is what I mean." Kelly then sat
down on the bed and took the woman's hand in her hand and went on, in the most
beautiful way I have ever heard, to describe exactly what the surgery was. (I wish I
would have had the tape recorder there so I could repeat it word for word) and how
the implant was done, and she explained that it would be 6 to 10 days before the
battery could be hooked up. I was watching the woman's face during this
explanation, and she had the most trusting look in her eyes. I don't know whether
the woman felt better afterward, but it was apparent to me that she was physically
more relaxed. I noticed her other hand, the one that was lying on the bed. It had
been somewhat clenched before; in fact, I had noticed that her hand was clenched
all during the discussion with the physicians, but now it began to open up and was
just lying there in a very relaxed position. The furl in her forehead was also
smoothed. She was still smiling (she had been smiling before), but now she
generally looked much more relaxed. She lay back in bed and patted Kelly's hand
and said, "Thank you, dear." Kelly and I left.

When we returned to the nursing station, the team leader on Team Two was
there, and Kelly immediately told her that Mrs. M. could get up but that it was very
important that someone be with her the first couple of times because her blood
pressure was low, and that the team leader should be sure to look and see if the
blood pressure was dropping any as Mrs. M. got out of bed. The team leader then
asked Kelly if she had noticed that Mrs. M. was sort of "two-faced." One of the
LVN's chimed in and said that she had noticed it. Kelly asked Vickie (the team
leader) what she meant by two-faced. "She's smiling at you, but if you turn around
quickly, she looks tearful and depressed," said Vicki. "Or sort of wistful," said the

9

LVN. Kelly then said yes, she had noticed it, but that she hadn't thought of it as being two-faced, but rather that the patient was always trying to be cheerful. There then followed a 10-minute discussion during which these three discussed the patient's behavior and decided how and what they would do about it. I particularly watched the interactions during this discussion, rather than following the content. First of all, there didn't appear to be a leader per se; all addressed each other by first name, and all reported on observations they had made and corrected what they thought were erroneous opinions or conclusions of others. They were interrupted at least three times (phone, people coming into the station, lab technician, and so on) during the discussion—and Vicki was pouring some of her 9:00 AM meds during this—but the amazing thing was that they always got back to Mrs. M. It was a viable discussion about a very real problem, and like a dog with a bone, no one let go until they were satisfied.

In general, I must say that everyone on this unit seemed to be on a first name basis, including the physicians. Kelly called some of the physicians by their first names, some she addressed by the surname. There had been a steady procession of physicians all morning. Some of them went about their own business and didn't say anything to Kelly or the nurses; others made it a point to talk with her. (In between all this, Kelly was checking the charts that Jo had done.) Kelly addressed almost everyone who came into the station by either their given name or their surname. She didn't rise for the physicians, but she did make some effort to hand them their charts.

Some time had elapsed during which Kelly continued to check the charts that Jo had done. Sometimes, Kelly didn't wait for Jo to take the orders but did them herself. There didn't seem to be any pattern regarding which ones she did and which ones she left for Jo—I thought at first that it depended on who the patient was, but as I watched longer, it seemed much more happenstance—whichever chart just happened to be lying in front of her. During this period, the amount of activity on this ward and in and around the nurses' station would be enough to boggle the mind of a field marshall! The interruptions—personal and phone—were almost continuous. For the most part, Kelly ignored the phone and had Jo answer it, but virtually all personal contacts were made with Kelly.

In the course of a half hour, there had been eleven physicians on this floor, not to mention several house officers, and numerous interruptions from the various staff members. There was also a constant stream of interruptions from x-ray, lab, and EKG technicians, and also from family members. Kelly's manner with the latter came across to me as friendly and sincere. She went out of her way to get them coffee, sugar packets, and so on. One thing I noticed was that she always got up and approached them. This style was different from that with staff members, physicians, or other hospital personnel. Here, her manner was light and informal, friendly, but with only a small amount of bantering. In fact, I was somewhat struck by the lack of bantering observed on this ward. It was much less than I expected. People were friendly and informal, but quite serious. The moments of levity were

10

very brief and seemed to be restricted to one or two comments, but they did reveal past knowledge and off-the-ward contacts. For example, one of the doctors, with a twinkle in his eye, asked Kelly how she thought George had fared in the bedroom the other night. Kelly's eyes crinkled, and she retorted, "I bet a good time was had by all." And that was it. Both immediately got down to business, discussing the patient, and so on. (Perhaps it was my presence on the ward.)

The only other general thing I will say about interactions is that Kelly seemed to adopt a definite teaching posture with the staff—this posture was directive—I wanted to say somewhat condescending but I have no data to support that. Here's an example: Vicki was discharging a patient to a nursing home (not the same patient as was discussed earlier) and was writing on the summary record a description of the patient and care plan. When she had finished, she showed it to Kelly for approval. Kelly read it, said, "Fine," and handed it back. Then Vicki said, "Oh, I forgot to put in about the condom catheter," and picked up the pen to write. Kelly said, "Oh, no, don't put in about that. He is so proud of himself when he can use the urinal; don't put in about the condom. They'll put that on him right away, and then he'll never have a chance to have some control over his own bodily functions." Vicki nodded her head in agreement. Then Kelly said, "You know, maybe we should call them about that, and explain to them why it's so important to give him a chance." Vicki, Kelly, and later, another nurse came into the station—and a little bit later, one of the house officers—and before I knew what was happening, an impromptu conference was being held on the subject. Would it do any good to call, why was it important, and so on. The intern or resident, in particular, asked lots of questions as to what nursing homes were like, what went on there, and what kinds of patients were sent to nursing homes and which to their own homes with visiting nurses and so on. This was the second one of these informal, impromptu conferences I had now seen held—actually there had been more than two if you counted the ones just between Kelly and the physician, but only two that involved more than two people. It seemed to me that in a way, these conferences accomplished in short order what is usually done in more formal team conferences. Anyway, the outcome of the discussion was that Vicki got on the phone with the nursing home, and the intern got on the extension to listen in and ask questions and also make comments. (Again, I want to say that this impromptu discussion was also interrupted several times. People were either diverted, they joined the discussion, or else they received a brief answer from Kelly, and she rejoined the discussion.)

Kelly had returned to taking off orders again. She took care of drugs for home-going patients, she took care of a pneumoencephalogram test, she phoned the social worker to make arrangements for some patients, and after a while she asked if I wanted to go to coffee. At coffee Kelly talked mostly about her private life.

Shortly after we got back from coffee, Kelly said she was going to begin rounds and asked if would I like to join her. We went into Mr. R.'s room. Mr. R. was a Caucasian, about 40 years old, and he had Hansen's disease. His leprosy was quite far advanced. He had neither hands; both were just sort of stumps, although the left stump had an indentation where he could hold a pencil. His color was rather pale and sort of gray looking. He certainly didn't look the picture of health, and there was a characteristic odor about the room. Kelly welcomed him very jovially. She did not gown or carry out isolation techniques when she approached him. She put her arms around his shoulders and asked him if he were ready to go to surgery. Mr. R.'s face was grotesquely misshapen. I'd say there was a smile on his face, but unless I had seen Kelly's smile in response to his, I would never have known it was a smile. One half of his face was sort of eaten through by the leprosy, and he was almost just a caricature or a shell of a human being. In a guttural response he said, "Yes, I am looking forward to it and can't wait until it's over with." I was overcome with my own feelings at this time and was disgusted and ashamed of myself at the same time. I had awe, respect, and also fear for Kelly; I had never been as close to a leprosy patient as this before. Although I know it is not highly contagious, I am afraid of the whole idea, of personal and intimate contact, and was quite repelled by the sight of this poor man. Kelly did not introduce me to Mr. R., nor did he even seem to recognize my existence in the room. Kelly told him that people from surgery were there and ready to take him, and so she helped the surgery people get him on the cart. As we left the room, I realized that although I had these other feelings, I was not uncomfortable being in the room, even though neither Kelly nor Mr. R. acknowledged my existence. (I wondered if a number of people sort of came into the room and looked at Mr. R. and if he were sort of accustomed to being "looked at." I didn't know; I would have to check this out.) But anyway, as he went to surgery and we left the room, I asked Kelly what he was going for. Kelly related that he had been a resident of the leprosarium out at White City for something like 15 years and that he had his own business and took care of his own accounts. He was able to write with the stump of his hand. He was going to surgery because one of the things he wanted to be able to do was to eat, and to eat food, he had to chew. He had a pair of false teeth, so now he was going to surgery to see if they could reconstruct his mouth so that he could use his false teeth and be able to eat.

I also talked to her a little bit about whether leprosy patients were common on the ward and found out that they were quite common. If any patient with leprosy were coming to the hospital, they would come to her ward, and they almost always had one or two patients with leprosy on the ward. There were also a number of standbys as she called them—patients who repeatedly came to their ward for care of some type or other.

Kelly stopped to see a few more patients (I retreated to the bathroom to take notes), and then we met back at the nurse's station. In the meantime, some other physicians apparently had been in, because there were a number of charts lying on the desk, and Kelly went through them and began to check again the orders that the ward secretary had posted. Kelly seemed to spend a good deal of her time checking on the orders that the ward secretary posted. Sometime I would have to check with her and find out why this was.

During the entire course of the morning, the phone had rung very frequently, but Kelly had only answered the phone personally three times. The first time, it was some physician requesting the prothrombin time on a patient; the second time, it was to take a message regarding some overtime for the staff; and the third time, it was a personal call for her. The majority of the time when the phone rang, even if Kelly was at the desk, she ignored the phone and had the ward secretary answer and take care of it. So, in actuality, the time that Kelly was at the desk was apparently spent checking orders that the ward secretary had posted or giving or receiving information from other personnel. (Four additional days of field notes followed this day but are not included here.)

Day 2–1971

It was now almost 1 year later—June 21, 1971, and I was going back to Mercy Hospital to continue my observations of Kelly and her staff. I had several goals in mind. First of all, I wanted to see if there was consistency in my field data—perhaps this was as much to convince myself of the reliability of the data as it was to see if Kelly's behavior was consistent. (I guess maybe I'm still too much quantitatively oriented.)

Kelly, however, could and would be a different nurse now than when I saw her a year ago. At that time she was a new head nurse, having been in the position for about 3 months. By this time, she should have had sufficient opportunity to operationalize her goals as much as she was going to be able to do.

I also realized that I had formed some tentative hypotheses about this nurse and her performance. My 5 days of field notes from last year show her as a nurse who is a collaborator with physicians, as a teacher and leader of her staff, as a nurse who seems to enjoy and who *gives* direct patient care, and as a nurse who spends a great deal of time checking the ward secretary's posting of orders. She is an individual who is goal oriented and who assesses her progress toward her goals. She is actively involved in the maintenance of the organization, but at the same time, she disregards some of the rules and regulations of the organization—apparently with impunity. How does she accomplish this? Other tentative inferences: Kelly generally seems to have control and influence over her staff, but there is some difficulty and perhaps jealousy with Shirley. Kelly's concern and involvement with patient care is focused mainly and almost solely on the patient alone, which seems incongruent with her other values and beliefs. In many ways she seems to encapsulate many of the current ideals of comprehensiveness and continuity of patient care promulgated by nurse educators, but her lack of family inclusion is inconsistent. Why?

The above observations and tentative inferences led to another goal of these follow-up observations, and that was to check out these inferences and look for negative instances that would help in confirming or negating these hypotheses.

•   •   •

I had written to Kelly and the Director of Nursing several weeks in advance to reinstitute the field study, make arrangements, and so on. No difficulties here;   **13**

Kelly responded in a warm, friendly, personal letter, and I also received a more formal letter from the Director of Nursing. I checked with Kelly to ascertain how much of the work situation and personnel would be constant over my two observations. (Actually, I found this out before I decided to make the second set of observations.) Factors and personnel that would be the same: Kelly Bye, was head nurse on Ward B; Vicki was now the charge nurse (Margie having been promoted to head nurse on another unit). Jo was still the ward secretary, and Shirley, a three-year RN, was still a staff member on the unit. One of the nurse aides was the same, as was one of the LVN's. Several of the evening and night RN's were also the same as last year. Major differences between this year and last: the kind of patients serviced by Ward B had been changed from medical-isolation to straight medical; Margie, the charge nurse whom Kelly admired and respected very much was gone, replaced by Vicki, who was Kelly's choice; several weeks after this field observation, Kelly and about half of her staff would be opening up a new Medical ICU on Ward 3, the new wing of the hospital.

I arrived on Ward B about 8:15 AM —it looked pretty much the same as it had the last time I was here except that it was less cluttered. There weren't as many bedside stands with isolation material sitting in the hall. I found out subsequently that the reason for this was that the isolation patients had been moved from this ward. So this ward was now a 23-bed unit for chemotherapy, hematology, and general medical patients.

As soon as Kelly saw me, she recognized me (and I recognized her—thank heaven!). One of the first things that was obvious was that they were very busy that morning. There were about four or five doctors around a respirator in the hall, the desk was stacked with charts, and the nurses were bustling to and fro. Kelly said something about being with me in a moment and kept on with what she was doing. I sort of stood off to the side and watched. (Much to my surprise I was not feeling too uncomfortable. The surroundings were very familiar and I found that I even recognized some of the physicians.) What she was doing was admitting a patient who was a GI bleeder. He had apparently come to the ward about 2 or 3 minutes before I arrived and was actively bleeding, so she was quite involved in this. She drew blood for a pro time (I wonder why she did it, since the physician was standing right there), helped to change the patient's bed (he had a copious black, tarry stool), and then participated in a discussion between the physician and the patient's wife. (There were no interns or residents on the unit—I wonder why?) After this, Kelly gave a quick report on this patient to Sandra, and then she turned her attention to me, welcoming me, and so on. "Just make yourself at home," she said, which again made me feel very, very comfortable. Just about this time, a bevy of doctors appeared on the scene (there were already three or four in the nurse's station), and I thought that this might be a good opportunity to particularly zero in on Kelly's relationships with the physicians. One of the things I was going to particularly note was the quality of the relationship—whether it was a social

14   relationship, whether it tended to be more a master-servant relationship, or whether

it was a true colleague relationship. The first physician who approached Kelly was the private physician of the patient who had just been admitted—the GI bleeder. He asked Kelly to get the intern up there, and Kelly told him that the team service was closed. The doctor said, no, it ·wasn't and that he wanted an intern to work up this patient. (A little background on this situation—this [June 21] was toward the end of the intern rotation. As of the following week, the interns would be going off and the new group coming on.) The private physician was a little put out that the team service was closed, and he fussed at Kelly about it. She got on the phone, checked downstairs, and told the doctor, "It's closed." He frowned angrily, grabbed the phone from her, said a few words, and the next thing that happened was that the patient was on the team service and the intern was subsequently notified. (This relationship seemed rather of the master-servant type to me.)

The next physician who came up was a younger man—about 40. He greeted Kelly, and one of the first things he said to her was, "What do you think of Mr. Robello, Kelly?" Kelly responded, "He doesn't seem to be getting any better; he seems quite depressed and doesn't have much appetite." The doctor asked her if the patient was on cortisone, and Kelly responded, "Yes, he is," and gave the doctor the dosage and schedule.

A few other physicians approached Kelly; most of them addressed her as Mrs. Bye. She addressed the physicians by name, and most of the interchanges had to do with transmissions of orders or explanations of orders to increase a patient's medication or to send him down to x-ray, or something of this type. Finally, another young physician came along and greeted her with an open embrace that was returned; it was obviously a warm, social relationship. This physician asked Kelly about Mr. M.—a 46-year-old Japanese man who had been brought in over the weekend with a possible subdural hematoma. The physician had talked to the PT and OT departments about working with the patient. At this, Kelly raised her eyebrows and said, "Isn't that pushing it a little?" The doctor looked thoughtful and said, "Maybe so. Let's go see him." Kelly went into the room with the physician, and I trailed along right after them. Kelly did not introduce me to the doctor or give him any indication of who I was or what I was doing. He looked at me a couple of times, and I did feel somewhat uncomfortable about this, but the time was just not appropriate for me to explain. The physician stood on the left-hand side of the bed, Kelly was on the right, and I stood at the foot. Mr. M. lay sort of crisscross on the bed, and he really looked bad. He had an IV running. His color was ashen, and he was quite lethargic. He was only sort of half covered, but the day was quite warm; he didn't look as though he were chilled. The physician did a neural check on him, and even at the foot of the bed I could see that there was very little response. The man seemed to be completely paralyzed on the left side. His eyes would not deviate to the left at all. He could barely talk or respond even when stimulated. He responded with his right hand by squeezing the doctor's hand, but not with his left, and it was obvious that the doctor was becoming more and more concerned and worried as he was examining him. The physician looked **15** up at Kelly and asked, "Is he on any sedation?" Kelly told him the medication he was on and when the last time was that he had had a dose. Kelly didn't volunteer any more information; in fact, during this entire inspection of the patient, Kelly just stood there, except that after the examination she and I repositioned Mr. M. in bed and covered him with a sheet. (In retrospect, I don't know what else I would have expected her to do; maybe I was going overboard looking for negative instances.) As we left the room, the doctor commented to Kelly that he really looked much worse than he had yesterday, and Kelly agreed but didn't volunteer any additional information or observation. The physician sat down and started going through the chart. He looked at the temp chart and immediately commented on it, wheeling his chair around so that he could show it to Kelly. "He's been spiking a temp periodically," he said in sort of a surprised tone. I got the impression in terms of his body movement and in terms of his tone of voice that this was something he didn't know and would have expected Kelly to have pointed out to him. I was disappointed that she did not respond. She asked no questions and offered no kind of supporting information. Earlier it seemed to me that she had had an open, friendly, social relationship with this physician. I wondered why she was now so reserved and unresponsive.

Other physicians were coming up to the desk and usually handing Kelly a record; some of them commented to her and some didn't. I would say that in a period of 10 to 15 minutes there were at least eight private physicians on the floor. The private physician who was admitting the GI bleeder told Kelly to be sure to have the doctor see the patient—this was a consultant—and that he wanted her to call him the pro-time at his office. Much to my surprise, Kelly suggested a stat CBC on the GI bleeder; the doctor agreed and ordered it. (Wow! This was confusing! This doctor treated her like a "dog" [do this, do that], yet she made suggestions to him. The other guy seemed to be "sweet on her" and she didn't even give him *obvious* information!) A little bit later, a relative of the man who was the GI bleeder came into the nurse's station and asked the doctor if the patient might have some water. The doctor addressed Kelly and said that the patient could have a little water. Kelly got up, went in, and gave it to the patient.

At this point, which was only about an hour since I had arrived, Kelly had been in to see two patients—the GI bleeder and the patient with the subdural hematoma. She had seen the GI bleeder twice. On both occasions she had given active personal care to him.

I sat at the desk for awhile checking the orders that the ward secretary, Jo, had posted. (To review the procedure: the physicians ordered things; the ward secretary filled out the forms, requisitions, and so forth, put them in the charts, and then slid the charts over to Kelly. Kelly checked on the accuracy of the ward secretary and this sort of thing and then routed the slips on their way.) I was checking the charts before Jo slid them to Kelly to see if I could figure out why Kelly spent so much time doing this.

As Kelly was checking charts, Sandra came up to her and asked if Kelly would come and look at her patient. Kelly agreed, and both Kelly and Sandra, before they left the nurse's station, went briefly to the Kardex on this patient. (I wondered if they were both looking for the same thing?) I made a mental note to ask Kelly about that later, but at any rate, both Sandra and Kelly checked the Kardex for a few minutes; then Kelly took a thermometer and stethoscope and went with Sandra to look at the patient. I followed along behind them. One of the first things that I noticed was that as Kelly walked into the room, she had a marked frown on her face. (That certainly would increase my apprehension, if I were a patient.) Sandra walked into the room first, went to the right-hand side of the bed, and stood between the bed and the wall window. Kelly stood next to her, and I stood at the foot of the bed. The first thing Kelly did was to address the patient by name. She took the patient's hands, squeezed them a little bit, and immediately took the patient's pulse.

Let me stop a moment and describe the patient. This was a 50-year-old Japanese or Oriental woman with a very tightly pinched face and very loud, labored respirations. It was really hard to understand how her wheezing could become that severe without any lead-up to it, and it made you wonder why it wasn't noticed earlier. Sandra said that she had noticed the wheezing when she came in to give the patient her medication. (There was another RN who had been bathing this patient.)

The patient was becoming cyanotic, and it definitely sounded as though her lungs were very, very full. She was coughing and sounded as though she were drowning in her own fluids. Her fists and hands spasmotically clenched and opened, and she was picking nervously at the bed covers every now and then. She pulled out paper tissues and tried to cough and spit up into them; meanwhile it was very evident that she was fighting for breath. (This patient was fighting so hard for breath that I found that my own respirations were becoming labored and that I was sort of trying to breathe for her.) One of the other things I noticed immediately was that the bed was only elevated about 10 degrees. (I was fighting with myself to keep from raising it. If someone didn't do it soon . . .) Well, almost immediately after Kelly had taken the pulse, she helped the patient into a sitting position. (To be accurate, this was probably done within a minute or so after we had entered the room.) Kelly then listened to the patient's chest in the back and in the front; then she took the patient's blood pressure. While she was doing these things, Kelly's manner, voice, and tone were gentle and reassuring. One hand was almost continually stroking or patting the woman's shoulder. But, she was frowning severely the whole time, conveying, at least to me, that she was very concerned and worried about the patient. Kelly asked the patient a few questions—what was she doing immediately before the attack? (Eating breakfast.) Had she taken much fluid with her breakfast? (Her usual, juice and two cups of tea.) Had this ever happened to her before? (No.) Following this, Kelly inspected and palpated the neck of Mrs. Y. a bit (neck veins were obviously distended), and then without a word to the patient, she mumbled to Sandra that she would call the doctor, and left the room.

As we were going down the hall, I asked her if the patient's blood pressure had

17

been a problem. She said, yes, it had been high, but that this time she couldn't hear it very well because of the wheezing. The blood pressure was 130/90.

Kelly located the intern almost immediately and got him in to look at the patient. She went immediately to the nurse's station and began to draw up some Adrenalin. She didn't have an order for this yet; she just figured that this is what would be needed. (I checked this out with her later.) Kelly went back into Mrs. Y.'s room, showed the intern the Adrenalin, checked the dose with him, and administered the drug. Sandra was still in the room with the patient, but didn't appear to be particularly alert to the situation. She was straightening the bedcovers, putting the room furniture in order, and clearing up the basin, bedside stand, and so on. Kelly said, "I'm going to see if I can find another pillow so that we can sit Mrs. Y. up more." She told Sandra to stay with the patient. Meanwhile, the physician had completed his wordless examination of the patient and had left the room. (The intern was a young, sloppily dressed fellow, with the gangly awkwardness characteristic of adolescence. He looked tired and groggy, although he had only been on duty for about 2 hours. His reactions were a bit slow; I was singularly unimpressed by his speed and diagnostic ability, particularly for an intern who was within days of completing his internship.)

Kelly was out at the nurse's station drawing up some aminophylline for Mrs. Y. The intern was looking through the patient's chart. When Kelly finished, the intern took the medication and said he would give it IV push in the IV tubing. He looked quite quizically at Kelly as if to get her approval, and she nodded, "Yes." (Kelly and this intern were about the same age, but the intern definitely appeared to be looking to Kelly for direction. Kelly did not treat the intern with any particular measure of respect. She was not rude to him, but she didn't particularly respect him either. I confirmed this by asking Kelly later.)

We were back in the room. Kelly was standing on the left side of the bed; I was at the foot; the doctor was on the right side. Shortly after we entered, Sandra left. While the intern was administering the aminophylline, Kelly was standing there with her hands at her sides and a marked frown on her face. (I was wondering why she didn't make any attempt to establish touch or voice contact with this patient who was obviously extremely apprehensive. She's very good at this; I've seen her do it so often before.) All was silent for about 3 minutes, and I was getting terribly uncomfortable. Besides, it was very hot in this room, and the air conditioning was off. I was thinking that with the labored breathing, Mrs. Y. must also be very hot.

Finally, the "silent" intern, in rapid staccato-type questions (that Mrs. Y. had little breath to answer that rapidly) began to elicit a history. The general nature of his questions suggested immediately that he was thinking that Mrs. Y. was having an allergic reaction of some type. He asked Kelly what medications the patient was on, whether she had anything new, whether she had received any albumen that morning, and so on. In addition to asking Kelly these questions, he also asked the patient the same questions. Mrs. Y. just rolled her eyes and looked at Kelly, continued wheezing, and didn't say anything. (I checked with Kelly later—when she checked the Kardex before going into the patient's room the first time, she was looking to see if the patient had been placed on any new drugs. I checked with Sandra, also; she was looking for an elevated temp, but couldn't explain to me why.) The intern continued to pursue this allergic theme—looking for rashes, and so on. Kelly pointed out the distended neck veins to him, and mentioned the quantity of fluid the patient had had IV in the previous 24 hours, but there was no visible evidence that this had registered with the physician. Soon, the doctor left the room without a word to anyone.

At this point, the patient asked Kelly to button the front of her gown, which was open, exposing her breasts and large, protruding abdomen. As difficult as it was for this woman to breathe, she was very concerned about her modesty. There were so many small nursing comfort measures that could have been done; I wondered why Kelly seemed oblivious to them. On previous occasions, I'd seen her give a great deal of attention and focus to them. Now, she seemed to be completely wrapped up and attuned to only the diagnostic and therapy problem and getting through to this intern. It was also noticeable that Kelly was very concerned and worried about the GI bleeder patient because she made frequent forays into his room—in fact almost everytime we passed it.

Some of the comfort measures I noted were needed (but remember, I was not in the heat of battle, and perhaps my perceptions were less tunnelled); Mrs. Y.'s lips were very dried; she had this white frothy stuff on her lips; there were beads of perspiration on her forehead (the air-conditioning had still not been turned on in the room); and she looked miserably uncomfortable in a very disheveled bed.

At this point Sandra came back into the room, and Kelly suggested that they start oxygen on the patient. Sandra went to get the O_2 equipment. Kelly was still buttoning up the patient's gown. Sandra came back with the O_2 equipment, and they set up. Sandra checked with Kelly about running it at 4 liters a minute. Kelly said, "Yes," and then it seemed they needed another tube, and Kelly left the room to get the other oxygen tube for the patient. I was waiting out at the desk for Kelly to return from taking the tube in because I wanted to check with her to find out what she thought was wrong with the patient and what she thought the doctor thought was wrong. (My inferences: Kelly—left-sided failure and pulmonary congestion. Intern—allergic response. I checked this out with her. She thought the patient's lungs were filling up with fluids, and it was also clear to her that the doctor was operating on the basis that it might be an allergic reaction—it is noteworthy that the doctor didn't write any kind of note on the chart, so we had no way of knowing what he was thinking, and he was off with the GI bleeder, so I couldn't talk to him.)

Kelly looked at one or two charts and worked on those for a few minutes. Within the next 5 minutes, Kelly jumped up and said, "I'm going to check on her again." I went with her. Sandra was sitting on the bed with the patient, stroking the patient's arm. It was good to see a nurse doing this sort of thing. (I found out later that Kelly had suggested this to Sandra.) Kelly checked Mrs. Y.'s respiration, front and back, with the stethoscope. The patient looked much more comfortable and appeared to be breathing much better within just this 5-minute period. They had her propped up well on pillows so that her neck and head were extended back, and it really did seem to improve her airway remarkably. Kelly checked the blood pressure and pulse again and then said to Sandra, "I couldn't get much of a radial pulse on her," and then she checked the pulse again apically by stethoscope. Neither Sandra nor Kelly spoke to the patient the whole time. After doing this, Kelly said to Sandra, "I am going to check the GI bleeder." (It was amazing how warm and individualistic Kelly was sometimes, and how detached she was at other times.)

Kelly went and did this (I was exhausted and found that I could only handle the observations in one acute emergency at a time, so I didn't go with her), and a few minutes later the doctor came back and said that he was going in to see Mrs. Y. again; Kelly went with him. She stood at the end of the bed while the doctor listened to the patient's chest. Then he wanted the patient to sit up. Strangely enough, Kelly made no effort to help the patient sit up at all, so the doctor helped her sit up. He took the second pillow out from under her back, so he could have more freedom to check her respiration, and then he put the pillow back, but it wasn't placed so that her neck and chest were hyperextended the way they had been before. It was very obvious that there was a difference in her respiration when it was like this. The doctor said he wanted a chest x-ray done stat and left the room. Kelly stayed, readjusted the patient's pillows so she could breathe easier, and then patted the woman's arms, smiled, and said, "You'll be breathing easier soon." The patient responded with a weak smile and closed her eyes.

We went back to the nurse's station, and almost immediately, Kelly started to chart in the nurse's notes. (I had noticed that when she first gave the Adrenalin in the patient's room, she turned the patient's tissue box over and began to make notes as to what time she gave the Adrenalin, how much, when the physician gave the Aminophylline, and so forth.) Vicki came into the nurse's station. Kelly looked up and suggested that Vicki might want to see if she could help Sandra a bit, that Sandra had gotten sort of behind in her 9:00 o'clock meds because of this emergency. The x-ray people came. Kelly got up and made out the chest x-ray requisition, and before she gave the x-ray people the requisition, she said, "Just a moment, I want to go talk to the patient." This kind of surprised me, but it was something beautiful to see. Kelly got up from her charting, kept the x-ray people from going in, went down to the patient, walked into the room, addressed the lady by name, took her arm, and said, "I'm sure you've been a bit frightened, but your breathing is much better now. We are going to take an x-ray and see if your lungs have enough room to move so that you can breath more comfortably." It really was a beautiful thing to see! The patient sort of half smiled and said, "Yes." As Kelly left the room, the intern who had been working with her on this case was about to leave the ward, and Kelly said to him, "Did you remember to write the orders for the medications that were given?" He said, "No," and turned around and started back to do it.

20

While all this was going on, I made a few other observations: one was that it seemed as though one of the functions of the head nurse, Kelly, on this unit was to interpret things for other nurses, the ward secretary, MD's, and other departments. For example, at one point the ward secretary was checking through the doctors' orders and there was a urine culture ordered. She showed this to Kelly and said, "There was a urine culture ordered on Saturday that was sent down on Saturday. I wonder if the doctor knew about that." The doctor was right there, so Kelly spoke to the doctor and said that a urine culture was ordered on Saturday and it did go down, but the report wasn't back yet; did he want another one? The doctor said no, and Kelly said, "Well, I'll see if I can get the report of that one as soon as possible," at which point the ward secretary picked up the phone, dialed the lab, and asked them for the report of the urine culture. (It seemed to me that this was something the ward secretary could have done directly with the physician without having to go through Kelly. It would have saved Kelly a lot of time.) The same thing happened with an order for salt tablets. The ward secretary picked up an order to increase the salt tablets from one to two. When she went to check on this, she said to Kelly, "Well, the patient isn't on any salt tablets"; so they checked back and found out that the unit the patient had been transferred to had interpreted the salt tablet order of 3 or 4 days ago to be a one-dose kind of thing and didn't realize it was to be given all the time. So Kelly said, "Well, we'll just have to talk to the doctor." When the doctor came in, she checked with him, and again it seemed to me that this was something that the ward secretary could very well have done, rather than having Kelly get involved. The same thing happened with Sandra and a bland diet order for this GI bleeder. Apparently they had a bland diet 1 and a bland diet 2, and the physician was under the assumption that a bland diet 1 included Maalox. Denise talked to Kelly about this, and Kelly talked to the doctor and explained that the diet didn't include Maalox unless he ordered it specifically.

A few other observations I made from 9:45 to 10:05 AM: there was an old lady who was going down to PT, who had been put in a wheelchair and was sitting in the wheelchair crying. She was waiting to go to PT, and nobody came to get her. At 9:40, as Kelly was charting, she looked up at Sandra and asked her if she had used the emergency O_2 setup for the patient with the wheezing, and Sandra said, "Yes"; so Kelly said to the ward secretary, "Don't forget to charge the patient for the emergency oxygen setup." At 9:50 Kelly hopped up again to go in and check the patient. At the doorway she met the patient's husband coming into the room. Kelly drew him aside and explained to him what had happened. She comforted him and explained that it had been bad there for a bit (in fact, Kelly told me afterward that at one time she thought the patient was going to arrest and was going out), but that his wife was improved now. Kelly placed her hand on the husband's arm and really attempted to comfort him and explain to him what had been going on.

It was now around 10:00 o'clock. Kelly was checking charts. Sandra asked her how to mix the albumen for Mrs. Y. Kelly explained how to do this. (I was puzzled by this request; it's a straightforward mix. But maybe Sandra was a new graduate. I would have to ask Kelly about this later.) Kelly then received a call from the supervisor to discuss some request for time off that the staff wanted. A few minutes later, while checking charts, Kelly jumped up and went to answer a light; a patient wanted to get off the bedpan. Kelly did this frequently. If a light went on and no one was around, she always answered it. The same thing with the phone: Kelly would answer the other phone. This was the only time she answered the phone; otherwise she let the ward secretary do it. A few minutes later the supervisor called again and scheduled a meeting that Kelly had to go to on Thursday.

It was now about 10:30 AM Sandra was still fixing up the albumen for Mrs. Y., and she asked Kelly if she needed a filter for it. Kelly said to use a blood filter. The lab called up the pro-time on the GI bleeder patient, and Kelly called it to the doctor.

After a little while a relative came to the desk and said that her mother had been discharged and that her daughter was going to be at the front of the hospital at 11:00. Would the patient be ready to leave by 11:00? Kelly promised she would be. Then Kelly chatted a few minutes socially with an intern who was going to be leaving the next day and asked what he was going to be doing. (He was going to Yale to take up psychiatric residency.) The nurse's aide came and told Kelly that a patient needed something for pain, and Kelly said, "Have you told Vicki?" The nurse's aide said yes, but that Vicki was busy, so Kelly got up and gave the patient Demerol for pain. Kelly was checking charts, then we would go for coffee, and hopefully I would get some questions answered.

I asked Kelly to tell me about Mr. R. I wanted to check out my observations that perhaps Mr. R's physician was really attempting to establish a collaborative working relationship with Kelly on this case. Kelly said she had initiated the conversation by commenting to the doctor (when she'd seen him on the elevator) that Mr. R. (a patient with status asthmaticus) just wasn't doing well, that last night he had to have three Bennett treatments to get him through the night, and that the present dosage of cortisone seemed to be helping him somewhat. Apparently they had tried various other kinds of medications with him earlier. Kelly said the doctor listened very carefully and asked her a few questions, and when she commented that he just seemed to be getting worse, he said he didn't agree with her. He thought that the patient wasn't any better, but that he was no worse. Kelly went on to say that with some of the doctors you can really talk and collaborate, but others seem to like to lead you on but pay no attention to you. She also said that the nurse has to be the one to take the initiative.

Now, a few comments on some of the conversation I had with Kelly over lunch this day. Particularly noteworthy is the fact that Kelly told me about how the situation had been with her staff, that they had a big blowup, which was led by Shirley because they felt Kelly wasn't spending enough time with them and wasn't living up to their expectations. They also felt that she wasn't helping them enough with patient care. I was really somewhat shocked to hear this, especially the part about her staff telling her that they thought she should get more involved with patients. (I was going to have to think about this more through the rest of the week and see how and in what way this knowledge affected my future observations.) This kind of blew my mind because I thought that for a head nurse, Kelly was quite involved with patients. I would have to discuss this more with her later to find out exactly what the conflict was, and perhaps with the staff, too, to find out what their expectations of this head nurse were. (Someone joined us at lunch and we couldn't continue.)

SUGGESTED QUESTIONS FOR DISCUSSION AND ANALYSIS

For undergraduate students
1. What kinds of activities is this nurse primarily engaged in? Are these nursing, hotel-type, or system maintainence activities?
2. What seem to be Kelly's goals and purposes in her work? Does she accomplish these?
3. Do you think Kelly is an effective nurse practitioner? Why? Based on what criteria?
4. How does Kelly see her role as head nurse? Is it the same as or different from the way the patients, physicians, other nurses, and supervisor see her role?
5. How does Kelly handle patient care crisis situations? Are there other ways of handling these? What are the advantages and disadvantages of each?
6. Describe the nature of Kelly's relationships with physicians. What effect do these relationships have on the health care system on this ward unit?
7. Analyze the social system of this unit. Does the social system foster or inhibit meeting the health care needs of Mrs. Y.? Of Mr. R.?

For graduate students and teachers of nursing
1. Is this the role of the practitioner in nursing that is desired for today? For tomorrow?
2. Identify and list the values, skills, and behaviors that you think are desirable to transmit to basic nursing students.
3. Where in your present curriculum, or in curricula that you are familiar with, do basic students have the opportunity to learn the values, skills, and behaviors you have identified in the above question?
4. How would you describe Kelly's philosophy of nursing? What are her work goals?

section B

Two perennial problems

Nurses who work in hospitals confront many difficult problems. Not the least among these problems is how to act toward and around patients who are dying or who are in great pain. Nurses' reactions are, understandably, affected by their own personal feelings and experiences—whether they have encountered death in their own immediate families, whether a close friend has died recently, whether they have not yet thought much about death because, being young, dying seems so far off, whether they have themselves experienced a disease with lots of pain, or whether they have overidentified with a patient visibly suffering from terrible pain.

Compounding such personal reactions are those reactions that ultimately derive from two other sources: training and hospital organization. Until recently, the curricula of schools of nursing scarcely touched on the social and psychological aspects of dying, focusing rather exclusively on the procedural and physiological features of terminal care. Pain is still a topic that is approached largely in terms of its physiology and its relief through procedural or pharmacological measures, although it is now increasingly seen as also a psychological issue. Older nurses in our hospitals, however, have been little affected by the newer psychological and sociological emphases, although a growing movement to humanize and professionalize the care of hospitalized terminally ill patients has become apparent across the country. Another compounding factor, however, is the organizational one. Hospital wards are not organized so that social and psychological features of dying or pain are reported routinely back to the desk, put in the medical record, discussed in team conferences, and made part of careful nursing (or medical) plans. There are exceptions of course, but generally there is little accountability for these matters in the sense just described. This lack of accountability does not mean that individual nurses do not give superb terminal care or manage pain sagaciously and compassionately, but the ward as a whole is not organized to do so—an example is the excellent organization of one burn unit where a team of personnel acts concertedly and quickly when changing patients' dressings (so as to reduce the duration of peak pain), but where there is scarcely any talk on the ward between patients and nurses about pain or how the patients may feel about it.

2. Conversations with dying patients

Jeanne Quint Benoliel, RN, DNSc

The following selection is taken from a book written by a nurse researcher, who with a team of sociologists studied terminal care in several hospitals (in the Bay area of San Francisco). She also interviewed nursing students and nursing faculties in three schools (collegiate and hospital) and observed both on the hospital wards. Her focus in this particular chapter is upon the understandable difficulties that students encounter either when dying patients wish to talk about their dying or when the students feel that they ought to make themselves available to such discussion. As the chapter makes evident, the problems that mature nurses encounter in interacting with the dying begin by the common practice in schools of nursing of assigning students to patients in accordance with criteria other than their terminal condition, so that students may be giving terminal care—pregnant with possibilities for "conversations"—unexpectedly and sometimes very early in their training.

Students' encounters with dying patients can sometimes result in serious and upsetting conversations. Patients may know they are dying and wish to talk about it. Patients may suspect they are dying and be testing another's knowledge about it. Patients may be in error and still want to talk about it. They may not know they are dying; but if the student does, she must make certain that she does not say or do anything during conversations to rouse their suspicions. Patients who precipitate conversational dilemmas for students are not necessarily dying in the medically defined sense of "being terminal," although some may be. They are often persons who have a personal interest in death at that time.[1]

Reprinted with permission of Macmillian Publishing Co., Inc., from *The Nurse and the Dying Patient* by Jeanne Quint Benoliel, Chapter 4, pp. 77-112. Copyright ©, Jeanne Quint 1967.

Under some conditions talk with dying patients can be relatively easy. Under other circumstances it can be extremely difficult and typically it is. At best, however, conversations with dying patients are hazardous enterprises because of the unstable nature of these conversations. They typically take place under conditions which can easily change and alter either the context of the interaction or the subject matter under discussion—thus endangering the student's equanimity. Surprise is a frequent component in many critical encounters, and some incidents are meaningful to students precisely because there is no forewarning. In sharp contrast, other incidents exert an influence so subtle that it is not recognized either by the students or by their teachers. These latter incidents play an important part in the socialization process by which students learn how to define patients in general and how to control delicate work situations which threaten to get out of hand.[2] (The students are not always successful in maintaining the control, as will be pointed out later.) Before turning to the specific influence brought about through early encounters with dying patients, it is well to consider first the relative importance of conversation with patients in general, and the rules which govern this aspect of nursing practice.

RULES GOVERNING PROFESSIONAL CONVERSATION

All professional schools provide sets of rules governing practitioner-client relationships, and schools of nursing are no exception. Such rules derive from legal, ethical, and authoritative sources governing "accepted" standards of good practice, as well as relationships with other professionals and the society as a whole. Some rules are explicit and set well-defined limits of responsibility. Thus it is the physician's prerogative and responsibility to tell the patient his diagnosis and prognosis. By comparison, other rules are generalized and vague; for instance, the directive to provide psychological care is subject to somewhat different interpretations and methods of implementation.

The rules governing conversation with patients are less explicit than the rules governing physical care and technical procedures. There are some exceptions, of course, but generally speaking the management of conversation is left to the commonsense determination of the nurse. Even specific directives—such as the commitment to teach patients—emphasize the content to be taught, but include few well-defined statements on how to proceed or when to start.[3] Some teachers stress the nurse's role in encouraging patients to express their feelings, but offer few explicit guidelines for determining when this action is or is not appropriate for the nurse.[4] Some teachers do offer specific advice about talking with patients, often to facilitate the students' performance of other nursing tasks. One teacher commented about the matter,

> I think that the students do have difficulty learning how to talk to patients as a whole, and how to phrase conversation so that they can be more or less the leader of the situation. This is something that I try to help them develop. When they say to a patient, "Do you want your bath now?" I suggest they try something like, "Well you've had your breakfast, let's

get along with your bath." In some instances the younger students have difficulty in learning to say no to a patient. They want to do everything the patient wants.

Often, however, the directions given by the teacher are vague, with the exception of those rules which clearly specify the doctor's obligations to the patient.

Initially the teacher is perceived as a major resource for information about handling conversations. In the beginning, students are concerned about what to say if the patient asks about his diagnosis or his treatment. The concern about what to say is commonly triggered by an early assignment (sometimes the first) to a patient with cancer. One student reported her first encounter with a cancer patient in this way.

> One of the first statements she made was that the patient next to her had cancer. She looked at me and whispered, as if it were something to be dreaded. Yet she had already gone through this. She also indicated that the person across from her had cancer, and she was a little concerned about that. She talked about her previous hospital experience, and once said that she hadn't seen the doctor in two weeks. There was a note in the nurses' notes that she was anxious about it because she didn't know. I was kind of worried that she would ask about it because I wouldn't know how to answer.

As was common practice when patient assignments were just beginning, the student turned to a teacher for explicit direction.

> Yes, I went to her (the teacher). I concluded that if she (the patient) did ask, I was to try to find out how she had been told. I would just have to say that I didn't know very much. I don't know too much about patients with cancer. If it were me, I think I would be afraid if I didn't know.

Rather than consulting on an individual basis, the students sometimes bring the subject into a class discussion to get answers on the proper ways of talking with such patients. There are four general strategies that the teachers present: (1) Disclosure of the diagnosis (and dying) is the doctor's prerogative, and "you'll have to ask your doctor" is the chief method for handling direct questions about such matters. (2) Because health teaching is an important part of nursing practice, an emphasis can be placed on preparing the patient to leave the hospital. (3) The nurse can also help patients keep their minds off their troubles by encouraging them to talk about their families or their life outside the hospital, or, perhaps, by initiating some form of occupational therapy. (4) Rather than diverting them from their troubles, the nurse can instead provide them with emotional support by encouraging them to express their feelings at a deeper level. The specific ways of implementing emotional support are not always clear to the students, as the following comment suggests, "Once the patient knows his diagnosis, the nurse supposedly is to help the patient talk about this, come to terms with it, and somehow feel the feelings and thoughts. How you do this, I don't know."

Few teachers are experienced in coping with the delicate conversational nuances which prolonged contacts with dying patients may require, nor are they comfortable in such situations. Consequently, they can offer few suggestions for talking to patients who may be frightened by the prospect of dying. The teacher's direction may even deny the possibility of dying, as the following example clearly shows.

A student was assigned to a man with a myocardial infarct during the critical period following its onset. She was aware of the danger of certain physical complications and defined this assignment as a challenging one, with the important nursing tasks being to keep his mind occupied and to plan for his hospital discharge. In discussing her plans with the teacher, the student asked if it were giving the patient false hope to tell him "things will be better, and you can do more for yourself later." At this time the patient's activities were completely restricted by the doctor's order. Even though the teacher was well aware that the patient's prognosis was viewed as highly unfavorable by the physicians in attendance, she answered "no" to the student's question.

Not only are many of the "rules" for talking with dying patients decided by the individual student, but many of the "rules" for deciding when a patient is dying are also decided by her.[5] During the first year in school, assignments to dying patients play an important part in the development both of the "rules" for knowing when a patient is dying and of the strategies for managing conversations when the patient knows (or does not know) that he is dying.[6]

THE ASSIGNMENT CONTEXT AND RECOGNITION OF DYING

When students first begin their patient assignments, they are often concerned about what to say if the patient starts to talk about a subject like dying. A student made these comments about the first day on a ward.

> One girl does have a cancer patient, and it doesn't look too promising right now. The patient's had previous operations on this. Our group, the three of us and the instructor, discussed this when we left the floor. I think all of us were concerned about how to handle the patient's apprehensions and anxieties because evidently the patient doesn't know the real definition of her condition. Not knowing how much she knows, we don't know how much to convey to her that we know.

The students are actually concerned about two problems—recognizing that a patient is dying and being able to cope with conversations about difficult subjects (of which dying is only one).

In the beginning, assignments are usually chosen to protect the students from extremely difficult nursing problems. At the same time, these experiences offer them opportunities to learn conversational strategies through direct practice and through observation of others. During the first year much time is devoted to formal class work and less time is given to clinical practice. What few hours the student does spend with each patient are likely to be focused on technical practice, and faculty supervision is frequent. The custom of assigning students to patients for only one or two days limits the opportunity for serious conversation by restricting the time available for it. However, these brief periods give students the chance to test different conversational approaches and to evaluate their worth.

New students are prone to seek advice on what to do from others whom they see as "knowledgeable": older nursing students, students from related fields (medicine or dentistry), classmates, nurses in practice, and family members, particularly if they are nurses or doctors. Not uncommonly, the students check out in advance the "rules" given in the hospital procedure book or in the standard nursing texts.

> We have a nursing manual, and it has a page on care of a patient after death. I think this was very interesting to all of us about realizing what the responsibilities of a nurse are—preparation of the body, tagging, and escorting to the morgue, proper position, and things you really don't think about in relationship to death in our culture. That's why I see it as a formal kind of ritual you might say. I think this starts right after death in preparation by the nurse to escort the body—it was interesting. You really don't think about it.

Another kind of planning is in the form of speculating about what to say if a patient asks an awkward question. This type of strategy session usually takes place in the residence hall in preparation for the following day.

> We were talking about it last night, as to what she could possibly say. We only came up with the fact that we would all have to be patient until the testing results came through, and then we could find a definite course of action. Other than this, there's not much you could really say.

Classmates who have worked in hospitals prior to becoming students are considered particularly knowledgeable authorities, and some find themselves serving as "mother hen" to less experienced colleagues. Once in the hospital, the student can observe the words and actions of others. She can overhear other nurses talking with patients and can profit from their mistakes and successes. She can listen to the teacher talking with another student and can pick up useful cues about what to do and what not to do. No longer does she rely principally on the instructor, for she can now turn directly to the hospital staff for assistance.

The patient assignment has a characteristic which permits students to engage in a wide range of conversational experimentation. A great many conversations between students and patients take place when others are not present. Conversation between any two people is generally quite different from that which occurs when others are in the room—and particularly "others" who represent authority to one or both of the interactants. Because these conversations with patients are often not observed, the student has considerable control over what she does and what she reports; she can decide whether or not to share it and, perhaps equally important, with whom. The one-to-one conversation is important for yet another reason. It is in this context that the student is most likely to encounter conversational difficulties with patients who are dying.

Some important "rules" became apparent during the early weeks on the wards. The students learn that instructors, for the most part, do not hold them accountable for their conversations with patients. When a student approaches a teacher for advice about a conversational problem, she is likely to be told, "You'll have to do it yourself," or, "Every case is individual." She may be referred to a book on interviewing. Occasionally the students can see and hear their teachers interacting with patients, and the reactions are favorable: "It was so easy for her to get the patient to talk." On other occasions, the student is disappointed: "She

29

wasn't any more comfortable or any better than other nurses." There is a progressive shift away from asking instructors for advice and an increased reliance on staff nurses and other students. The students soon recognize the need for getting advance information about patients, and ward personnel who can fulfill this function are readily identified. Sometimes the information is shared through the student grapevine.

The assignment context in which students are introduced to patient assignments often helps prevent the student from recognizing when a patient is dying. Although the student is expected to know the patient's diagnosis, she is left to draw her own conclusions about the likelihood of death. Under these circumstances the student slips easily into the practice of considering patients recoverable. Certain early encounters with patients and staff play an important part in fostering the practice of keeping oneself unaware of the possibility that a patient can be classified as dying. In the beginning, students are prone to ask the doctor directly about a patient's prognosis and can be shocked to learn that nothing more can be done. A student reported these reactions after talking with a physician.

> It was just a feeling as though the whole floor had been taken out from under me. He told me that the cancer had gone all the way. I had suspected it, and I had even discussed the case with a medical student who suggested this. But I just ignored it from him. But this confirmed it when the doctor told me. It really hit hard–hit home.
> That whole day I was more sensitive to everything that was going on around me. Which is unusual for me. When I was in psychology class, I felt more. I was more sensitive to the emotional picture, and it wasn't until that evening that I snapped out of it.

As all nurses know, it is one thing to read *cancer* on the chart; it is quite another to hear the doctor say *there is nothing more we can do.* Many students discontinue this practice of querying the doctor because it is upsetting to know that no cure is possible, and teachers seldom hold them accountable for knowing it.

The first assignment to a patient with cancer is often an important one. To their surprise, students find that patients with cancer do not necessarily initiate conversation about cancer or dying. Other students find–as did one–that asking a patient what the doctor had told him brought forth a surprise announcement, "Things don't look too good." To avoid this unforeseen situation which is likely to be both upsetting and difficult to manage conversationally, students are likely to make minimal use of the direct question. From these assignments students can also learn strategies for coping with unexpected remarks. Quite rapidly they find that silence can be a particularly effective way of deflecting the unwanted question or comment. Sometimes an innocuous comment can successfully parry a penetrating question. In one situation a man with a grotesque skin cancer tested a young student by asking her how his wound looked. She found that the comment, "It doesn't look bad. I would rather look at that than a skinned knee," averted further discussion of the topic.

Not all encounters provide such simple answers. Sometimes students decide *what not to do* as an aftermath of an incident, as the following episode shows. A student was assigned to a cancer patient shortly after the doctor had informed the woman of her poor prognosis. The student encouraged the patient to talk and on the second day of the assignment found herself quite unprepared to handle the situation when the woman began to cry. As a consequence, this student decided that it was better to let patients take the initiative in deciding what to discuss.

Students also find that patients who are defined as dying do not always "look dying," nor do they necessarily act as though they are about to have their lives brought to an end.

> We had a fourteen-year-old boy with a terminal diagnosis. He came in for a biopsy of a tumor of the leg, which was cancer and had metastasized. They were originally going to do radical surgery but decided that it would be foolish to do because the boy had not long to live. This was very difficult because he was extremely healthy looking, and a healthy acting person. He enjoyed talking about sports. He wanted to fix up the student nurses with his uncle for a date. He was marvelous with the other children, and he didn't seem ill at all.

Out of experiences such as these, some students become aware of the protective value of knowing in advance that a patient is categorized as dying.

It is not only patients with cancer who provide these kinds of experiences, but they provide a great many. From these and similar incidents students construct a picture of how patients generally behave in hospitals and what kinds of surprise conversations can be met. Concomitantly, they find that certain techniques are effective for avoiding conversational difficulties or for cutting them short. Social conversation is a useful technique for eluding talk about distressing topics and is generally successful unless the patient is terribly upset and forces the issue. Such an unexpected encounter can happen to anyone at any time, but students learn early to guard against the possibility in several ways—getting advance warning about patients, avoiding extra time with a potentially dangerous talker, bringing someone else into the room, directing the patient's attention to the procedures to be undergone. As young adults they are already familiar with many ways of controlling awkward conversation, and they can easily put these into practice. Also, the assignment context permits the student to make many choices which control the amount of time spent with patients.

Obviously the students cannot completely protect themselves from awkward or difficult conversations with dying patients, but they have many conversations which are not in the least troublesome. Sometimes the nondifficult conversation occurs when the student knows that a patient is dying. Often, however, the student is quite unaware that the patient falls into this classification. As will become clear later, the degree of vulnerability to conversations which pose problems for the student is less a function of awareness of dying *per se* than of the *timing* of becoming aware and the *mode* by which knowledge about dying is conveyed.

AWARENESS AND NONDIFFICULT CONVERSATION
The student does not know

Students do not encounter conversational difficulties with some patients simply because the students do not know that the patients are dying, and nothing happens to change their awareness of the situation. Sometimes the patients themselves do not know they are dying. In some instances when they have been told, they do not care to talk about it. Frequently students move out of the picture quite unaware of the death potential. The hopeful atmosphere common in hospitals serves not only to play down the importance of dying but also to keep its presence hidden, especially from newcomers. The conversation may represent no special problem to the student—though the extent to which some patients talk about their personal problems often comes as a surprise.

> Then she began to tell me about her marital problems. She told me that she hadn't been able to get pregnant and had gone to the doctor. She tried to get her husband to go to the doctor, but he wouldn't—"Just a big, dumb Swede." I was surprised when she talked to me about this. I didn't expect it.

Many conversations, however, are quite social in nature and easily forgotten.

The inexperienced student may not suspect dying because her limited knowledge prevents her from recognizing the possibility. On the other hand, the advanced student may not suspect because she is already in the habit of treating all patients as recoverable. In either case the student is likely to remain unaware of the dying status when the patient assignment is of short duration and her attention is directed to other matters. Students are assigned to many patients whose diagnoses and prognoses carry "death anticipations," but these patients are usually not defined as dying by the nursing staff or by teachers. Persons facing major surgery or extensive diagnostic testing, for example, are often concerned about what the doctor will find and what the future holds for them.

Sometimes the student may not know the patient is dying, but the patient does and makes efforts to talk about it. The student may not recognize the patient's words either as a clue that death is a possibility or as an invitation to talk about the matter. A specific example will illustrate the point. A first-year student was assigned to a patient facing cardiac surgery on the following day. The student was primarily concerned with teaching the patient how to breathe during the postoperative period, when deep breathing would be a difficult and painful process. During the discussion the patient commented, "I know that God meant this operation to be, that he wanted me to live through it." The student did not know what to say in response and returned to her teaching. The student did not recognize this statement as an indication that the woman might want to talk about the possibility of dying.[7] Furthermore, the patient's statement did not increase the student's awareness that this woman conceivably could die during the surgery. Her death on the operating room table came as a complete surprise. The student learned of the death only when she called the intensive-care unit several days later to inquire about the patient's welfare. The student was not expecting such an outcome, and described her reaction in this way.

> I think it was probably because I hadn't had any contact before with someone dying on the operating table. A lot of times these things happen, you know. I think that death is something that you sort of figure, it's there but you don't exactly figure that it would happen to your best friend or to a patient you have taken care of. She seemed so well and walking around. I think I would have had a different attitude if it had been a patient, like

one on a medical floor, or someone who I had taken care of who was slowly slipping. But the idea that she was perfectly well when I left the floor, and I wasn't back for three or four days before I checked it. When I finally found out that she had died, it didn't register particularly. It's unreal. And I had assumed that she would be in ICU anyway, so there would be no reason why I would have found her on the ward.

This kind of situation—failure to recognize the possibility of dying—is likely to happen under several circumstances. The student is new and lacking in experience. The patient looks healthy. Neither teacher nor staff warn the student of the possibility of death. The student's attention is directed to other matters. The assignment is extremely brief. In the preceding instance, the student learned of the patient's dying status as a postassignment phenomenon. Many students engage in conversation with dying patients under similar circumstances but never realize that the patients are trying to talk about their fears of dying. The assignments change and the students move on uninformed of the patients' desires (or dying status). The context of awareness remains "closed" (with the students as the innocent parties).

The student knows

Sometimes the student knows the patient is dying, but the patient does not know (also a closed awareness context). This situation can occur when patients with such potentially fatal diseases as cancer have not been told the diagnosis and are not yet sick enough to ask questions which might be difficult to answer. Patients themselves can make talk easy by chatting about social matters or by expressing interest in the nurse's affairs. Students in this context not uncommonly guide the conversation away from talk about the illness, or they limit the time spent with the patient.

As long as the patient does not suspect or is content to let things be as they are, conversation can be relatively easy. The more clues the patient has to arouse his suspicions, the more unstable the situation is conversationally, and the more the student must guard her words (suspected awareness context). This situation may be easy to maintain for short periods of time, but it can be extremely difficult when an assignment is extended and other conditions change concurrently.

Sometimes both the student and the patient know that he is dying, but they engage in mutual pretense and talk about other matters.[8] This type of exchange is likely to occur when the student and patient are new to one another, when the patient has come to terms with his impending death, and when the patient is not distressed by pain or upset by other matters. In such an interaction, neither participant makes an effort to find out directly what the other knows, although both may suspect; nor does either openly acknowledge his own state of awareness. One student described an assignment in the following words.

This was just sort of conveyed between us. I didn't come right out and say, and she just sort of knew. The next four or five days she had progressively gotten worse. She was in bed most of the time, and was vomiting a good deal. The nurse had told me that she probably wouldn't have long to live, even though the doctor had said that she had six months. There wasn't much verbal communication from that point on, because she was extremely tired and

> weak. Due to all this vomiting, she didn't have much time to sleep. She told me one time that it was more comforting to her to have someone just there, rather than to have someone to talk to her. So I just stayed there as much as I could, and maybe put my hand on her shoulder just to let her know that I was with her.

Because the circumstances underlying the situation can change rapidly, and frequently do, the game of mutual pretense has limited chances of continuing when assignments are prolonged. For one thing, it simply becomes extremely awkward for two people to behave as though everything were fine when both know otherwise and see each other day after day. Again, both patient and student may know that the patient is dying, but the patient may not be sure the student knows and does not discuss it with her. Alternately, he may simply act out of compassion for the student who is "so young."

In the situations described thus far, the conversations were relatively easy because they did not focus directly on dying or its possibility. Even open talk related to death is not necessarily difficult if the topics raised by the patient are not troublesome for the student. A student told the following story about an assignment.

> Afterwards I had a great sense of achievement with her. She was a young woman of about forty-four, and she had a young daughter of ten. I had her for two days (two mornings), and the first day I kind of, you know, felt my way along in the situation. My instructor had me do what we call a process recording. That night I went over it with my instructor, and we looked at the patient's needs and all, so I had a pretty good idea of the patient's emotional needs and questions and recurrent scenes and all.
> The second day she talked quite frequently about after her death—who would iron her husband's shirts and how her daughter would go to college. She wanted her daughter to be sure to go to college. I was able to give her suggestions about the college facilities that apparently she was not aware of. I felt a sense of accomplishment here.

Open talk about death is not difficult if the patient is relaxed about the matter, and the topic is a peripheral one—in this instance, a mother's concerns for her child's future. Also, the same student was able to perform a concrete act of assistance, a factor which reduced the sense of hopelessness so commonly felt by students when they talk with dying patients.

Protection through short and multiple assignments

The preceding assignment might have changed in character and in emotional tone had it continued beyond two days. Once more, the significance of the short assignment as a prime condition for "easy" conversation becomes apparent, though other conditions may vary.

When students are assigned to many patients, the short assignment offers few conversational risks. The student has less time to devote to each patient, therefore less time for talk, and she has access to many strategies for removing herself from potentially difficult situations. Student interest is frequently focused on learning nursing techniques and on completing assignments within a prescribed time period, and instructor supervision is likely to be spread thin to accommodate the needs of other students. Not uncommonly there is less emphasis given to the significance of nurse-patient conversation in this assignment context, and students are not pushed to experiment with it. Obviously, troubled patients can initiate "death" conversation under these circumstances, but students have many avenues available for avoiding situations they cannot handle. They have other patients to serve, other tasks to finish, and classes to attend. As a last resort a student can always ask for an assignment change. Under the multiple-patient assignment, which is like the staff nurse work assignment, students less frequently get into conversational dilemmas of their own making.

AWARENESS AND DIFFICULT CONVERSATIONS

Each situation previously described carries the potential for difficult conversation if one or more conditions change. Thus the patient may learn the truth and announce his dying status to the unsuspecting student. The surprise announcement is difficult at best, but can be worse if the patient's behavior is also disturbing. The following incident illustrates this point.

A young student was giving morning care to a man who quite suddenly blurted out that he was dying, that there was nothing more she could do. He brusquely told her to leave the room. Taken aback, the student went to her teacher, who told her to do whatever she thought best. Returning to the patient, the student tried to explain that the treatment was necessary. He responded, "Don't fool me; I don't want it." The student completed the treatment, but the assignment was a "terrible experience" because he never stopped telling her to get out of his sight.

The patient who does not know may become suspicious when he notes certain physical changes in himself and may ask the student probing questions that she finds difficult to parry. The doctor may tell the patient he is dying, yet the student may not know this has occurred and may continue to block the patient's conversational overtures. The patient who knows he is dying may change his behavior pattern, as can happen when pain becomes worse or family pressures impinge on him so heavily that he must blow off to someone. He may no longer pretend that he is getting well, but begin to talk about death in general, or his own in particular. The patient who has talked serenely about leaving his family behind may suddenly start talking about his fear of dying or his concern about pain and what the end will be like. He may become very agitated and openly talk about suicide. Whether influenced by a change in awareness of his dying status or by changes in other circumstances which affect his living, the dying patient may need to talk about matters that are important to him. These topics, however, can be very upsetting to the student.

Some difficult conversations take place because students initiate talk which gets out of hand. The student herself may unknowingly precipitate a crisis by asking the wrong question or by making what she thought was an innocent comment. In the middle of an assignment the student may learn that the patient is dying and then find herself speechless in a situation which formerly posed no problems. Students who encourage dying patients to verbalize or to express their feelings can find themselves very upset by the unforeseen consequences of using this approach. Thus even a short assignment can be conversationally hazardous for any student who encourages patients to talk about their real concerns.

Sometimes an assignment is difficult not because of the conversation but because the patient will not talk at all. Similarly, a student may find it difficult to carry on when a patient is openly hostile, highly critical of her actions, or constantly complaining. A student reported these reactions to her first patient assignment.

> I was shaking so much by this time that I was having a little trouble with the thermometer, so the instructor stayed with me. When I inserted it and told him I would have to hold it in place for five minutes, she left. Well, I was too concerned with myself to attempt any conversation with the patient, particularly after such a rebuff that I had gotten. He just turned his face away and made no conversation whatsoever. It wasn't until about a week later, in a conference in which we were discussing how one determines levels of illness and wellness, that I found out this man was a terminal patient about to die. At this time I felt guilty for thinking he was such a terrible old man, nasty and so on.

This type of interaction is difficult for any young student, and particularly one who is unsure of herself. It can be a traumatic event when it takes place as part of the first patient assignment.

As can easily be seen, the conversation becomes hazardous whenever a patient attempts to shift from one awareness context to another, whether this be from closed to open or suspected, from mutual pretense to open, or from suspected to open. In addition, an open awareness context without danger can unexpectedly become a perilous enterprise. The student can also cause a change in awareness context, sometimes purposefully and sometimes inadvertently, thereby suddenly finding herself faced with a situation that has gone completely out of control.

The shifts in awareness context occur with greater frequency when prolonged assignments are used. Even when the multiple assignment (usually low in risk) is employed, the conversational hazards increase when the assignment time is extended for several weeks. A student is less able to define a dying patient as nondying through such a lengthy period, and she is not well protected from personal involvement with the patient and his family. Prolonged contact increases the possibility that a patient may initiate efforts to talk openly about his dying. Maintaining the pretense that the patient will recover becomes increasingly difficult for both him and the student as physical signs indicate otherwise.

CONVERSATIONS DESCRIBED AS DIFFICULT

It is now easy to understand why there are two general classes of conversations students find very difficult. First, there are the conversations to be handled when the student is assigned to a dying patient who is not to be told the truth about his condition, yet he suspects the truth. Then there are the hazards when patients want to talk openly about their own deaths, and the students cannot tolerate either the topic being discussed or the patient's behavior, or both together.

Conversations and the nondisclosure assignment

When the student is assigned to a patient who is not to be told his diagnosis, she is faced with several distressing problems. She must converse with the patient without giving him any clues which might reveal his true condition. This task becomes extremely difficult, if not almost impossible, when the patient suspects and asks direct questions. One student described the problem in this way.

> When I would walk into her room, she would say "I wonder why I have pain in this region or that region." If I knew that she was aware of what her diagnosis was, I would be able to explain a little bit, but she didn't. I was almost afraid to say anything because I didn't know if I would slip.

The much-used phrase *you'll have to ask your doctor* may not stop the patient's efforts to get information from the student. Frequently the student is primary recipient of a patient's concerns because the hospital nurses tend to withdraw from patients who press them for the "facts." Conversational pretense becomes particularly awkward when the patient's physical condition is obviously deteriorating, or when relatives gather in the room as though preparing for a wake. A student commented about an assignment which was a "great strain."

> She kept referring to all those purple bruises, and every time you'd walk in she'd say, "Why do I have these bruises?" She had two conditions (I can't remember what the other one was) but it certainly wasn't something that would cause these bruises. It just didn't correlate to the point where, if it were you or I, we would suspect something was seriously wrong. She was always asking questions. You always had to be on your guard.

In addition, the student may have trouble with her own feelings if she thinks patients have the right to know what is happening to them, as the following incident suggests.

> Some of my friends are taking care of this man since I left. His wife refused to let him know he is dying, and I think it is pretty wrong. She has him so subjugated and she has done so many things. I think he might want to do things a little differently if he knew he was dying.

Like the ward nurses, the student often finds herself caught between the patient and his doctor and family. Sometimes the patient, informed by signs and symptoms, may well suspect a certain diagnosis and will ask pertinent questions which must be answered by not saying anything which would disclose his condition. As one student observed, "Here you have a fight between the doctor who doesn't want you to tell her and the patient who wants to know. Where do you talk first?" The student who does give information to a patient, either accidentally or purposefully, may have the added problem of facing an angry physician.

Nondisclosure problems can be even worse if the patient is emotionally disturbed, as the following episode illustrates. A first-year student was assigned to a woman who had gone to surgery on the previous day for a breast biopsy. The patient had previously had one breast removed for cancer and was suspicious of what the doctors had found. The student knew that the biopsy was positive for cancer, but she also knew that the surgeon had not yet talked to the patient. This

37

student had been told by a teacher that she could not use the word *cancer* until the doctor himself had used it with the patient. One of her classmates described what took place.

> Anyway Mary attempted to talk to this woman about it, but the woman was incapable of it. She just kept saying, "I want to die, I want to die, but I cannot ask you to do this. I can't ask you to let me die because you are a student, and you can't do it." Then she began to cry and Mary was completely dismayed. You know, what will I do now? Well, she had to leave the room and go and cry herself. Then she returned and asked the woman if she wanted to talk about it. The woman said "no" and started to cry again. Mary said, "I will stay with you, if you would like," and the woman said, "yes." So she just stayed with her and held her hand.

The student herself found the assignment a very upsetting experience, and she did not know how to cope with it. Part of her difficulty stemmed directly from the paradoxical assignment with its two conflicting directives.

Tension-producing topics of conversation

The preceding incident clearly demonstrates the two conditions which make open talk about death a difficult problem—the upset patient and tension-producing subject matter. When patients aware of their coming deaths talk about peripheral topics, such as reminiscing about the past, students have little difficulty either in listening or in engaging in repartee. However, the student and many others find themselves at a loss for words when the patient focuses directly on the central issue of his personal death—for instance, when he says, "I want to get it over with now." The student is faced with handling her own reactions (feelings of helplessness and hopelessness, or a sense of frustration) when a patient openly expresses the wish to die. As one student commented, "When she talked about death, I always got anxious."

Another particularly distressing assignment is one in which the patient talks openly about his death on one day, yet makes plans to leave the hospital on the next. In this situation it may not be talk about death which poses problems, but rather deciding what to say in response to the erroneously hopeful plans for recovery. When the patient swings from hopeful talk on one occasion to deep despair the next, the problem of maintaining conversational equilibrium is a strain. The student may well feel inadequate and uncomfortable. She is likely to remember the assignment as an unhappy and emotionally draining experience.

The topics which give students the greatest difficulty are those that are likely to be extremely important to the dying patient—the time of his death, the manner of his dying, and the desire to bring closure to his life. The patient may wonder when he will die, and whether he will be conscious until the end. He may worry that the pain will get worse, with no relief available to him. He may want to die quietly without the use of extensive life-prolonging measures as the end draws near. He may want to talk openly about dying so that he can say good-bye to his family and the staff, or to make plans for what will happen after he is gone. A student reported this conversation with a patient.

She was talking to me in this general area, and finally we got around to the fact that people shouldn't be afraid. I said, "Well, are you afraid?" She said, "Well, I'm afraid but not of death." I said, "Well, what are you afraid of then?" She said, "of the pain," because she felt so much pain now and she was sure as she got worse, she would have a lot more pain. She said the actual dying didn't bother her.

The patient may ask for help in making critical decisions, and the student can view this request as an inappropriate one. A terminal cancer patient was faced with the alternative of going home to die or of taking an experimental drug with no guarantee of cure. In talking with the student assigned to her, the woman kept repeating, "What shall I do? What shall I do?" The student thought that the patient was asking her to make the decision. The student reported her own reactions thus.

When she said, "I want to die," I kept thinking, "Well, *I* don't want to die—you *couldn't* want to die." I was always thinking that she *can't* mean that, and tighten up. A lot of her comments were what-should-I-do types of things and asking my advice on what choice I should make, which made me anxious because here was somebody who was older than my mother, who was very intelligent, and who I would normally think of myself as looking up to, she was asking me for help.

To the student this assignment was an exhausting experience.

In some ways, I guess it was a drain on me because I got to like her so much, maybe more than I should have, and I just felt too much I *wish* there were some way I could help her, but I didn't know how. She wanted some answers, and I couldn't give them to her.

Being this close to another person's experience of dying can indeed be an emotionally depleting experience. The tension can be heightened even more if the patient talks about killing himself or makes a direct request to "put me out of my misery."

It should now be abundantly clear that difficult conversations with dying patients have degrees of difficulty depending not so much upon awareness of dying *per se* as upon other features—the timing of the awareness announcement, the conversational constraints imposed by others (the doctor, the family, the teacher), the subject matter pursued, the emotional states of the interactants, the prior experiences of both, and the length of time they are in contact. As was noted earlier in the chapter, prolonged contact between the student and the patient is a critical precursor for conversational problems. There are several other conditions which also lead in this direction.

CONDITIONS FURTHER MAXIMIZING DIFFICULTIES
Prolonged contact

Prolonged contact does not only occur through lengthy patient assignments, but also takes place when students continue to visit their patients after the official assignment has terminated (a practice which is noticeably less common among senior students than among their less-experienced colleagues). Some patients are also in and out of the hospital several times before their final stay, and students can become well acquainted with them under these circumstances. These points are important because the longer a student knows a dying patient, the more likely she   **39** is to learn of characteristics that are not observable on brief contact. In the United States such values as youth, beauty, or talent are highly esteemed, and dying patients who embody these characteristics tend to produce feelings of loss in those who are around them. Like others, the student can become vulnerable to feelings of sadness associated with a person's loss to society or to his family, and thereby can increase her susceptibility to involvement in his dying.

Social loss reactions

In any society people are esteemed on the basis of personal and social characteristics which carry high value. In this country age is an important condition for assigning high social value. The death of a child or young adult is generally perceived as a greater loss to society than that of an older person who has lived a full life. Each individual has many kinds of characteristics; social class, ethnic group, sex, education, occupation, family background, accomplishment are some that are important. As is true with nurses in general, students respond to patients in terms of the values ascribed to their social characteristics.[9] A person who is young talented, and personable tends to be more highly valued than one who is old, useless, and disgruntled. When the patient is dying, these characteristics determine the extent to which his death is perceived as a loss (to society or to the family), thus producing feelings of sadness and regret.

A cluster of high social-loss factors usually carries more impact than a single factor, but even one characteristic can assume singular importance if it is personally meaningful to the student. Patients with these highly valued characteristics are potentially risky assignments because student reactions to them can intensify the tragic feelings of *this person's death*. A student reported these reactions, "There was a boy not too long ago—he died of leukemia. His family was completely upset and cried a lot. I found the best thing to do is to cry along with them." By comparison, the same social characteristics can be relatively unimportant factors if the student is unaware that the patient is dying.

Sometimes a combination of traits can produce a social-loss "story" which is sad and disturbing. One student described a three-week assignment to a young mother dying of leukemia. The woman's last baby was also in the hospital, where he had been placed when the mother's disease had exacerbated. Much of the patient's conversation centered around her family and stories of the new baby, as relayed by the patient's mother who visited the nursery daily. The patient did not openly talk to the student about dying, but on one occasion burst into tears. The student could only respond with the words, "Is there anything I can do to help?" She described the assignment as "terribly hard" because "there isn't anything I can say or do." She was reacting to a tragic death: a young mother leaving behind small children and a loving husband.

This incident is important for another reason. It illustrates the compounding of involvement which takes place when a student responds, not solely to social loss, but also to factors which are personally significant. In this instance the student was married and had children of her own. She had first became interested in the patient while assigned to give care to her baby. In the student's words, "I think I am closely associated with her. She has a young family."

Certain situations carry a special poignancy, and one of these is talking with children who are dying. In many instances, the youngsters have not been told what is happening and may even be given false information. While visiting each day, the mother of a boy with cancer metastases in the lungs would say, "When your pneumonia gets better, you can come home." Later the boy asked the nurse student, "Why don't I get better?" The student could say nothing, but she wept when she got home.

Personal-loss reactions

Personal loss by itself can be troublesome, as when the student identifies with someone her own age. It can be magnified tremendously when the patient is someone she knows. For instance, she unexpectedly finds herself assigned to the boy next door, for whom "nothing more can be done." An entire class can feel the impact of tragedy when one of its members falls victim to an incurable disease.

Inexperienced students in particular are prone to respond to personal and social-loss characteristics by continuing to visit their patients. A student assigned to a fourteen-year-old boy with a malignant leg tumor kept returning to the ward. As another student commented, "She is never able to do what she wants to do, and I don't think she knows what she wants to do, but she is drawn back." Extended contact through such visits does not necessarily lead to disastrous outcomes, and the student may well come through such an experience with a sense of reward for having been able to give support to the patient or to his family. However, these visiting habits can lead to upsetting consequences if the patient dies unexpectedly and, even more so, if the student was involved in serious conversations with him.

For example, a young man facing heart surgery became very dependent on a student who permitted him to talk about how frightened he was. He wanted her to be with him following surgery, but because of other commitments the student was unable to grant his request. When he died several days following the operation, she felt that she had betrayed his trust by not being present during the postoperative period. Students are frequently unaware of the potential hazards in their encounters with patients, and they cannot predict the impact such experiences will have on their feelings. It is the patient's personal and social characteristics which attract the student and are likely to pull her into a close involvement. It is the conversational dilemma, sometimes left unfinished by sudden death, which can perplex and trouble her.

Accountability for conversations with dying patients

An assignment which frequently leads to conversational difficulties is one in which the student has only one patient—known to be dying—with the commitment to focus conversation on the patient's concerns. Graduate students who are assigned to terminal patients for the duration of their hospital stay (often a matter of weeks) invariably encounter problems either in handling the conversation or in coping with their own feelings, but usually both. Basic students can have similar experiences with short assignments if they happen to be assigned during a period when the patient is undergoing an emotional upheaval. It is the commitment to talk with the patient which makes this assignment a particularly dangerous enterprise. When the teacher holds the student accountable for what goes on between her and the patient, the student cannot easily avoid spending time with the patient. (There are, of course, those students whose facile imaginations can manufacture conversations which please the teacher and save the student from painful first-hand experience; but few students are so blessed.) During this assignment the student tends to get into conversational territory which is new for her, and she often makes matters worse by an inappropriate response.

A specific illustration can clarify the latter point. A student was taken by surprise when a patient said, "I think it would be so much better if the doctors would give me a shot and put me to sleep now." Quite unprepared for this comment, the student responded by saying, "But why should they do that. Look at the way you've been joking." The student felt "horrible" when the patient patted her on the hand and said, somewhat sarcastically, "Oh, you're developing a good bedside manner. You'll make a good nurse." The student said of this assignment, "Emotionally it was the hardest week I've ever had with a patient."

THE MANAGEMENT OF CONVERSATIONS WITH DYING PATIENTS
General tactics

It should now be easy to see that the students must develop tactics for coping with several distinct problems. They need strategies for knowing when patients are dying so that they can be prepared for a variety of eventualities—patients who know they are dying, those who suspect they are dying, and those who do not know they are dying. Stated differently, the students learn ways of discriminating between potentially "safe" and "unsafe" contexts in which they are expected to talk with patients. With experience the students become aware of important resources for getting advance information—the seriously ill list which contains the names of "unsafe" patients; the patient's chart (not always a reliable source, as students rapidly learn); the reports between nurses at change-of-shift time; and staff members who are usually knowledgeable about such matters.

Another problem is that of learning how to prevent safe assignments from becoming unsafe. This means knowing what to do when an awareness context starts to change—for example, indications appear that a closed awareness context is becoming a suspected awareness context. The student needs two kinds of strategies for controlling this type of interaction problem, contact management (ways of minimizing the time spent with the patient) and expression management (ways of managing conversation which threatens to get out of hand). As far as managing contact time, the student can spend little time with the patient, leave the room when the conversation becomes threatening, or have a third party present if at all possible. The conversation itself can be managed by effective use of both verbal and nonverbal interaction techniques—the nonspecific comment, a change of subject, a selective use of the direct question, referral of questions to an authority (the doctor, staff nurses), the plea of ignorance (readily available to the student and the new employee), the use of social conversation, the depersonalization of the patient by not talking to him, or the professional manner which "puts the patient in his place."

Finally, there are guarding tactics that are necessary for dealing with the assignment which is definitely an unsafe enterprise. The same strategies previously listed can be readily used for avoiding some conversational problems. In addition, the student must be wary of other dangers. Among the additional hazards to be avoided are involvement with a patient whose death would be terribly saddening and conversation which provokes feelings of helplessness, hopelessness, or anger. The effect of prior experience on the development of protective strategies clearly shows up when one contrasts the management of patients by experienced and inexperienced students when they are assigned to a ward with many high-risk patients.

The experienced student

Experienced students, when confronted with high social-loss patients, behave so as to minimize the possibilities of personal involvement. On one pediatric ward, which housed a high proportion of children with fatal illnesses, these students successfully kept themselves detached by using the following methods. The assignment was defined as nonterminal. Little conversation was initiated with parents about the child's illness. Personal contact with the child and his parents was limited, and extra assignment time with the patients was avoided. Conversation was focused on everyday matters. Instructor help was seldom sought. Even with children who showed obvious signs of physical deterioration, the students were able to keep themselves uninvolved with the children personally by focusing their attention on the disease or treatment process. The students were aided in the process because assignments were short and instructor supervision was scanty.

Although these students were told that support for families with dying children was an important nursing function, they had little direct help from their teacher, and many chose to minimize their contacts with family members. Such behavior was commonly justified by the rationale that it was not fair to families to start something and then not to be present at critical moments. The practice of minimizing contact with families was also used by the hospital staff, e.g., they frequently held staff conferences during visiting hours. Thus these students were supported in their choices by the nurse models they saw in action.

The inexperienced student

The inexperienced student in this setting was likely to get herself into trouble because she did not recognize the warning signs of potential involvement, nor was   **43** she adept at ignoring them. A specific incident will illustrate the point. A student was assigned for two days to a twelve year old boy with lymphosarcoma. She became so involved that she continued to see the boy and his parents in follow-up clinic. There were a number of factors which led to the involvement. During the assignment the student encountered several conditions she was unable to ignore. The patient's swollen neck was an observable sign, and she chose to define him as "terminal." Twice the boy raised questions about why he was admitted to the hospital. The mother was extremely upset and spoke to the student about her fears that his classmates might "tell him something" when he returned to school. The student responded with sadness to the tragedy of a child facing death.

Caught up in these concerns, the student discussed her goals with a teacher who encouraged her to continue working with the family. The student's primary concern was that no one had given the boy a realistic appraisal of what was happening to him. She wanted to protect him from the chance of hearing the bad news from his classmates. The patient was discharged before the student had "accomplished everything," and she felt compelled to see the family again.

While the youngster was hospitalized, the student had several awkward moments during her conversations with him. She wanted very much to ask him questions directly but was afraid he might put her on the spot. In her words, "It is not my place to tell him." In the clinic she found he was "different than in the hospital" and not receptive to talk. However, she did not spend much time with the boy at this time but chose to talk with his mother, because she wanted the mother to tell the boy that he had a serious blood disease. She never knew whether her effort achieved success because other commitments and new interests assumed priority, and she did not maintain her contact with the family.

Compensating for helpless feelings

There are several ways by which students counterbalance their feelings of helplessness and inadequacy when talking with dying patients. Although the counterbalancing does not help them manage actual conversation with patients, it does help them get through unavoidable interaction with patients. Some students learn that referral to the chaplain may give some patients the opportunity to talk about their concerns and to come to terms with their impending deaths. The students find, however, that not all patients find comfort in talking to ministers and that some clergymen have difficulty in providing this kind of help to dying patients. Sometimes a social worker is available for referral when a patient indicates he wants to talk more openly about his coming death, and the student makes use of this service. The student can compensate for her personal inadequacies by bringing another human resource to the patient.

Conversation with family members is another technique which seems to assume a special importance when the dying patient is a child, perhaps to atone for the impact of social-loss feelings. The value of this device is that helping the family provides a sense of helpfulness to the nurse student where hopelessness prevailed before.[10] In the example previously described the student tried to help a twelve-year-old boy by encouraging his mother to give him some definite information. These conversations were not easy, and the experience was described as emotionally depleting. At the same time the student had a sense of accomplishment, and she stated, "I helped the parents more this time than I did in the hospital. Not that I could give them any solutions; this is impossible. But they could express some of their feelings, and I could show them that I cared." Such a strategy can indeed help a family through this period of strain, but the outcome for the patient may be to isolate him further from involvement in and discussions about his own death.

Sometimes a student is well aware that she has helped a dying patient by bringing him into contact with the "right person." For example, she tells the doctor that the patient seems to be asking for more information, and the patient appears more relaxed with himself after he has talked with his physician. However, sometimes the student is unaware that she has provided assistance. . . .

SOME CONVERSATIONAL CONSEQUENCES FOR STUDENTS
The search for support

When students encounter conversational difficulties, they often turn to persons other than their teachers for counsel. Even those instructors whom students recognize as good listeners usually have little concrete advice to offer. Some may even withdraw from listening because they cannot tolerate talk about death and the strong feelings which tend to be engendered in them by the student's reactions. When students turn to hospital staff for advice about handling certain patients, they are likely to get one of two responses—agreement with the decision the student has already made, or "You seem to be doing fine by yourself." A few students seek out the clergy for support, but eventually most students turn to classmates or boyfriends, using them as sounding boards. Thus, the advice they get and the decisions they make are based primarily on commonsense determinations, combined with trial-and-error experience. Some students pick up tactics vicariously by listening to student colleagues describe their successes and failures, and many finish the first year quite adept at avoiding distressing conversations with patients. Students without an early exposure to the interactional problems associated with dying develop few cues for judging potentially dangerous situations. They are, therefore, prime candidates for encountering conversational difficulties when they are assigned to seriously ill patients at a later time. They are also ill prepared for the emotional impact these experiences usually bring.

The aftermath of conversations with dying patients

As has been indicated, students can have very positive experiences in talking with dying patients, and also some very difficult ones. The former are frequently remembered with exhilaration, as moments of great success in providing help or comfort. The latter can run the gamut, from being recalled as mildly upsetting or

45

surprising to being remembered as very traumatic, leaving the student with doubts about herself and uncertainties about what to do in the future.

It is not uncommon for nurse students to attach a cause-and-effect relationship between their conversations with dying patients and the events which take place following them. Some may even blame themselves for the patient's death. In one instance, for example, a patient with inoperable cancer pushed very hard to learn the truth about her condition from the student. The latter took this request to the physician, who then told the patient about her incurable condition. When the patient suddenly developed complications and died within three days, the student blamed herself for having instigated the announcement. Another student can blame herself if a patient who knows he is dying indicates a readiness to talk, yet he dies before the student is psychologically ready to talk with him.

These conversational experiences are upsetting at the time, but they can also serve as important turning points if the students have someone available to help them live through these difficult periods—and particularly when the listeners clarify the positive as well as the less positive consequences of interactions with patients. The few nurse students who learned to talk more openly and comfortably with dying patients had someone to whom they consistently turned for support and guidance when they encountered these difficult problems. As a result, and with the passage of time, they were able to view their actions within a more realistic and less self-critical framework.

There is another reaction which the students do not anticipate, the intensity of their feelings of grief when they become involved with a dying patient. Not only are these reactions personally disturbing, but also they often cause the student to experience conflict within herself because the social role of bereaved person is incongruent with the social role of nurse, as defined by the norms of hospital culture.[11] Just as students were helped by talking about difficult conversations, so also were they helped when they could openly express the many and varied feelings which accompanied and followed these critical experiences.

Many students did not have access to this kind of help when they encountered difficult conversations or intense grief-provoking experiences. Some were openly chastised for becoming personally involved with their patients when such incidents took place. Others became cautious in their conversational ventures because of conversational *faux pas* which occurred during the early weeks, when vulnerability to failure was acute. Still others felt guilty when they could not use the "right conversational techniques." As one put it,

> I was always in trouble. It came out, I ruined my process recordings and felt guilty. That was what it produced—a guilty feeling about what I was doing to the patients. . . . I would either come out with guilt feelings that I didn't use the techniques, or I would come out with guilt feelings that I did use the technique but I didn't get anywhere, or I don't know what is going on really.

It is not surprising that the majority of students became skilled at avoiding conversations which offered more penalties than rewards, and more discomfort than satisfaction.

As this chapter has indicated, variations in awareness of dying, conversation under stress, and student experience play a major part in determining what happens to nurse students when they talk with dying patients. Both the conversational guidelines for providing psychological care and the anticipated results of such conversations are unclear to many students—thus they use their commonsense judgements in deciding what to say and when. In general, they learn many strategies for managing conversations which threaten to get out of control. They also learn ways of compensating for the helpless feelings which are engendered when they are assigned to dying patients. It is true that students have many positive experiences in talking with dying patients. It is also true that under some conditions the less positive conversational experiences can have far-reaching effects on the student, as a person and as a nurse. So also can assignments in which the student is brought into direct contact with death itself. . . .

NOTES

1. More appropriately, this chapter is concerned with conversations between nurse students and persons who are living with a disease carrying fatal connotations or who are threatened by the possibility of sudden death or of a particular way of dying.

2. As used here, the term *socialization* refers to a process whereby an individual learns to perform in a given role. Rence C. Fox, in *Experiment Perilous* (New York: Free Press, 1959), p. 235, defines the term as follows, "Stated in more formal sociological terms, 'socialization' consists of the processes of learning through which an individual acquires the knowledge, skills, attitudes, values, and behavior patterns which will enable and motivate them to perform a role in a socially acceptable fashion."

3. The critical importance of such factors as the timing of instruction, the assignment of a specific person to do the job, and the basic "facts" which help patients to understand what lies ahead for them has been explicitly detailed for one group of patients. The results of a systematic method of preoperative instruction for patients facing open-heart surgery are described by Filomena Fanelli Varvaro in "Teaching the Patient About Open Heart Surgery," *American Journal of Nursing,* 65 (October, 1965), pp. 111-115.

4. Bursten and Diers suggest that the literature on patient-centered nursing may have given undue stress to the importance of helping the patient clarify and express his feelings, without concomitant attention to the value of other aspects of the nurse-patient interaction—hereby fostering the danger that communication with patients becomes a new kind of ritual. Ben Bursten and Donna K. Diers, "Pseudo-Patient-Centered Orientation," *Nursing Forum,* Vol. 3., No. 2 (1964), pp. 38-50.

5. For a more general discussion of the sociological perspective on dying as a definitional problem, readers are referred to Barney G. Glaser and Anselm L. Strauss, *Awareness of Dying* (Chicago: Aldine, 1965), pp. 16-26.

6. The interaction which occurs between a nurse and a dying patient is guided by the patient's and the nurse's awareness of his dying state. There are four commonly recurring situations (referred to as awareness contexts) observed in the hospital. They are (1) *closed awareness*—the situation in which the patient does not recognize his impending death though everyone else does (or when the patient does, but the nurse may not); (2) *suspected awareness*—the situation in which the patient suspects that he is dying and tries to confirm his suspicions; (3) *mutual pretense awareness*—the situation in which both the patient and the others define him as dying, but each pretends that the other does not know; and (4) *open awareness*—the situation in which both the staff and the patient define him as dying, are aware of the other's definition, and are relatively open in their conversation and actions. See *ibid.*, pp. 9-13.

7. What this comment actually meant to the patient can only by conjectured.

8. See Glaser and Strauss, *op. cit.*, pp. 64-78, for a general discussion of this kind of interaction.

9. A more complete discussion of these points is given by Barney G. Glaser and Anselm L. Strauss in "The Social Loss of Dying Patients," *American Journal of Nursing*, 64 (June, 1964), pp. 119-121.

10. This statement does not mean that students do not encounter problems in dealing with the families of dying patients . . .

11. Volkart has suggested that in American culture the role of the bereaved person, with its emphasis on loss, grief, and the open expression of these feelings, may be in conflict with the expected behaviors associated with other roles, e.g., the role of adult male. He adds further, "But to the extent that social and cultural conditions encourage interpersonal relationships in which overidentification, overdependence, sense of loss, hostility, guilt, and ambivalence are bred in profusion, and to the extent that the social role of the bereaved person does not take account of these feelings and the needs they inspire— to that extent bereaved persons may often be uninitiated victims of their sociocultural system." Edmund H. Volkart and Stanley T. Michael, "Bereavement and Mental Health," *Explorations in Social Psychiatry* (New York: Basic Books, 1957), p. 301.

SUGGESTED QUESTIONS FOR DISCUSSION AND ANALYSIS

For undergraduate students

1. What does the author indicate about the relationship of students' assignments to their problems with terminal patients?

2. Not all conversations with terminal patients are difficult for students. Which kinds are easiest and why? Which are particularly difficult and why? What has been your own experience?

3. What does "awareness" have to do with the whole issue of talking about terminality with patients—and their kinsmen?

4. What is "social loss," and how does it enter into the problems of talking with people who are dying?

5. What are some consequences of trying to give terminal care to patients who wish to talk about death—consequences for the patient and for the student? What has been your own experience?

For graduate students and teachers of nursing

1. How would you redesign the typical assignment system so that students (undergraduate or graduate) would have more graded experiences with terminality and suffer less potential trauma from giving terminal care?

2. What sort of training should nursing faculties have in order to teach the conversational aspects of terminal care more effectively—or to teach it at all?

3. If nursing students were taught to talk effectively, or listen effectively, to terminal patients and their kinsmen, what impact might that have on the staff nurses? And what consequences for relationships between the latter, on the one hand, and students and faculties on the other?

4. How could terminal care be improved, in its social and psychological features, by means of in-service training for hospital and clinic personnel? How much do you think that training would improve terminal care without also changing ward and clinic organization? How would one go about doing the latter?

3. Pain

Barney Glaser, PhD, and Anselm L. Strauss, PhD

The following is a summary of part of a case history of a patient in pain and the problems that that pain (and that patient) set for the staff. The patient, Mrs. Abel, entered the hospital in September, went home after a few weeks, and like other cancer patients soon reentered the hospital. The account of the events presented here is based on the observations of one nurse researcher (SA) and an advanced nursing student (SY) who was involved in giving some nursing care to Mrs. Abel. The account was written by the sociology professor (AS) who both supervised the nurse researcher and extensively interviewed the student nurse. In reading this narrative, one should take into account that pain is always connected with particular courses of illness or treatment (including giving birth, recovering from an operation, living through burns and their aftermath, or dying from cancer). This particular case history just happens to deal with cancer, but its applicability to nurses' work and nursing care with regard to patients in pain is much more general than merely to patients who are dying from cancer.

SA: There are no children from either marriage. She had been taking care of her mother for a long period of time just before her own illness and had actually nursed her through a final illness. Now there was no one left other than her husband.

Mrs. Abel spent quite a bit of time weeping off and on, telling about these things. Also she said the nurses didn't come in to see her very often: she frequently put on her buzzer, but no one would come. When I went out to have the nurses tell me about this patient, they told me she kept a notebook: everytime she had medication, she would jot down in her notebook what she had had—the kind of medication, the timing, and whether it was an injection or pill. She was getting

Reprinted from Strauss, Anselm L., and Glaser, Barney: *Anguish, a Case History of a Dying Trajectory,* Mill Valley, Calif., The Sociology Press, pp. 33-113, 1970.

both. At that time she was on methadone, percodan, and darvon. She would alternate them. She had a schedule she regulated so as to get something every hour for pain. When one nurse told me this, I realized she was rather annoyed about this. There were frequent notes in the cardex in these first two or three weeks about Mrs. Abel wanting her pain medications around the clock. Finally Dr. Colp wrote orders that she could have the medications. But the nurses didn't want to wake her up at night. Then Mrs. Abel got to setting an alarm clock so she could wake up to receive pain medication. This, of course, never goes over very well with a group of nurses who feel you should not wake up patients to give pain medication: if they're sleeping through all this, then they don't have pain! Mrs. Abel's explanation was that if she waited until morning to get the medication, the pain got such a start that the medication then didn't take care of the pain. She wanted a consistent dosage of medication; she was very frightened of pain. The nurses said the first thing in the morning—6:30—Mrs. Abel was on the buzzer for her medication. This was a real problem to them. They were annoyed, they were irritated, and they were complaining among themselves.

This had been her first admission prior to her final admission. She'd been here about three weeks. But she had been in and out of the clinic associated with the cancer ward. The ward staff frequently see these patients before they come in to the ward.

AS: In other words, when you first saw her she was merely another patient who was somewhat bothersome.

SA: Yes. The nurses were irritated and annoyed, and they wanted her to stop using the notepad for writing down the medication.

SY: The head nurse apparently told her not to use this book, and it was then that Mrs. Abel began to set her alarm clock.

SA: When I went in to listen to a nurses' "team conference" report one afternoon, they were describing Mrs. Abel. They talked of another patient who was in a room with Mrs. Abel, and a nurse said, "I wonder what she thinks of Mrs. Abel?" Another said, "Well, she just sits and looks at her"—you know, as if the patient didn't know quite what to make of Mrs. Abel. One nurse said, "Well, Mrs. Abel keeps talking about suicide," so the other patient really doesn't know what to think. There was discussion as to "do you really think she's seriously considering suicide?" The nurses didn't think so. But the aide said, "I think she means it. She wouldn't even watch television or read this morning. She seems very low this morning. She is married but doesn't have any children, and she's fifty-four years of age. She's just kind of given up." This is one of the few times the aides have said anything about this patient at the meetings.

During this early two-week period, the next thing was that the nurses stated, "She is on the buzzer all the time." There was a note about this in the cardex, but the patient told me that the nurses "keep holding off." The girls described this tactic as: "We try and get her to hold off for at least two hours between medications." Mrs. Abel was trying to get them to come right on the dot when the medication was due. She was handling her medications—ordered every three hours—and arranged her schedule so that she would get it once every hour.

Also, she was complaining about a private doctor whom she had originally seen about her illness. "I went to see him, and he told me to go home and exercise my arm." She had gone to him for a lump in the breast; he had told her to go home and exercise her arm and it would go away. So she waited for about four months and went back to him—this is a man she had been going to for a long time. Then he sent her immediately to a surgeon, because the lump had continued to grow. She complained bitterly to me that he had not done a biopsy, that maybe if he had done something she would have been spared all this. If only it had been caught in time. She said, "I have an adenocarcinoma which is one of the fastest growing tumors." This is one of the first things she told me. When I first went to that floor, it was news to me that the patients there all knew they had a cancer; but she said very openly, "I have cancer, and it is one of the fastest growing kinds, but they think they can stop it with medications." She showed me at that time, too, her radiation wound lesion which had not healed. It was open and raw and irritated, ulcerated—a very ugly thing. Later on her shoulder became very painful looking, very black.

She also said she had had a whiplash injury from a car accident. She was involved in getting the lawyers to arrange for a lawsuit to get some financial remuneration. (This becomes part of our story later.)

Soon after, she went home for a week. When I talked to Dr. Colp—I talked to him the first time she was in, too—we talked about pain thresholds. I asked, "How did you determine this?" He said, "I used a No. 25 needle and she jumped. This patient has a very low threshold, and so she will need medication. I also told her she is on narcotics, hoping that she wouldn't take very much. I tend to discourage patients from taking narcotics and will tell them that I have so many patients who are in for the same problem and only two out of twenty are on narcotics. This isn't, usually, anything that is painful and therefore, I say, you should not need very much." He hoped that Mrs. Abel would stop taking medication but she didn't. This didn't even faze her.

At the same time, there was a note on the cardex to use a No. 25, a very small needle. Mrs. Abel was getting IM injections and should have had a larger needle than a 25, but they were using the smaller. She was still jumping and complaining about how much the injections hurt.

AS: Did you pick up that the nurses had some questions about how much she actually hurt?

SA: They *were* beginning to have this feeling because, normally speaking, a patient does not jump over a No. 25 needle. Its tiny enough. But certainly there was not the degree of the questioning which came later.

During this early beginning phase of her hospitalization, I really have very few notes about her. She was not mentioned much—you know—if you asked about Mrs.

Abel, the staff people would say something, but she was not constantly on the tip of their tongues.

I went back to the floor on the 20th of October and discovered Mrs. Abel had been readmitted on the preceding day. The head nurse said that Mrs. Abel was still constantly complaining and "has returned because her husband cannot take care of her"; also, the doctor admitted her in spite of his turning away of others because of his diminishing budget. There seemed to be a great deal of feeling by the RN's that the doctor was in a bind. The head nurse was sort of questioning, you know, why he had readmitted this patient. This isn't usual. She also told me the patient was admitted specifically for reasons of pain.

She was still complaining, still waking, still asking the night nurse for medication throughout the night. She was still waking up at 6:30 and asking for her shot. Dr. Colp said to keep her comfortable but don't wake her up, and this was the bind—how to keep her comfortable when she was constantly complaining. The night nurse said: she sleeps all night and sets the alarm to wake herself up, and yet she wants the medication during the night. The doctor says to give the medication to her but don't wake her up. He's telling the patient one thing and he's telling us another. He's telling Mrs. Abel, "They'll keep you comfortable," and he tells us, "Don't wake her up." So this was causing real problems then.

She was also beginning to complain of drowsiness from the amount of pain medication that she was getting, and beginning to sleep most of the time. One of the things by which nurses determine the amount of pain that patients have is how much they sleep. Are they sleeping through the pain? If so, they don't have a great deal of pain, or at least are fairly comfortable at the moment. Mrs. Abel was still keeping her medications timed so that she was getting them right on the dot of the three-hour schedule. The head nurse said, "The doctor has now ordered the medication for every two hours, but we haven't told Mrs. Abel that and so she's still running on the three-hour schedule." She was on sparine and morphine at the moment. While a staff nurse was talking to me, the head nurse went to give the medication to Mrs. Abel. It's not unusual for the head nurse to give medication. Normally the staff nurse who is medication nurse for the day will do that. But the head nurse took the medication down—a shot—and the staff nurse indicated that the patient's crying down there now because Miss Lee just gave her a shot. She also told me if you talked to Mrs. Abel, just stood there and talked to her, that she would forget about needing the medication.

AS: Did she also sleep the night through without medication?

SA: Unless she set her alarm clock.

AS: You mentioned that nurses believe if the patient sleeps the night through then the pain can't be quite that bad. Did this enter into that nurse's judgment?

SA: Yes, it did, very decidedly so. On the 20th of October, I also talked to Mrs. Abel. I had her tell me something about her week at home. Her husband had some problems in giving her medication—in controlling the amount and the time when she received the medication. She had a disagreement with her husband about the

52

amount of dosage: he had actually given her an overdose. He had gotten confused over the doctor's orders. There had been a refill of a drug order, and he got a different dosage. So this had been a real problem at home; there had been a lot of disagreement over medication.

Then she began again to complain about the RN's forcing her to space the timing of her medication. Also, "They all give injections differently"; and some nurses hurt, some give better injections. And she had begun to play one nurse against the other, and one shift against the other. She did this by complaining about one nurse to another when the latter was standing there giving medication, or by saying, "You do a better job of this." So she would try to manipulate or coerce the girls into giving her the medication. And by trying to make friends also, siding with people. She said the doctor had told her she didn't really need to worry about medication because the drug has an effect of at least six hours; but it never works that long for her, and she has to have it more frequently.

AS: Did she have great faith in her doctor, in his being able to handle the pain?

SA: Yes, she did. But she questioned whether the nurses could; she felt that they weren't giving her the medication.

AS: But the real control was in the hands of the doctor and he could, in the end, manage it?

SA: Manage the pain, that's right. She said, "I'm on three different drugs and I'm alternating them by the hour again."

The same afternoon, when the evening shift arrived, a bull session developed at the desk between the two shifts around Mrs. Abel. The evening girl said, "I just can't get along with her. I just don't get along. I never had a patient who rejected me so." She felt Mrs. Abel had very much rejected her. I think this was connected with Mrs. Abel pitting one nurse against the other, and one shift against the other. The nurse said Mrs. Abel complained about everything she did; and when she gave the injection, Mrs. Abel would say it was the worst one she had ever received. "Mrs. Abel told me she just didn't understand why some of the girls hurt and why some didn't. When I was redressing her, she finally got to me and Elaine had to go in." Elaine is the other evening nurse, so the other girl had to do the dressing because the first girl just couldn't take it any longer.

AS: There was no indication that she had been inept, less competent than the other nurses in giving the injection?

SA: No, I don't really think she was. I would say both nurses are competent in nursing skill. As a matter of fact, the whole staff on the floor is exceedingly good. I would say rather that Mrs. Abel was playing one against the other.

The nurse also said Mrs. Abel is still complaining to the doctor that they're still using too large a needle, even when they're all using a No. 25. So now he's written an order that they have to use a No. 25.

AS: We know that Mrs. Abel is negotiating very hard with the doctor.

SA: That's right. It was Fran, the night nurse, who was talking to me. She mentioned again the bind they all felt they were in—which the doctor was putting

53

them in—and he was in one himself with his relationship with the patient: the patient trusting him, telling the patient one thing (he could manage the pain, he could control it), and telling the nurses another thing (to keep the patient comfortable but don't wake her up, and so forth). Fran said, "Certainly she is in pain." There was not really much question that she was, although the staff had begun to question whether this was legitimate in terms of the amount of pain she had. But they all had the feeling that this woman was certainly in pain. "I should be able to do better," was what Fran was telling me.

During this bull-session, Elaine was saying Dr. Colp had gotten to where he was saying: you girls can't do anything right. He got to complaining the nurses couldn't even collect 24-hour urine correctly. The beginning of poor communication began, right at this point, between the nursing staff and the doctor. Until then there had been a fairly good communication between them. They had worked together for at least a half year.

Around that time, Dr. Colp complained about being called at night. "Why don't you call me earlier in the evening if you know a patient is going to need something or other?" Dr. Colp's way of handling it was to write a whole list of medications that would cover everything Mrs. Abel might possibly need, so he would not be disturbed at night or wouldn't be called on a weekend. This was just normal habit of doing things; but this becomes much more significant later in Mrs. Abel's hospitalization.

AS: What you are describing up to this point is the unfolding of routine tactics used when patients have "normal" pain. The doctor does this, and the doctor does that; the nurses do this, and the nurses do that. The complex of tactics probably would not vary much from patient to patient, although the staff might use one specific tactic with one patient and not with another; but combinations of routines are building up around Mrs. Abel—and more now than say a week ago in her hospitalization.

SA: On October 21, the next day after Mrs. Abel's return, the head nurse told me Mrs. Abel had set her alarm clock at 4:00 AM in the morning. That pretty much is all the nurse had to say about it. So, although the nurses were still being frustrated, they felt they were still in control of the situation.

AS: Can you summarize where you stood at this date?

SA: You and I had just begun to look at the phenomena of legitimation of pain and manipulation by patients for medication. We were to look at Mrs. Abel as an example of these things.

AS: We said there was some ambiguity for the staff concerning their reading of the degree of her pain. There seemed to be some difference between her definition and the staff's. We were raising the question of "how do they read the signs of degree of pain."

SA: We had begun to look at a physician's viewpoint and the nurses' viewpoints.

On the 23rd, I went back up on the floor. They said Mrs. Abel did not set her alarm that night. The day shift felt if Mrs. Abel had done so, the night float would have blown her top, would have been very angry. Since she hadn't mentioned it, they were sure Mrs. Abel had slept the whole night through. I don't know if this was the first time, but that was the beginning of her not using the alarm clock.

The mood of the nurses was irritation and annoyance—with a patient who sets an alarm clock or who keeps a schedule. And they were frustrated. They were not sure what was going on. They didn't know what to anticipate; I'm not sure I would call it surprise because you run into this in varying degrees with one patient or another.

AS: Were they puzzled?

SA: No, because then she began to fall asleep more in the daytime and when she was eating.

That's the last time anybody mentioned her setting the alarm clock. She had been setting the alarm clock since the 19th, when she was originally admitted. But now she had gone from methadone and percodan up to morphine. She had begun to sleep more, and sleep through; so she stopped setting her alarm clock. That was the 23rd. She wasn't especially mentioned in ward conversation until the 28th.

During this period, she was one of many patients with problems of pain whom I was seeing. In fact, the staff was more concerned with and had a great deal of sympathy and empathy for another patient who couldn't swallow and who had a great deal of pain while eating. (Also, at this time, you and I began to understand how a patient's pattern and routine affected the whole ward's routine. We were thinking about patients who had difficulty in swallowing and eating who upset the ward's routine. This is significant in terms of later problems which Mrs. Abel ran into.)

On the 28th the nurses said Mrs. Abel was still the same. Nothing new was happening. "We were running at an even keel. Now she is getting morphine every three hours, and her last dose was at 5:45 this morning." The night nurse told me Mrs. Abel said to her she didn't mind dying because she was afraid of too much pain. She had talked about suicide to me before, but this is the first time that I began to pick up that the patient didn't mind dying so much but couldn't tolerate the pain.

Later in the afternoon I was talking to another nurse who said that Mrs. Abel is now euphoric, that it must be due to the amount of morphine she is getting. The nurse and I tried to evaluate this europhia: how much was due to organic reasons and how much to psychiatric reasons and tensions that might be within Mrs. Abel, leading to the amount of pain that she had and her reaction to pain. It was then, too, that she was put on ritalin, which is sort of a mood elevator.

(The other thing that you and I were looking at then was "stockpiling" of drugs by patients, and Mrs. Abel was an example of a patient who would ring the buzzer a few minutes before she was actually due for the medication to make sure that she got it. Also to make sure that she got it every three hours, so that she would never run out of medication and therefore experience pain.)

Most nurses had seen me around the hospital before this in the capacity of a graduate student nurse. Also they were interacting with me as a beginning researcher for the first time. So they played two roles with me. Part of the time I was in uniform, and the other in lab coat or in street clothes. So off and on again we switched between two roles.

On the 28th, Elaine and I were talking to Dr. Colp about sending Mrs. Abel home and about the possibility of teaching her to give her own injections so she could go home. She was requiring so much medication that a nurse would have to be there 24 hours a day. Mrs. Abel's finances wouldn't quite allow this. This was the beginning of the problem of what were they going to do with Mrs. Abel, and how they were going to get her home? This was nine days after her re-hospitalization. The nurse was concerned: at that time they hadn't tried teaching Mrs. Abel yet to give her own medication, but she felt Mrs. Abel had the capacity—partly because Mrs. Abel had given medication to her mother during the lady's last illness. But the nurses were a little concerned about the possibility of an overdose of medication.

AS: The nurses had given up on the husband already.

SA: That's right. In fact, I hadn't seen the husband yet. But he's a traveling salesman.

My feeling about Mrs. Abel's self-medication was probably pretty similar. I felt she had, probably, the capacity to learn and to give herself injections. I, too, had wondered about whether she would give herself an overdose since she had expressed the desire for suicide. I was aware of her desire to hurry the process of dying. She knew she might eventually become terminal.

AS: Did you bring this up with Elaine or the doctor?

SA: No. They were thinking in terms of over-medication and overdose, but not the full picture. They didn't really start looking at this until quite a bit later. I went back a few days later. As it turned out, Mrs. Abel was not able to give herself the injections. Since her right arm was so edematous, she could not manage a syringe to give herself the injection. This put them in a final bind because she simply couldn't give herself medication, and she was not getting any relief from anything oral.

AS: If she were left handed, would they have sent her home?

SA: I question it because I had already begun to pick up the feeling of the physician, as had the nurses, that he didn't want to send her home. A couple of days later, I actually talked to him about what on earth he was going to do. But I already began to get this feeling, and the nurses began to get this feeling. This was why they were feeling the *bind*—I think. They did not actually talk about it, but the mood was there, and the feeling was there.

By this time, Mrs. Abel was on increased amounts of morphine and also on leritine, a synthetic narcotic. She could have each every two hours, alternately: morphine every two hours and leritine every two hours. So she was getting them every hour and still keeping track of everything in her book. The nurses began to say that Dr. Colp was making sure there was a whole raft of medication for the

56

weekend, so that they wouldn't have to call him about pain medication for Mrs. Abel.

At this point June and I talked about medication. She asked what were we finding out that might begin to help them solve the problem. She felt Mrs. Abel was more afraid of pain than she was afraid of actually dying. For the nurses, the psychological aspects of death were becoming a part of the picture. Dr. Colp, as was his usual custom they felt, was side-stepping the issue and not really being honest with the patient—about her real prognosis and outcome. They felt he was clouding the picture.

AS: Do they expect the doctors on that unit to give straight stories to the patients?

SA: They expect this, but on the other hand the philosophy is that you hold out as much hope as possible, and they are very optimistic on this whole service, so that it is sort of an ambivalent kind of expectation.

SY: In talking to the resident, Dr. Colp pointed out it's like tight-rope walking, trying to hold out hope and at the same time have the patient face reality that his life expectancy is two years.

SA: However, about then Dr. Colp told me that he was holding out hope for her but telling her that she had very little hope. Yet the nurses still felt he was really clouding the issue in making her feel that she had more to hope for. He was actually giving her a ten to twenty percent chance.

At this point I started to look at how pain may affect care, stemming from June's description to me about Mrs. Abel having to have things done in certain ways, since she was never satisfied with anything. June described: "I tried to cut her fingernails and ran into such a problem that I couldn't do *anything* right for her. It had to be done *her* way, and just *exactly* that way." June added, "I just don't know what to do with her," and was very frustrated. Mrs. Abel was on leritine and sparine around the clock, every two hours. They didn't have the alternative of choosing at night whether or not to give it to Mrs. Abel. They had to give it by order.

This dosage was contrary to the usual feeling on this floor that there is—as they say—very little pain connected with cancer. Patients are started out on gradual dosage—aspirin and so forth. Here on this floor we have a group of doctors with a particular philosophy of giving pain medication. Yet this specific patient was getting massive doses of narcotics and also sedatives. She was getting these medications on or around November 4, but she lasted for three and a half months thereafter.

The nurses were extremely busy during the month of November. There were quite a few critically ill, terminal patients then. A note on the chart said Mrs. Abel could have whatever kind of schedule she wanted for pain medication at bedtime, and by the doctor's orders she was allowed the privilege of scheduling things—to some extent. A penciled note in the nurses' planning care sheet, on the cardex, noted that the patient is very frightened about pain and keeps a schedule, and she was to be given medication every three hours. The note read, "Awake and use No. 25 needle" and also "Please awaken for meals and check her as she falls asleep during meals."

I ran in to see Mrs. Abel the night of November 4. At the same time, the nurse came in with the pills. Mrs. Abel asked if her pain medications were among the pills she was about to receive. The nurse said no, and that she would be back in about a half hour with the pain medication. I stayed about an hour and a half, but she did not mention the medication again for a while. About half an hour or forty-five minutes later she finally said, "Where's the nurse?" She hadn't realized that it had been forty-five minutes over the time she was scheduled to get the medication. I had been standing there talking about many things. As previously, she had been crying off and on.

The same evening Mrs. Abel and I got into a lengthy philosophical discussion— and this is the reason why I thought maybe she had forgotten the medication— about the meaning of reincarnation and about her religious beliefs. She had been reading some articles on the Essene.

Mrs. Abel also began to tell me about the increasing appearance of new nodules, particularly around the region of her neck, and she began to point them out to me. Her shoulder had begun to look very black and necrotic looking. There was a patient in the bed next to her, Mrs. Holt, who was also experiencing pain. She was requiring a lot of medication.

I then, on November 6, saw Dr. Colp and asked him about what he was going to do with Mrs. Abel. Was he going to send her home or was he going to keep her in the hospital? What were his plans? We were in the hallway. He spent a half hour explaining. He seemed to find a need to talk to somebody about this problem. He really was up a creek. He didn't know what he was going to do. He told me that he was going to see his supervisors and the social worker and find out what could be done, because there wasn't anyone at home to give her medication—the husband was a salesman and was away from home most of the time. When Mrs. Abel had been given insulin before, they had used an automatic injector syringe which the husband was going to bring in; and possibly, although mechanically she couldn't use her right arm very well, she could use an automatic injector type of syringe to put in the medication. He told me, "I *know* she's having pain," and that you could just look at her and see it—"all those nodules on her chest and arms." He gave a very graphic description of how horrible this was. He knew she was having pain, and he felt something had to be done. She just couldn't go home with no one to take care of her, and he didn't want to just send her to the County hospital or any place like that because nobody would take care of her there. So he wanted to keep her in this hospital. He didn't know *what* he was going to do, but he was at least going to talk to his supervisor and find out what could be arranged. He had gradually increased the sedatives and the leritine. He kept increasing the leritine rather than the morphine in order to keep her comfortable. He'd been explaining to her that the nurses couldn't wake her up to give her medication, because she still was sleeping a great deal; she had begun to sleep more and more during the day and night. He was trying to tell her "we can't wake you up to give you medication," and Mrs. Abel kept saying, "But I need the medication." So he was beginning to have problems around this issue.

The nurses were still feeling he was not aware of the basic problem. The problem was Mrs. Abel was *asking* for medication and *he* was telling *her* that they were going to keep her comfortable—but sort of ignoring that she was sleeping through the schedule yet still demanding medication and still complaining. But as we spoke, I became aware that Dr. Colp *was aware* and actually attempting to say something to the patient. The nurses were not seeing clearly what he was doing.

AS: This was the beginning of genuine animosity between the two sides. It is also the first time we really catch him in a moment of desperation, as he faces up to what he's going to do with his patient.

SA: That's right—what am I going to do with her, as she only has ten to twenty percent chance of cure? He was estimating roughly six months, in his prognosis . . . Almost a month will pass before the nurses realize Mrs. Abel is really a terminal patient though they do know her prognosis is poor.

Then we started looking at Mrs. Abel as a person who we would observe regularly. We began to predict some problems that *might* come up around her hospitalization.

At that time we thought she was going home. They were still looking for ways of getting her home, but even as Dr. Colp was telling me about this, he was planning a way of keeping her in the hospital because he couldn't see how he could send her home. Up until then we thought she might remain a week or two, or three weeks at the most, since he was using research money to keep her in the hospital *only* because her husband could not take care of her.

Then I began to focus closely on her. She was beginning to become the "patient-of-the-day" for the staff (i.e., the patient who gets the lion's share of the staff's attention). My notes become much more concerned with *Mrs. Abel*.

AS: In other words, it wasn't that you were just focusing on her in your notes. As you went around the unit, her name began to pop up everywhere when you talked with nurses. That's important to remember. It is also important to remember that we read the system wrong: we thought that it would not be able to contain Mrs. Abel for more than two or three weeks. How wrong we were! We didn't bank on research money or the anguish of a conscientious doctor. And the powerlessness of the nurses . . .

SA: . . . to be able to do anything about it. Remember, too, that we began to look at her as a patient whose whole attention was centered upon pain; the nurses' attention, too. This was the beginning of an expanding mushroom of staff focus upon the pain of one patient.

On the 8th of November, I talked again to Dr. Colp to find out what actually had transpired in the interview with his supervisor. The only way we could keep Mrs. Abel in the hospital was by making her a research patient, because the budget was getting so low they just couldn't keep her in simply because she had pain. There was no bed space, and there was no budget for her. This is the first time that he mentioned the possibility of having Dr. Tree—who was doing research around new drugs for control of pain—do research on Mrs. Abel. This would legitimate her stay in the hospital. So within two days' time, he had this arrangement made for Mrs. Abel so she could stay. He even knew what Dr. Tree was going to study with his new drug. Dr. Tree was going to compare new drugs, testing them against morphine. He would substitute his new drugs in place of morphine. Dr. Colp had tried to convince Mrs. Abel that she would stay just as comfortable with the new research drug. She had gotten very worried about the possibility of pain but took his word for it, he said. She still had a great deal of faith in him. In fact, I think she never did lose that.

He had to persuade her into this research because she was so deathly afraid the new, untested drug wouldn't keep her comfortable. But he had promised her that she would be comfortable. Also, he had to persuade her by saying: "This is the only way I can keep you in the hospital." He had no other choice. It was either make her a research patient or she had to leave. It was that simple.

But he did give guarantees that he would keep her out of pain. He said, "I kept persuading her and telling her that I would do this." I wondered at that time whether he would have to cut the medication to just percodan and the other sedative. But he said no, that they were just going to keep the medication as is.

It was the first time I had ever heard of this tactic to keep a patient in the hospital, and I began to wonder what his motivations were for keeping this patient in, because maybe other things could be done which might keep her comfortable. Did she really need to be in the hospital? And you and I had begun to recognize, first, it was pain that had first brought this lady *to* the hospital; second, pain was keeping her *in* the hospital; and third, one man now had control of *keeping* her there.

Then, too, a brief side issue came up. The nurses' notes reported the nurses had heard Mrs. Abel saying, "The doctor promised to keep me pain-free, but he hasn't." Mrs. Abel had begun to be very sleepy and to complain that she was never really pain-free in spite of the medication. Also, Dr. Colp said, "I keep her on high levels of sedation and high levels of morphine, and I'll keep increasing." He didn't know what else he was going to do, because I asked him: "What are you going to do when you reach the limits of morphine? What's happening? What can you do for this woman"? I was envisioning that he was saying to Mrs. Abel, "I'm going to keep you comfortable," while she was saying, "But he isn't keeping me comfortable now." And I thought, how much morphine can you give a patient? He began to indicate to me—this is the second time—feelings of guilt about the massive dosage of narcotics and medications that she was getting. This amount was very unusual—this much already at that point of illness. By this time he knew she was terminal, but he was still looking at her in terms of his six-months' prognosis rather than as immediately terminal. And he never was concerned with her becoming an addict.

AS: Also, you were not concerned because you thought she was terminal. We will soon see that the nurses get very much involved in the idea of narcotic addiction.

SA: Throughout the whole course of her illness her tumor growth was noticeably obvious. She was getting more nodules. They became more apparent, on the skin surface. Dr. Colp mentioned this too, in terms of legitimating her needs for medication. (Later she had increasing numbers of nodules, particularly right at the end again, so he kept changing the medication and apparently was keeping the obvious growth—which was apparent as soon as you walked in—controlled.) So now she began to have more trouble.

I began also to watch the nurses, each spelling the other. They'd walk into her room and do something or other to get the other nurse out of the room. Get them off the hook. They were getting caught in there and couldn't easily get out, so one girl would call the other girl out. She was making more and more demands, utilizing everything she could think of to keep them *in* the room. She began to take a long time swallowing her medication. In fact, a couple of times when I was there, it took a half hour. Mrs. Abel began to use methods to manipulate the nurses so that they would stay in the room. The nurses really began to be unable to tolerate her.

They were saying that they couldn't stand to take care of her because she needed to do certain things in a patterned way, ritualistically. They couldn't tolerate her—as Fran mentioned, she couldn't tolerate Mrs. Abel and had asked June to take over. And June had said, "We can't tolerate working with her for more than a day at a time." They worked out a pattern of who would take care of this patient: The aide was in on it, and so forth. They assured me that they all rotated an equal amount of time, so that all would spend some time with her.

When I talked to Mrs. Abel that night (about the 10th of November), she was very depressed. She was crying a lot, and she said, "I've been out of bed since 9:30 this morning." The nurses had gotten her out of bed and taken her down to the window. This was when they started the tactic of getting her out of her room and down to the view window—they'd take her out and she'd sit there all day long. She was still getting out and in bed fairly well by herself, but the tactic provided more things for her to watch: they were hoping that she would focus less on her pain.

About now Mrs. Abel really began to say that she was not being kept comfortable, that she was never out of pain. Most of the pain was during the day; she didn't complain much of staying awake at night. The sedatives were keeping her fairly comfortable at night. She began to describe this pain as a tight, drawing sensation, mostly in the right arm which was very edematous. She began to say, "I don't want to live. The few moments I'm free of pain aren't worth living for."

The nurses were feeling that this patient was demanding more attention and more medication than she probably needed—because she slept a great deal of the time, even sleeping through meals. She'd sleep down at the window, and the girls had already begun to feel they couldn't tolerate her, and Mrs. Abel was not

61

legitimating her pain completely. They knew she had some pain—they all say this—but the amount was doubtful.

The girls would often be in Mrs. Brands' room. She was a very severe and critical patient, a highly valued patient, a young, beautiful Italian woman with children. I noted that the staff was spending more time and help, even more than they normally would with a highly valued patient, to legitimate staying *away* from Mrs. Abel.

The doctor knew she was terminal but was not yet accepting it. We were predicting they would either have to keep her happy or comfortable; and were already beginning to predict they were going to be unable to do either.

In reviewing my notes again, I have realized certain changes occurred over the months. Mrs. Abel in September began to tell me about her husband and some of her family problems and how she had gotten into the hospital. By November she had completely stopped talking about that and began focusing on "how large my arm is, how much pain I have, and the increasing number of nodules" that were becoming apparent. After that, she strictly focused on pain, that they were unable to keep the pain in control.

We had been talking about the period around the 14th of November when Mrs. Abel wanted to be pain-free. But she didn't want to be snowed or so sleepy and had asked Dr. Colp to cut out or at least decrease the sedation that she was getting. I think he decreased the phenobarb. I began to think about the phenomenon of a patient being able to tolerate a certain amount of pain in order to be awake. A patient would tolerate so much for something she valued.

The nurses had varying feelings about her. They described how part of the time she was tolerable, and part she was not. They were still rotating her care. The aides were supposed to be rotating one day at a time: an aide would take her during the day, and one of the nurses on another day. They could tolerate her for one day at a time. The evening girls were having more problems, probably because there were only two evening girls on, and therefore they couldn't rotate as frequently. They began to have mixed feelings about her too. Mrs. Abel was complaining very bitterly about the staff. One day she was crying and complaining that on the preceding night although she was supposed to be getting medication every three or four hours, she hadn't gotten it even though she had repeatedly asked for it. In the report, it came out, the night nurse had gone back to check but Mrs. Abel was asleep, so the nurse hadn't given the medication to her. But the next morning Mrs. Abel was complaining that they weren't giving her the medication.

Dr. Tree, by the way, supposedly had come into the picture but had not appeared. In fact, he hadn't appeared after almost a week and a half. There was never any clearcut reason as to why he didn't appear, and he had never met the patient, so I don't know what the problem was. We never did find out why he had delayed.

The nurses on the floor said they were expecting him to come about a week and a half late, but varying people were expecting him momentarily, and Dr. Colp did

not know why he was late.

Since they were in the process of rotating, I talked to the aide about Mrs. Abel. I don't think the aide was as much involved really as the nurses were—although she did say they don't like to have her crying, and they were bothered by this. She said Mrs. Abel always cried, in order to get procedures done the way she wanted them done. She also described how she had to give Mrs. Abel's bath exactly the same way every day. This bothered her. She said, "It isn't as if I didn't know how to give a bath." (It has just occurred to me that maybe the reason why the aides weren't so involved is that they didn't have to fuss around with the pain medication; they weren't involved in the responsibility of giving or not giving the medication.)

On about the 17th Mrs. Abel said that now she was asking for pain medication about ten or fifteen minutes ahead of the time she was actually supposed to receive medication. It took the nurses that long to get there, she said. And she wanted to make sure that the medication actually was *there* on the appointed hour, so she would ask *at least* ten to fifteen minutes ahead of time. She would begin to put the buzzer on for the nurses, to remind them just in case they had forgotten. They were then supposed to be giving it every three or four hours—it was not a "prn" order. They were actually supposed to be giving it. She said, "I like to give them advance warning."

This was actually written for every three hours. I think by then the physician had changed to morphine, and the order was written for every three hours. "Prn," I think, at night, but an automatic order for the day time.

AS: The addiction question had not yet come up.

SA: Not for the nurses. The nurses never really talked about this.

On the 17th, Mrs. Abel was on 15 mm of morphine every three hours and was on percodan "prn." Helen said then that Mrs. Abel had put herself on a one and a half hour schedule, so that every hour and a half she got something or other. (You and I began to look at whether this is the area of contest that could occur between a patient and a nurse over the routine, and *who* was going to set up the routine at that point.) Helen was still complaining that Dr. Colp was telling the patient one thing and telling the nurses another about how much medication she could get and how often. And so Helen said, "We've sort of given up, we give her anything she wants."

Now the patient is setting the pace and not the nurses. They've given up arguing with her, are now following her routine, and she's pacing her own medication.

AS: On the cancer unit the patients often set the pace when it comes to deciding what to eat, when to take a bath, when to have their temperatures taken. But this patient is also setting the medication routines.

SA: Now on the 18th of November, Dr. Tree started doing his research with Mrs. Abel. This was when the nurses really began to really question whether she was responding realistically to pain. They always had been giving her IM injections with a No. 25 needle; but Dr. Tree was giving injections with a No. 22, which is the normal procedure. The girls said, "I don't understand how he can get away with it. She wouldn't ever let us do it." They began to question Mrs. Abel's tolerance to pain by using some objective facts. Dr. Tree was giving her the medication,   **63** increasing the amount of research drug and comparing that to the response of morphine and the response she was getting. He was also using placebos. On the day when I was there, he used the placebo without telling her. She thought she was getting the research drug. However, this followed his use of the research drug about three hours prior, and so there was some question about whether he could interpret whether his research drug was still having a lasting effect, or whether she really did not have the pain, I mean whether the placebo drug reacted the same as the research drug did. When I talked to him about a week later, he felt that she actually had pain, but that he really hadn't been able to evaluate this too clearly—other than by way of her blood pressure drop and in pupillary reaction, and there were some differences in changes. But he felt he could say she had given a good response to his drug.

I spent half an hour standing with him and his assistant at the bedside watching her reaction and watching Mrs. Abel's reaction to him. Her mood swings were alternating. She would cry one minute and then ask to have the window either open or closed, or talk about how awful her condition was and how much pain she was in. She was using the same tactics on him that she had on the nurses. He listened to her, but from my vantage point, he was listening with one ear open and one ear closed—so as to speak. He heard what she said but he really wasn't listening to her. He spent a half an hour in there and then left his assistant to spend the other half hour with her. When talking to Dr. Colp and me immediately after, he said, "I just can't stand a whole hour with her." He said, "I leave my poor assistant." So that *he* also pulls out! He made no attempt to reach her psychologically or assuage anxiety. He was strictly focused on how one research drug compared with the large dosages of morphine she was on. Although he planned to do further work with her later, he never did.

AS: Did her talking get in the way of his own research observation? Did she drive him out of the room so that he could not spend the other half hour in further observation?

SA: (laughing) He just literally left. They were watching, not so much her reaction—emotionally—but her blood pressure. The assistant followed through on that. The only way, Dr. Tree said, you could really interpret whether she had pain was the amount of emotional response that she had. And, of course, with Mrs. Abel this was almost impossible to assess.

AS: It sounds like the research doctor was having essentially the same trouble, although on a more technical level, that everybody else was having when trying to decide how much pain she really did experience.

SA: That's right.

AS: It's as if everybody was saying, "She's having pain, but we don't know how much"!

SA: That's true, they didn't ever know. The common lay perspective that everybody uses involves the idea of tolerance—how much people can stand in relationship to pain. Talk to anybody and they'll tell you that some people can tolerate more than other people can tolerate or that people react and behave differently to an identical amount of pain.

AS: Would you say that running through the confusion as to how much pain Mrs. Abel could stand was the assumption that "it's hard to tell exactly what her tolerance is"?

SA: Yes, that's right, but the nurses did not use the word "tolerance" for her. The chaplain did. They never really talked about her in terms of how much pain she had. They just didn't know how much pain she had but said that she complains constantly.

AS: Yet we have heard nurses talking about this with regard to other patients: how much they could take?

SA: That's right, but not in terms of Mrs. Abel. It's not in the notes *any* place.

SY: That's true, I have not heard the nurses talk about tolerance of pain. Not in relation to Mrs. Abel.

SA: In the middle of November, Elaine was complaining about the nurses' inability to tolerate Mrs. Abel, and the rotation of people going in to answer her light. They even took turns answering her light, then. "My turn, your turn," kind of thing, you know. Then they actually had a team conference. The girls got to discussing their inability to tolerate Mrs. Abel and that she always irritated them so much that when they walked out of the room, they took it out on the next person, whoever it might be: the aide, the other nurse, or what have you. So they finally got a team conference to discuss this situation because they were all getting mad at one another since they couldn't openly get mad at Mrs. Abel.

AS: Did the nurses feel that the team conference helped?

SA: Yes, in terms of their own inter-relationships. In fact, although there was a breakdown in communication between them and Dr. Colp, there was no real breakdown among the nurses themselves. You started the next week, Shizu, and by then Dr. Colp was really pulling out of the situation. The communication between him and the nurses *really* stopped then.

I think the actual final break came when he just would not dismiss Mrs. Abel from the hospital. That was in December. The nurses got to the point where they asked the supervisor to get rid of Mrs. Abel, the the physician said, "No." That was just prior to Christmas vacation, when I took the message back to Elaine that Dr. Colp was going to keep Mrs. Abel in. But the real break came over with their getting the supervisor "in" on the situation.

AS: Had the patient now become what we ourselves call "the patient of the year" or "the patient of the month"? That is, whether day by day she preoccupied the staff members, providing the major talk and gossip among them?

SA: She had: almost all my notes are completely about Mrs. Abel. This started about the beginning of November, in spite of the fact that Mrs. Brands, who was a terminal and very highly valued patient, lay dying in the middle of December. Also Mrs. Holt and another patient died. So there were three deaths on the floor, but Mrs. Abel preempted my notes!

65

AS: Even the highly valued patient got less ward conversation?

SA: They were spending *time* with Mrs. Brands. In fact, they involved me in her patient care. I was in street clothes one night, taking care of Mrs. Brands. There was also a staff nurse on the floor at that time—and she spent all of *her* time with Mrs. Brands, too. Although she indicated that she felt Mrs. Abel was a patient who if she couldn't tolerate death and talk about death ought to be snowed. She was the new night nurse.

It was in the same conversation that I had with Elaine that she began to look at how miserable things were for both the evening and night nurses. Elaine then was the assistant head nurse. One head nurse had left about the first of November and another had come in, Mrs. Twist. The girls had forgotten to tell me this, but Elaine was now the full assistant head nurse who had replaced the one who left around November 1. Elaine later, in fact still, is really running the floor.

AS: When the new head nurse came in did you see any impact on the relations with Mrs. Abel right away.

SA: No, I didn't. It was in reverse: Mrs. Abel had an impact on the staff. I had a hard time setting up a relationship with the new head nurse. In fact, I really had none, although I told her who I was and she was familiar with Mrs. Abel, and we were all heavily involved in working with Mrs. Abel. (This was about the beginning of when the girls couldn't tolerate *me, too*.) I just never seemed to be there when Mrs. Twist was on the floor and never really talked with her. So I always talked to Elaine. Elaine was not only my main informant among the nurses, but she was also essentially running the floor at the time. The supervisor first began to appear near the beginning of the year. I talked to her *after* Christmas—there were two or three supervisors ill at one time and so there was a lot of confusion in the administrative staff. She didn't get to the floor too often, but told me she'd like to spend time with Shizu talking about the care of Mrs. Abel. Toward the end of December she tried to spend some time with Mrs. Abel.

AS: Tell me about the nurses beginning to pull away from you.

SA: By and large, I talked to Elaine and June. Helen was off for a little while. I usually could talk to Helen, but I could catch Elaine and June sort of on the sly. They were still talking to me. Previously June had spent quite a bit of time talking to me about "what can we do for this patient?" But also they were really ventilating their frustrations; they're no longer asking "what can we do?" By the beginning of December, they would make a brief comment to me and suddenly get very busy with medications, or go off down the hallway, or some other place, so that even *they* began to pull out. But I have the notes from Helen, Elaine, and June about their frustrations, and they just couldn't tolerate . . .

AS: We might note here that June is a graduate of a university school of nursing. I interviewed her within four months after she'd arrived on this unit (about two and a half years ago). She was then struggling with how to handle dying patients—by herself since nobody had given her any real techniques for doing so. Then about a year ago, she was on a panel of experienced people that the Nursing Service set up, talking about the handling of dying patients.

66

SA: Really? And she's the one who sat down and talked to me in terms of "what can we do" for Mrs. Abel—the psychological care of Mrs. Abel.

AS: She's aware of this as an issue even though she's never really succeeded in answering it.

SA: Well, to continue: Elaine was talking in November of her complaints about Dr. Colp and the misery that all the nurses were going through, and the anticipated misery that was going to develop for them because of the research study. They did not know quite how Mrs. Abel was going to relate to Dr. Tree. They didn't know enough about the research project that he was on, but neither did I, then, to know whether this was going to affect Mrs. Abel's routine schedule. And wouldn't the research pull her off some of her medications? Would she, therefore, become more complaining, more weepy, and so forth? Was this drug going to be as effective as morphine or wasn't it? If it wasn't, Mrs. Abel was going to be in real trouble and would cause many more problems for the nurses. Elaine said, "Next week it's going to be awful for the patient *and* for *us*." The emphasis was on *us*, and "we" are going to get her constant complaints.

AS: Had they tried to talk to Colp to find out the nature of the research?

SA: No.

AS: Could he have told them?

SA: He knew that a drug was to be used instead of morphine but that all the other drugs used on Mrs. Abel would remain the same. But he didn't really know how this research was to be carried out. I had to go see Dr. Tree to find out myself.

AS: Could even Dr. Tree have told the nurses what would be the effect of their own tasks of his research? Was there any way of knowing then?

SA: Not at that point. I don't think they had done much similar research. In fact, that drug had not been used here before. This was the first patient he had used it on. When he pulled out later, he wanted to use it with a patient who had never been on the *amount* of morphine that Mrs. Abel had: he was looking for patients with fewer problems.

AS: Even if there had been adequate information between him and the nurses, it would still be very difficult to predict Mrs. Abel's reactions.

SA: That's right. He wasn't sure. But *he* was very difficult to find! In fact, I made several trips to his office, and since Dr. Colp and he didn't seem to have much communication, I became the person who had most of the information. The staff nurses were picking up information from me about what was going to happen. . . . This was around the 18th of November . . . .

I think I mentioned before that Mrs. Abel had mood swings. When I was there, she complained about the pills that now were due but she hadn't gotten them—and with the next breath asked the nurse who had come in to water the plant. The nurse started to water the plant with water from the pitcher, and Mrs. Abel said, "Heavens no, not with ice water." It was as if she said: "Even *I* know that you don't water the plants with ice water." So she went from one thing to another, complaining about how much pain she had and then she worried about her plant. I think this is where the nurses started to question, "How much pain does Mrs. Abel   67 really have?" Of course, when the affair with the placebo began (and *they* were supposed to make descriptive notes that Dr. Tree could use as a reference for his research, which meant that the girls had now to spend much time in Mrs. Abel's room), then they really began to question the amount of pain that Mrs. Abel actually had.

On this same day I spoke with friends who came to see Mrs. Abel. It's interesting that only once that I know of did a friend come. I saw the husband at least two times, a friend only once. She was a next-door neighbor. Although Mrs. Abel had been crying and complaining about her arm, the friend said to me: "This is the first time that Mrs. Abel has been willing to show her arm; before she has always hidden it and thought it was a disgraceful kind of thing." Mrs. Abel was happier *in* the hospital, than at home, according to the friend. I think it was because she was getting more attention in the hospital; and also because of problems at home. That Mrs. Abel and her husband did not get along together was apparently common knowledge in the neighborhood. There had been a lot of fighting and feuding over pain, and so forth.

As Mrs. Abel's edema became worse, the right hand got puffier and puffier, and she couldn't even straighten her hand. She would say, "Do you think I'll ever be able to straighten my fingers out again?" Her arm looked as if it was ready to split the skin, it was so edematous. She would focus on her inability to use it, along with the amount of pain, and the heaviness, the weightiness, of her arm. So I began to notice how localization of a particular body part should so engulf her attention that virtually her total life was focused around it.

AS: So what she was doing openly and publicly was to draw people into an orbit that circled around this particular body part.

SA: Yes. My note of November 8 says that it showed, even at this date. Although the nurses couldn't tolerate Mrs. Abel, the aide said, "She's in a lot of pain, poor thing." So the aide stuck with her at least up to then.

During Dr. Tree's research, Mrs. Abel was beginning to complain about the tension building up: "I just have to cry." She began to talk about crying as a way of relief from pain. I remember the nurses talking about how *they* began focusing on the pain, too. In fact, June said, "With some people, crying helps, but with Mrs. Abel it doesn't." But it was Mrs. Abel's feeling that crying actually relieved her tension, pain, and the whole frustration that she had built up. She said, "It's within my chest," where her lesion was anyway.

When June said this, she had a great deal of feeling in her voice, because she had begun to tell Mrs. Abel to stop crying. The nurses began to change: instead of tolerating Mrs. Abel's crying, all of a sudden they were beginning to be very aggressive toward her. "Look, crying just doesn't help you, so stop it!" It is unusual for a nurse to stop a patient in this fashion from reacting.

AS: What was their justification for this pure invasion of a patient's privacy?

SA: Feeling that they were more helpful if they became authoritarian, and very openly so. There was an interchange between June and Elaine and between June and me, particularly in terms of: we just *have* to make her do things and become very authoritarian. June wasn't using the word "authoritarian" really; what *did* she use . . . ? "Setting limits"—they had to set limits for this patient.

Actually, although they talked about it, they never really did set limits. In some sense they were going to set limits concerning her taking her pills, and so forth; that she had to do these things; she had to move around and get up. But they really stuck with her pattern. They had become used to her routine ritual and did realize that they were sticking with it. But they always talked about how it would be better for Mrs. Abel to be moved off this floor so that limits could be set. Yet Mrs. Abel had them wound around her finger, so to speak.

AS: Did they talk about stopping her crying because of her disturbing other patients?

SA: I believe this was mentioned in reference to one night when Mrs. Abel had disturbed other patients. Somebody told her that she just had to stop this: "You're upsetting other people."

AS: Were they under pressure from other patients to intercede?

SA: No, I don't think so. Unless they were picking up some cues from the patients. Nobody expressed conversation from other patients to do something, which is what happens on other floors when patients say, "I can't stand this, move me out of here." No one ever did this about Mrs. Abel. The thing the nurses couldn't stand was that Mrs. Abel even had other patients' visitors wound around her finger to the point that one went to the Stonestown Shopping Center across town and bought some shoes for her. This was a special trip—and Mrs. Abel had her take them back to exchange them!

Mrs. Holt was her roommate during this period, but she was terminally ill and most of the time she was comatose. This was the time when Mrs. Abel would snag Marilyn, who was a special student nurse for Mrs. Holt. She talked to Marilyn and Marilyn thought, "Ah, this patient is just beginning to 'ventilate' to someone. All she needs really is some attention, and so forth." Marilyn felt that she really had accomplished something with Mrs. Abel, that Mrs. Abel had sort of unburdened, and cried, and "the whole works." But I felt this wasn't helping Mrs. Abel because she had also done this with me. She had done it with the other staff nurses too, and this is why they felt that this really was not helping the patient. She was doing it to everybody she could grab hold of.

Also, there was some kind of experimental study going on in which undergraduate students were being taught interviewing techniques, and Mrs. Abel was one of the patients interviewed.

This was something that the floor just couldn't tolerate. So many people were hearing Mrs. Abel talk about her problems, therefore she was focusing too much on problems. So they pulled out the experimental interviewing. This is also why the staff couldn't tolerate me: they thought that because of my project I was asking Mrs. Abel to talk about pain. They didn't stop to find out what I was doing, where I was or wasn't; but thought too many people were causing her to focus on pain.   **69**

AS: One question: When the girls are talking about moving in to set limits on her crying, is there a tone of desperation? What is the mood? Is it anger, is it desperation, or is it . . . ?

SA: Anger. They've *had* it up to their teeth and they're going to stop this. It's, "I did this and found it worked, and I've *had* it." In fact later, but not this particular week, June describes herself as doing something when Mrs. Abel had finally gotten to her. She called Dr. Colp one night after Mrs. Abel had pushed and pushed her. So June thought she'd better check with him about symptoms. So the next day, Mrs. Abel was not bothering any other nurses, but she was calling for June and pushing her to ask Dr. Colp for more medications. June said, "I laid the law down again. I'm not going to do it." So June had begun to set limits because she felt she *had* to or this patient would use her.

AS: Did other nurses at any time, or aides, talk in terms like, "She's using me as an agent to get something"?

SA: June is the only one that did. I don't think the other girls were even that aware of what was going on. They were mad and they were angry, but not completely aware of why. They had the beginnings of awareness, but not to the extent that June did. . . . I washed Mrs. Abel's hair, too, at this time in order to chat, to see whether—well, I had a two-fold reason: one was that Mrs. Abel's hair needed to be washed again, but they just hadn't had time to do it. So I thought, I'm spending time with Mrs. Abel anyway and this would help the girls, and also my relationship with the floor staff, if I actually assumed the function for them. A second reason was that I wanted to see how Mrs. Abel would react to me. The girls would say, "I can't even cut her fingernails without her telling me how to do it." And she complains afterward. I wanted to know if she was doing this just with nurses or with anybody. So I washed her hair, and she told me once how to do it and continued to talk to me; but even though I couldn't follow exactly what she had wanted me to do because we didn't have enough curlers and things, she never complained about how I did her hair or anything about the entire process. I had to go back the second day to finish because it was late and she didn't want to go to bed with curlers in her hair. I didn't find that I had the problem that the other nurses did. Of course, she wasn't "buying" medication from me though.

AS: Who did she see you as? Who were you to *her?*

SA: A nurse doing a study, by and large, that had no connection with *what* she got. This is just a person who came in and talked to her—at that point.

AS: If you were to summarize your feelings, as you then looked at things, can you say what you believed was going on?

SA: I was seeing both sides of the issue. I could see what Mrs. Abel was doing to get her medication, and I could see that she was having trouble getting medication. She was complaining that they never brought it, that they never came on time, that they didn't believe her about her pain. I could also appreciate the communication problems that the nursing staff was having with the physician *and* with Mrs. Abel, and its inability to tolerate these problems. I think I identified with both sides.

Also, this is the night that I saw her husband for the first time. He was in the room when I came in. She began to talk to me about not getting any relief from her medication, not getting her pain pills, and she began to cry. The husband *got up* and *left*. He just couldn't tolerate this. He came back in a few minutes. She had continued crying. He sat down without saying where he had gone or what was going on. He asked, "Are you having pain now?" And she very angrily said, "Yes, I told you, I'm always in pain." Almost within the next breath after that, as she waited for her pills, she reached into a box of Kleenex and pulled out a ballpoint pen—to give to me. She's crying and talking about one thing, and the next thing is: "I sent my husband to get something or other for the nurses. We decided not to give candy because you know that doesn't last very long, so he bought this ballpoint pen."

When I walked out to the desk, I said to the girls, "Mrs. Abel is giving you pens." Fran said, "Oh, yeah, I see you have the latest status symbol. I had one to start with." It was her pen that Mrs. Abel had seen, and she had thought it's so useful because the pens are blue and red, and the girls alternate between using red and blue ink for charting. So Mrs. Abel thought this was a real nice gift. Fran indicated that she already had one, therefore she didn't receive the status symbol. She was almost sarcastic and disgusted with Mrs. Abel, that Mrs. Abel would use this kind of mechanism. It was with disgust that she said "status symbol." Because the girls, well, they've just "had it" by this time.

AS: Had the girls made much reference to her husband?

SA: No. When they did they indicated that they felt sorry for him, to be married to a woman like Mrs. Abel, that having to put up with her must be pretty awful. Most who spoke of him, spoke in those terms, assuming she was like this outside the hospital too.

Fran felt Mrs. Abel was very angry at her at this point. Fran was the nurse who believed that Mrs. Abel considered her not competent to take care of her. Mrs. Abel was constantly complaining. This bothered Fran because she wanted to feel that she was a competent nurse. She said, "She's so angry with me, Mrs. Abel will probably make me swallow a pen instead of giving me one." I remember Fran's emotional tone. It was "loaded" when she said ball points were the new status symbol.

AS: Did Mrs. Abel make other nurses feel a sense of professional inadequacy, dishonor that they couldn't live up to being a nurse with her?

SA: Fran was the only one that really expressed that completely. She did that way back, early, when Mrs. Abel was complaining about infections, and it comes up again later: that she just cannot work with Mrs. Abel, and Mrs. Abel is constantly complaining about her ability. In the next breath Fran's saying that she feels sorry for Mrs. Abel, that she wants to help her but can't seem to. "Everything I do for her is wrong." This was about the 20th of November, and Dr. Colp was saying that because of Dr. Tree's coming up, he himself could escape a little more. He said that to both Dr. Tree and me.

Mrs. Abel was not, at this point, talking about death as such. June said, "She's not focused on death." But the nurses thought that her pain was heightened by her feeling that maybe the pain was related to death. We ourselves had begun to ask the question, "Is the pain and her suspicion of death correlated?" But Mrs. Abel was more concentrated on her disfigurement.

In fact, Mrs. Abel didn't then feel that she was terminal and neither did the nurses. The doctor knew it. In some sense the nurses knew that he was going to keep her in the hospital. But he never really expresses a decision that openly.

AS: The nurses, then, expected that some research would be done on her?

SA: And that she would go home—it's that simple!

We remarked earlier that the nurses did not talk about Mrs. Abel's pain tolerence. Mrs. Abel herself says, "My pain tolerance is different than other people." And I hadn't looked at it in terms of *her* talking about tolerance. It really wasn't used around her. This is something she was talking about by herself with the common knowledge that everybody reacts differently to pain. So she said, "I just can't tolerate this much." She said this back in the middle of November. As a field worker, I was assuming that she picked it up from the nurses. But it's not until now that I realize the nurses didn't use it. Mrs. Abel wanted to know, too (she was having a lot of trouble with her pain), why couldn't the nurses give her medications earlier. You know, fifteen minutes earlier, what difference would it make. She was bargaining for more medication. June said, "She asked me for it. And I just wasn't going to give it because the three hours was not up."

AS: Did Mrs. Abel ever show a genuine comprehension of what the nurses were going through and their difficulties with timing, and so on?

SA: No. . . .She took a good half hour to take medication one night when I went in with June. June slipped me the pills so that she could go on to her other jobs. You're not supposed to leave pills at the bedside at any time with a patient, particularly if they are narcotics. She could stock-pile them. I don't think the nurses were too careful about that with Mrs. Abel, and they would leave medication at the bedside. June left knowing I was a nurse, saying, "You'll be here anyway, won't you?" I said yes. So she passed over giving the medication. Mrs. Abel was annoying her because she was spending too long taking the medication. Not until the middle of November did they actually start expressing this. Elaine was the one who told me the amount of time the patient consumed. They felt even after Shizu left that Mrs. Abel required more time. They said, "Look at the number of times we *have* to be in there, just to give her medication!" Somebody had to be in there almost every hour because Mrs. Abel had it scheduled so that at every hour she had her medication. Well, it took her a half hour to take the medication, so the medication nurse was in there a half hour of *every* hour. Then the bath would take longer than that, and Mrs. Abel stretched this out. There was very little time when Mrs. Abel did not have some member of the staff in there for legitimate reasons. There was very little time when she was actually alone.

• • •

We turn now to a theoretical commentary on the earlier "pain" phase of Mrs. Abel's trajectory. The commentary consists of an analysis of the events—and of the general story of Mrs. Abel's deteriorating relationships with the staff—during this phase. Our analysis is directed mainly by a theory of pain. . . .

Earlier we noted that when patients are recognized as dying, the staff organizes its activities in terms of the perceived dying trajectory. Similarly, when a patient enters a hospital ward, the staff members quickly begin to form estimations of how much pain a patient has, whether it will increase or decrease, and at what rate. In short, they have pain "expectations"—and perceive the patient as having a pain trajectory. Patients may also have such expectations. Leaving aside for the moment how these expectations are formed, let us note first that the nursing personnel who attended Mrs. Abel conceived of their ward as a place where patients usually die without much pain. Furthermore, patients with Mrs. Abel's kind of cancer—even when they are dying—tend to have relatively little pain. Consequently, the nurses and aides neither anticipated that Mrs. Abel would offer a great problem in pain management nor were ready to believe that she had as much pain as she claimed initially. The doctor gave her a little more credit than they, but also expected a relatively easy pain trajectory. The experiences of all the staff, especially the nursing personnel, with previous cancer patients played a major role in their evaluations of how much pain Mrs. Abel really had—no matter what she claimed—during the first months. To understand fully, however, why they were successfuly able to reject her claims it is necessary to analyze how pain is discerned and what a patient may have to do before his claims to pain will be believed.

Only the person who is experiencing ("feeling") pain can directly perceive it. Others must either rely on his report, trusting him, or use his gestures as indicators of pain. When the onlookers expect pain, then crying, groaning, grimacing, wincing, perspiring, or the clenching of teeth may easily convince them. If they do not expect him to have pain, then he must make his pain plausible. In effect, he must legitimate his pain. Under ordinary household circumstances, someone can remark that he has a headache and get others to believe him, but hospitalized patients are known to be unduly afraid of pain and quick to claim more than they have.

When Mrs. Abel began her attempts to convince the staff that she really did have considerable pain—crying and "complaining"—she only managed to persuade them that she had little or at least much less than she pretended. The more she attempted to legitimate her pain during these first months, the more she gave the impression of being "overdemanding," of not being honest about her assertions. After her readmission, when she was insisting on even greater pain, the nurses discounted this because she would sleep right through the night or would forget her so-called pain when she became engrossed in conversation.

In Mrs. Abel's case, the physician and the nurses assessed the amount of her pain somewhat differently, and this discrepancy began to lead to certain difficulties. We need to be clear on the complex division of labor which is involved in this multiple assessment. First of all, the physician is the legitimate person to assess pain—even if he is not certain and chooses to accept the assessment of the patient. Only he can legitimately decide on the proper means for relieving the pain.   73

Rarely does he carry out the relieving activity himself but delegates it to someone else: in the hospital he delegates the task to the nursing personnel. When he orders drugs, then the nurses can have little discretionary power, unless that is delegated to them as when they may reduce or increase dosage by agreement or by order. Because the nursing personnel spend much more time with the patient, they are or think they are, in a better position to reassess the patient's pain. Their reassessments are much affected by the patient's reactions while they are administering drugs, as well as by his reactions while they are merely working around him. If patients are too stoic or seem unrealistically "complaining," then the nurses can be misled.

Mrs. Abel, like many patients, adopted certain tactics designed to insure that her own assessment of pain got proper relief. Her tactics worked to some extent, but also irritated and angered the nurses. When her drugs were due, or even earlier, she got on the buzzer. She was preventing any possible increase of pain, or appearance of pain perhaps, that would arise because of a gap between drug administrations. She kept an account of the dosage in her book as they were given, presumably to insure that she got the proper amounts and at the correct times. She queried the nurses about what drugs she was getting. She attempted to prevent man-made pain, warning nurses when they injected her or complaining when they hurt her. The staff saw her as playing one person and shift against another. She also stockpiled her drugs against the day when she might need them desperately.

The personnel used standard counter-tactics, routine modes of dealing with patients like Mrs. Abel. They discounted her complaints, turned a deaf ear to criticisms, gave her drugs at longer intervals than she imagined the physician had ordered, and spelled each other in the onerous task of ministering to her needs and demands. But even in her first weeks on the ward these tactics did not work too effectively. One reason was that Mrs. Abel was doggedly persistent in her complaining and in reminding them about her drugs. Another reason was that she complained to her physician who in turn carried some of the message to them, to their understandable anger. Their anger was fed by their belief that he was putting them "in a bind"—telling the patient one thing (he would control her pain) and telling them another (keep her comfortable but don't wake her up for drugs).

For the understandings about pain control which grow up between physician and patient are crucial in their impact on ward events. Certainly they were in Mrs. Abel's case. In effect, Dr. Colp had promised her at first to keep the pain under control, believing he could. So his patient began with the expectation, trusting him. When he sent her home, neither she nor her husband could properly handle the medications, in order to control the pain, therefore he readmitted her to the hospital. The physician even allowed her some responsibility in her own control of pain, permitting her to schedule medications to some extent. However, he ran into a problem with her relatively early—the same one that he encountered with the nurses—because he tried to negotiate with her about sleeping through the night ("We can't wake you up to give you medication."), but she insisted that she needed the medication. Since, in fact, she did sleep through the night and later right through the scheduled administration, while yet demanding medications and complaining about not getting them, the nurses' anger toward her and the physician increased. The physician then is also in a bind: he is trying to keep pace, through increasing dosages of drugs, with the patient's genuinely increasing pain, but is well aware of the mounting strain between the nurses and himself. Meanwhile, as early as November 16, he is balancing two trajectories: a dying trajectory and a pain trajectory. He is estimating roughly that Mrs. Abel will live six months, with little chance that she might be saved, and yet he is aware that her pain may outpace his efforts at control—or if not actually outpace then at least Mrs. Abel would keep up her demands on the nurses.

Crucial in his calculations also was the absence of responsible kin. Had there been someone at home who could have administered the drugs, the physician would have discharged her. If she were sufficiently wealthy, private duty nurses could have been hired. Since neither condition was fulfilled, the physician had only the option of sending his patient to the county hospital as a welfare patient. At this point his personal feelings entered the story: because of certain events in his own past, he could not stomach the idea of sending Mrs. Abel to the county hospital. This in only the first of several times that his experiential career will crosscut the hospital career of his patient. All nursing personnel except one, however, have no such experiential career, so they begin what later becomes a virtual campaign, pressuring their nursing supervisor to rid the ward of Mrs. Abel. By now the patient had become what the researchers termed "the patient of the day." She was the staff's main preoccupation. The patient's claims to pain now flooded the staff much as the pain itself flooded Mrs. Abel.

In any event, the staff's efforts to get Mrs. Abel discharged failed because of Dr. Colp's tactic of making Mrs. Abel into a research patient. Thus her pain—as Dr. Colp perceived it—first got Mrs. Abel readmitted to the ward and then kept her there as a special patient. And again his promises to a trusting Mrs. Abel are important: he assured her she would be kept just as comfortable on research drugs as on the drugs she had been receiving.

Since pain as a general phenomenon not only has such properties as intensity, direction and rate, but also varies in when it "appears," it is important that Mrs. Abel claimed her pain was quite continuous. If not continuous, it was at least intermittently frequent—that is, every two or three hours, and generally just before her next drugs were due. Such continuity in pain symptoms and complaints about pain is hard on the nursing staff, even when complaints are uttered in low key and pain in minor. Since Mrs. Abel claimed intense and worsening pain and complained loudly for all to hear, the nursing staff found her an increasingly difficult cross to bear.

They reacted not only by spending less and less time within beckoning distance of the patient but by disengaging each other from her room when stuck there. They carefully arranged staff rotation, so that nobody would have to spend much time with her. They invented the tactic of persuading her to a window which looked out on the city, hoping that her attention would be distracted both from them and her pain. They also reacted by spending more time with a highly valued terminal patient than normally they would.

Then we began to see the appearance of an important phenomenon, which we shall term "the balancing of priorities." Thus a physician frequently will decide to withhold temporarily pain relief because medication might obscure certain diagnostic symptoms. Or he will balance the giving of opiates against the probability that their administration will hasten death. Or he will give a milder rather than a stronger pain reliever because the latter will make the patient too groggy or will decrease the respiration rate. During the course of a patient's decline, the physician will balance and rebalance pain relief against other priorities—and so will the patient, the nurses, and the family. In Mrs. Abel's case, we see her relatively early balancing her increasing pain against her life. "The few moments I'm free of pain aren't worth living for." Soon she is balancing being groggy or awake against pain, deciding in favor of a slight reduction in sedatives. It is worth emphasizing that such balancing goes hand in hand with negotiation. At the moment, Mrs. Abel is negotiating with her physician to cut down her medications; earlier he had attempted to negotiate a reduction of her narcotics, but she had refused him. Later they will negotiate about further balancing.

Around November 17, there appeared another important phenomenon: the nurses gave way on their management of Mrs. Abel's pain relief, ceding over to her a considerable measure of control. ("We've sort of given up, we give her anything she wants.") By now, she was regularly and deliberately ringing her buzzer for medications at least ten to fifteen minutes ahead of time they were due. The visible battle over who should control pain relief had been at least partly won by the patient—even though the nursing staff continued to discount the amount of pain. (Her positive response to the research doctor's placebo only furthered their disbelief.) The nurses' lessened control stepped up the process whereby Mrs. Abel became further insulated (or "isolated"), since the nurses spent less time with her—even time devoted to attempting to control her pain relief and her general behavior. Nevertheless the conversation among them turned frequently on Mrs. Abel: she was still a source of frustration and anger—which occasionally spilled over to color their reactions to each other and of course toward Dr. Colp. It also affected their relations with the nurse researcher, whom they began to reject because she was associated with getting Mrs. Abel to focus more on pain. That rejection continues for many weeks.

Although the nurses had partly yielded control of pain relief, by no means had they given up their attempts to control Mrs. Abel's inappropriate behavior. In anger, one nurse told the patient to stop crying. "Look, crying just doesn't help you, so stop it." Indeed, coming down sternly on her became a staff tactic during this period. Nevertheless, Mrs. Abel was pretty much getting her way with the scheduling of the medications, despite the frequent discussion among the staff about "setting limits." She was still attempting to keep the nurses at her bedside for the many minutes it took her to down her medications. (This had the consequence that the nurses sometimes left before the medications were taken, leaving her an opportunity for the stockpiling of drugs, an opportunity she possibly used.) In fact, Mrs. Abel continued to keep personnel in her room, if possible, by using stalling tactics such as dallying over her bath or making various requests. During this period, then, the contest over "presence" in the room continues and even increases, although the contest over management of pain relief actually had lessened. Thus Mrs. Abel's success at inducing personnel to attend her, plus the physician's instructions that because she was on massive doses of drugs somebody now had constantly to be in her room, meant she virtually had a private nurse. Whoever was in attendance was also engaged in a contest to reduce the number of her requests, which tended to come one after the other. In this contest the nurses were at a further disadvantage, for after the physician had given his instructions, they could not easily escape the room as before. Meanwhile Dr. Colp was increasing the bind they were in because he was, unbeknownst to anyone (except the researcher), postponing any further increase of Mrs. Abel's drugs, balancing the potential decrease of her pain against more important priorities. Nevertheless, he had given up thinking there was anything more he could do for his patient other than to keep her relatively comfortable. He will discharge her, he believes, after Dr. Tree has finished his drug research with her.

About this time, November 25, the student nurse elected to care for Mrs. Abel, and in effect becomes a private duty nurse, giving occasional care to her. Unlike the staff nurses, the student perceived Mrs. Abel as a terminal patient—time of death uncertain and perhaps some months off. She had also a different ideology of pain. Pain was meaningful to a patient, and so a nurse should listen closely to a patient's complaints and comments. Mrs. Abel's tactics, as they focused around pain, presumably were associated with her anxieties and other psychological reactions, not merely with any need to dominate the staff. Listening and spending much time with Mrs. Abel, the student nurse heard the same details as the nursing staff did, but interpreted the pain as having to do with Mrs. Abel's changing body images. Her reading of pain was quite different from the staff's. She was not concerned with how much pain Mrs. Abel actually had or how much pain she could tolerate. She would even have been willing to admit that Mrs. Abel might have had little pain and yet assign it significance. The staff nurses, of course, perceived Mrs. Abel as having relatively little pain and thought it insignificant. On the other hand, the nursing care given by the student was much the same as the staff's and Mrs. Abel's management of her was much like her management of the staff. Hence, she too found herself engaged in contests with her patient. Yet in describing Mrs. Abel's tactics, the student uses a more sophisticated—and ideological—language deriving from her training in psychiatric nursing. And since she saw her patient as dying, she had already moved ahead of the staff in defining her own actions as "terminal care."

By the time the student nurse had appeared on the ward, a collective story about Mrs. Abel had, of course, fully emerged. Details were continually added to the story, but its central theme remained constant: an immensely demanding patient, whose increasing pain was never fully legitimated. The student was heir to this story. She attempted to reinterpret its details; nevertheless from the beginning she too is caught up in its central theme. Her reinterpretaton of Mrs. Abel's acts and comments is more psychiatric, but her tactics do not work much better with Mrs. Abel than those used by the staff. Before long she also found that "nothing works." Both she and the staff were, in her words, "up a tree."

By now the staff was getting desperate because they envisioned that Mrs. Abel might be around forever, and yet could not get Dr. Colp to discharge her. They do not yet recognize that this frustrating patient is dying. They do not understand that the physician has disappeared from the ward mainly because he has nothing more to offer his patient.

By now Dr. Colp had gotten himself into financial straits because Mrs. Abel's prolonged stay was eating up his research budget. He was having to turn away potential research patients. To Mrs. Abel he also admitted that no matter what medications he gave, he could not stop the pain in her arm. He made a slight attempt to convince her that it was not really pain she was feeling, but of course was not successful. Shortly afterwards the student nurse accused him of merely dosing her and offering false hope—"and probably just relieving your own conscience." Their tempers were getting ragged because nothing seemed to work with this patient.

It is important to understand that the patient did not yet fully understand she was dying—or at least had not abandoned hope—and was still focused on her pain; whereas her physician and student nurse had moved to the next phase of concern with controlling pain in the context of dying. So had the chaplain, who though he now despaired of helping her psychologically or spiritually had not really abandoned her, anymore than had the physician and the student nurse. The nurses, however, could not yet feel the contradictory tugs of compassion and despair because they did not yet define her as "now dying." They do not yet perceive the pain as an indicator of death as an outcome. Since the social worker does not know Mrs. Abel was dying either, and does not understand Dr. Colp's attitude toward the County Hospital, she is confused and frustrated by his seeming vacillation about the discharge of his patient. Also, the chaplain and the student nurse were avoided by the nurses when each asked about Mrs. Abel, and both were much concerned about the nurses' avoidance of an increasingly agitated Mrs. Abel.

All these events were the consequence of a closed awareness context: some people did not know that others believed Mrs. Abel was dying, and the latter people intentionally choose not to reveal that their actions were based on those beliefs. The stage is now set for closed awareness to move into open awareness, when the nursing personnel will understand that Dr. Colp believes Mrs. Abel is dying. And so will Mrs. Abel. The closing scenes in Mrs. Abel's drama flow from a combination of open awareness and the staff's definition that the patient has reached the "nothing more to do" phase of her dying. Then there are new bases for disruption of the ward's work and sentimental orders—and of course for further deterioration of the relationship between Mrs. Abel and the staff.

A final word about the analytic commentary given in the above pages. Without a theory of pain, this commentary would have been much less pointed or specific, at least in the directions guided by the theory.

SUGGESTED QUESTIONS FOR DISCUSSION AND ANALYSIS

For undergraduate students
1. What do the authors mean by "legitimizing pain"? By "assessing pain"? By the "balancing of priorities"? By "yielding control of pain relief"?
2. What has been your own experience in "managing" patients who are in pain—and managing yourself, as well, while doing so? Are you better with some kinds of pain—also some kinds of patients—than with others?
3. Do you think pain management is different on different wards—such as OB, pediatrics, surgery, geriatrics? What different kinds of tactics would nurses have to use on those different kinds of units in order to give good nursing (including psychological and social) care while yet "managing" the patient's pain reactions?

For graduate students and teachers of nursing
1. Discuss some of the implications of the following statement: a great deal of pain that is seen in the hospital is actually inflicted by the nursing (and other) staff.
2. Various staff members are likely to have different ideas or philosophies about pain and pain management. What implications does *that* have for giving good nursing care?
3. How would you go about reorganizing a given ward (or agency) so that better nursing care would be given to patients with certain kinds of pain? (By better care is meant psychological and social as well as procedural, physiological, and pharmacological aspects of care.)
4. If you were a teacher of nurses, how would you set up a program for preparing students for better managing of both patients in pain and the students' own reaction to the pain? Include social and psychological aspects of management in your discussion.

section C

Some special wards

Even relatively small hospitals consist of spaces that are used for very different purposes, such as for surgery, for delivery, or for the dressing of minor wounds. Larger hospitals have highly specialized work locales, such as intensive care units, coronary care units, psychiatric units, gynecological units, kidney transplant units, and urology units. Some wards have a preponderance of older patients; some are only for young children. Nurses who work in these different settings necessarily do very different types of work—or so an independent observer would note if he cared to watch them at their work. In intensive care units, for instance, nurses are busy with machinery and watching vital signs; on psychiatric wards there is virtually no machinery, and nurses are busy with quite other activities; on cancer wards nurses are giving terminal care to patients who, as a rule, are dying rather slowly or are not yet classified as "dying now or yet"; on obstetric wards nurses are busy helping to deliver babies, and the process is generally a rather speedy one. In this section we shall read about the work on a variety of wards, as well as the types of problems that nurses typically encounter while working on one ward or another.

4. The nurse as care-giver — managerial agent vs therapist

Anselm L. Strauss, PhD, and others

The following selection is taken from a study of two psychiatric hospitals and their personnel. One of the hospitals (PPI) was a private hospital—actually part of a larger community hospital—in Chicago. It had about 90 beds and was divided into five wards, graded from "most open" to "most closed." None of the nursing personnel were "trained" psychiatric nurses in the sense of having had special training in psychiatric nursing; they all learned their specialization on the job-either at PPI or elsewhere. Even the head of the nursing service had not been specially trained. This feature of psychiatric hospitals was not unusual in the period from 1958 to 1963, when this hospital was studied, and indeed it is still fairly characteristic of most psychiatric hospitals and wards as far as the bulk of nursing personnel is concerned. As in most American hospitals, the physicians (psychiatrists in this instance) house their private patients on the wards. The resulting interaction between nurses and physicians and between nurses and patients is exceedingly complex—and rather difficult for the nurses. As at PPI, they tend to be caught between the requirements for keeping control over a potentially chaotic situation and playing a meaningful part in the therapeutic drama. It is worth adding that this psychiatric hospital was highly regarded, both locally and nationally.

THE NURSES AND THERAPY

The nurses would not consider themselves psychiatric nurses unless their work also included therapeutic action. At PPI, there is no public statement of the

Reprinted from Strauss, Anselm L. (with Schatzman, L., Bucher, R., Ehrlich, D., and Sabshin, M.): *Psychiatric Ideologies and Institutions,* London, 1964, The Free Press of Glencoe, Collier-Macmillan Ltd. pp. 213-227. Copyright 1964, The Free Press of Glencoe, a division of the Macmillan Co.

position that nurses play no part whatever in the therapeutic drama. The hospital's main business is to make patients well enough to function again in the outside world, and everyone in the hospital who works with patients is supposed to be contributing to the institution's goal. A sense of genuine colleagueship in a common enterprise is shared by all echelons, even the lowest.

The sense of common enterprise, however, shatters upon the shoals of certain critical events. Then the various personnel discover how far apart are their respective judgments of who is contributing what and how much to the therapeutic enterprise. Nurses are in a peculiarly perilous position: They take their therapeutic duties and prerogatives very seriously, but intermittently they cannot ignore the at least partial rejection of their specific claims by the psychiatrists. Furthermore, nurses have vested interests in therapeutic action sanctioned by a universal professional ideology, which teaches that they are psychiatrists' right-hand men, their auxiliary agents. When they fail to serve this function, it is supposedly their own failure and casts no doubt upon the tenet that nurses should be useful participants in the therapeutic process. Unfortunately for the nurses' peace of mind, this ideological teaching overlooks certain operational questions. Exactly *how* is the nurse an auxiliary agent? In what ways ought she to supplement or complement the doctor's efforts? What specific therapeutic roles should a good psychiatric nurse play? How can a nurse know when she is successful in helping the patient to improve? How does she determine the kind of credit she deserves for success in this co-operative venture with the physician? Across the nation itself, nurses do not agree upon the answers to these questions and reflect profound disagreement among psychiatrists themselves upon the same issues.

The worth of the nurse and her ward

Both the nurse's professional ideology and the hospital's general philosophy support her professional self-regard. In addition, psychiatrists often remark that her efforts have supplemented their own in helping patients, indeed may have been more important than their own therapy. Since many patients come directly to PPI without previous treatment by their physicians, the latter are freer to compliment the nurses. From time to time, psychiatrists encourage specific nurses to continue working with specific patients because they believe the nurses have been successful. Even when they do not single out special actions or personnel as helpful, they may indicate that the ward's environment has been beneficial. The patients themselves, either during their stays at the hospital or when they leave, may acknowledge that the staff has been very helpful, and of course the staff is not inclined to dismiss this kind of evidence.

But the nurses can also see for themselves how well they have functioned therapeutically. They may disagree with a physician's therapeutic program and note the beneficial effects of their own actions upon his patient. They may take action when a psychiatrist does not seem to know what to do or will not state his program, again noting how well their own program works. They may observe that a doctor is not "getting through" to his patient, although one or another of the nursing personnel is. Indeed, it is common knowledge that some patients cannot or will not talk to their doctors but talk freely to at least one member of the staff. Nurses tend to believe that they know the patients best, especially the patients of psychiatrists whom they little respect, for they see more of the patients and in more natural situations.

In addition, certain general procedures and conventions characteristic of PPI lend support to nurses' sense of therapeutic worth. A patient placed upon or transferred to an "inappropriate" ward becomes highly visible when it is clear that he does not "fit" and thus grows worse. To nurses, this change signifies that the ward cannot be therapeutic for that particular patient. Conversely, it implies that the ward is therapeutic for "appropriate" patients. Whenever a psychiatrist disregards the nurses' advice to order a transfer from a ward that is not benefiting his patient, then further retrogression of condition is likely to be heralded as confirmation of the disregarded advice. Conversely, nurses may obtain a psychiatrist's permission to work longer with a patient whose progress on this specific ward seems dubious; then if the patient shows improvement, the staff feels that its therapeutic efforts have been vindicated. Most patients do improve, and this success is underlined for the staff by the propensity of most therapists to transfer improved patients to more open wards.

All this improvement leads nurses to believe that their efforts are useful, sometimes very useful. They do not always clearly distinguish between therapeutic improvements due to their own individual or collective efforts and those due to the general atmosphere and physical structure of the ward itself. Sometimes, however, that distinction is clearly made—as when a patient "pulls himself together" with astonishing rapidity on the most closed ward after "falling apart" on a relatively open one. The closed ward itself is then regarded as having been beneficial. In other instances, the credit is given to specific nursing actions or programs. Distinctions cannot always easily be drawn. In addition, nurses believe that the quality of ward life rests not merely upon the physical attributes of wards but also upon how the personnel govern them.

The nurses' vulnerability

Nurses are accountable both for ward management and for therapeutic behavior. The second is the price that nurses must pay for recognition as important agents in the therapeutic process. Nurses are exposed to criticism from the administration and from colleagues for actions that should have been therapeutic but were not. They may be reproached by attending physicians for becoming "overinvolved" with patients and thus producing untoward effects on them. In fact, nurses are open to criticism and accusation by physicians—and by one another—on many grounds, quite aside from imputed laziness or simple error. These grounds are expressed in psychiatric terms: The nurse is compulsive or anxious or interjects herself so that her interaction with patients is ineffective or actually harmful.

83

It is important to understand that nurses stand exposed to this sort of attack, whether justified or not, from a whole host of critics, more than any other echelon in the hospital. A nurse may be criticized by her colleagues, by the aides, by her head nurse, by the nursing administration, by various psychiatric administrators, and by each and every attending physician with whose patients she comes in contact. The ward meetings themselves are sometimes seized upon by administrators as occasions for directing criticism at the nursing personnel, although usually at the personnel in general rather than at individual culprits. In addition, every nurse is open to criticism by patients, who may shrewdly find chinks in her protective armor or genuine deficiencies in her therapeutic performance.

The nurse as a single individual often accuses herself, blaming and scolding herself and feeling guilty, ashamed, or in other ways self-derogatory. This self-criticism is not couched in terms of mere error but in the same stinging psychiatric jargon that others use against her. She sees herself as culpable because she has "acted out" or been "compulsive" and so on.

She is especially vulnerable to accusations, her own and others', for at least two sets of reasons. In becoming a nurse, she has absorbed enough of the psychotherapeutic orientation to act and think in its terms. This terminology is a double-barreled gun: It can, and indeed should, be used on oneself, as well as on the patients. (Stanton and Schwartz note that this generalized use of psychotherapy as a weapon throughout the hospital is an extension of the psychotherapeutic hour.)* Nurses are generally much more vulnerable than the aides, because they are much more likely to assimilate psychotherapeutic concepts. By participating in the wider psychiatric community, they become what may be termed "minimal psychiatrists." Psychiatrists appear to be considerably less vulnerable to this kind of therapeutic criticism, both from others and probably also from themselves, because they are institutionally protected against it. In the hospital, they stand in superordinate relationships to most personnel, which affords some protection. They spend far less time at the hospital than do the nurses; they are principally assailable only by their own patients; and they are less easily reminded of criticism by having to remain all day long at the locale. The nurses have only the stations to which they may flee from patients, and it is difficult to forget the remarks of critical colleagues and administrators while at the hospital.

Perhaps nurses are also more vulnerable than psychiatrists (although this point is far more speculative) because they operate with a minimum of psychiatric knowledge. Having far less systematic and extensive psychiatric education, they have less conceptual equipment with which to defend themselves against criticism. They are more open to accusation about their motives, because they are less practiced in thinking about themselves in theoretical terminology and at a psychological distance. This observation by no means implies that nurses are always vulnerable to higher psychiatric authority or that they have no answering

*A. Stanton and Schwartz, *The Mental Hospital* (New York: Basic Books, Inc., 1954), pp. 146-50, 200-6.

rhetoric–far from it!–but only that, having learned a little psychiatry, they are then in the position of all beginners in that trade: somewhat shaky, if somewhat knowledgeable, about their own "true motives."

Communicative despair

If not shaky about motives, they are certainly often unsure of what therapeutic actions they should take toward specific patients. They are very aware that they may do little good for some patients and may actually harm others. If we put together nurses' doubts about certain of their actions and their vulnerability to potential criticism from psychiatric authorities, then we need not be astonished at nurses' intense preoccupation with wresting two things from attending physicians–adequate information about patients' illnesses and advice (or commands) on how best to act toward the patient.

The most common grievance against attending men is that they fail to communicate sufficiently. Nurses are always complaining that physicians do not bother to write down information about patients and proper–if any–orders, that they skip in and out of the ward, not stopping to transmit information. One of the nurses' major criteria for judging psychiatrists is ability to communicate well; that is, whether or not they let nurses in on therapeutic programs. Quite aside from the programs' relevance to ward management, nurses wish to know about them because of their hopes for patients; they wish to know because they consider themselves legitimate participants in the treatment process.

Nurses consider themselves much more instrumental in recovery when psychotherapy is being practiced than when the psychiatrist merely treats his patient with shock with little or no psychotherapy. In the latter instance, there is not very much for nurses to do therapeutically: Time and shock and perhaps the patient's isolation from his family are the main therapeutic agents. The psychotherapist who communicates well, who invites them into the treatment program, who "co-operates" is not only liked; he is also able to foster genuine *élan* among the staff-providing that co-operative effort results in improvement. Since the nurses' ideas about hospital practice are closest to those of the exPPI residents, it is among the latter that "the most co-operative physicians" are usually found.

The least co-operative–those who drive nurses to despair with their refusal to communicate–are to be found among the individualistic group.... These individualists are less likely to tell nurses precisely what they are doing, partly out of deliberate choice and partly out of tendency to use the hospital unconventionally. What is more, their attempts at communication are all the more easily misread as being no communication at all. Even with the best behaved of attending men, there are days or weeks when a wide communicative gap exists. The men also differ in the clarity of their expression; in the amount of time available for talking to nurses; in their estimates of the value of talking with nurses about certain types of patient or the stages of therapy they have reached, and whether or not they care to transmit their own sometimes slight knowledge.

It is not too extreme a statement to assert that despair over the communicative gap is ever-present among the nursing personnel. Aides share in this despair but can more easily shrug off the psychiatrists' silence, since the latter are much more distant from their world. Within the nurses' world, however, the psychiatrist looms large. It is to their charge that his patient is given over. Nurses are also much more dependent than aides upon the approval of psychiatrists. When the men show their appreciation of nurses' efforts, the women glow with pleasure and even with a kind of subordinate professional colleagueship. When the men seem to indicate that nursing effort is really of no importance for the therapeutic project, then the women find it difficult not to react strongly. They do not feel ashamed, as they might if they had committed therapeutic errors; they feel deprived of participation in the community of effort. They feel ignored, even denigrated or worthless. When angry at attending physicians for disrupting ward order or blocking ward management, they feel merely frustrated or indignant; when upset over rejection by therapists, they feel a blow has been struck at their professional identities. Communicative despair is only one step removed from the reactions that nurses experience when a psychotherapist lets a nurse know how little her therapeutic actions really mean in the sum total of his patients' improvements. Only rarely do the somaticists appear to evoke such responses, since the nurses do not regard themselves as especially important to somatic treatment.

Where does nursing fit into therapy?

This discussion leads to two related questions, whose answers are vitally important to nurses. How is what nurses do for patients different from what physicians do? Exactly how does the work of each group of professionals contribute to the patient's improvement? We turn now to the nurses' answers to such questions—and why their answers take certain forms. Actually, we shall discuss nurses' conceptions of the proper division of labor that should exist between themselves and psychiatrists—as well as how nurses judge the success and failure of current collaborative efforts.

The nurses realize that certain attending men utilize their services unequally and somewhat differently. The somaticists ("EST men") are a class apart, for they are recognized as uninterested in nurses' therapeutic efforts or permissive with nurses who wish to behave "therapeutically" toward patients. The remaining physicians have reputations . . . according to how much and how wisely they utilize nursing personnel. The men are judged by their expectations that nurses will give support, give contact, be firm, point out reality to the patient, be maternal, and so forth. Nurses refer to their own actions in such terms, which is understandable, since that is how attending men write orders or verbally transmit their desires for nursing care. Such terms are common coinage that passes among the staff, as well as between staff and attending physicians.

This language does not, however, serve very well to distinguish between what the physician does and what the nurses do for a patient. Nurses at PPI understand

86

that psychiatrists attempt psychotherapy with patients while their own therapeutic activity is either not psychotherapeutic or of considerably less depth and duration. But not all nurses have very clear notions of what psychotherapy is and how it differs from what they themselves do with patients. They understand that the psychiatrists' insights into and talks with patients may go deeper than their own; but this understanding is counterbalanced by a firm belief that nurses frequently know and handle patients better. When we asked point-blank whether the hospital could get along less well with psychiatrists or with nurses (therapeutically, not managerially), the nurses faced a difficult choice. While aides would unhesitatingly answer "us," nurses gave more scattered and sometimes more anguished answers.

What is unquestionably involved is the nurses' feelings that they cannot do without the psychiatrists, despite the absence of a clear conception of how their respective collaborative efforts actually combine in the total therapeutic enterprise. Nurses are pleased when invited into the drama of treatment, when the psychiatrist regards them as genuine participants, but they are scarcely more articulate about their respective therapeutic functions than at any other time. When nurses talk about a specific patient, they are frequently quite capable of formulating their presumed contribution to his improvement, sometimes using fairly sophisticated psychiatric terminology. To talk about their contribution to a specific patient's improvement is much easier than to talk about therapeutic functions in general.

Their lack of clarity in defining a "true" or desirable therapeutic division of labor is doubtless connected with disagreements among psychiatrists on this very question. Part of the nurses' difficulty surely is traceable, however, to genuine differences between the two sets of professionals over what actually constitutes and may contribute to psychic improvement and deterioration. Naturally enough, nurses turn to attending physicians for judgments of whether or not patients are "moving," but they also have their own eyes and their own standards for judging progress and retrogression. The obvious discrepancies between nurses' and physicians' perceptions and evaluations result in further muddying of waters.

Nurses are preoccupied with whether or not patients improve, for the daily life of each ward revolves around helping patients get sufficiently well to move along either to the outside world or to another ward. A visitor is struck by the nursing staff's constant reference to patients' "moving" or "not moving," to their "getting worse" or "looking better today." When recalcitrant sickness yields before devoted nursing, the staff may evince relief and even jubilation at the smallest signs of improvement. Patients who remain on plateau for weeks tend to depress the staff or to receive scant attention because the staff no longer feels that the effort is worth the candle and turns to more promising or newer candidates. Improvement in patients is a vital matter for the nursing personnel. Such improvement—whether recognized by them or the physicians—allows them to measure, to a considerable degree, their own success and failure at psychiatric nursing. (Their only alternative measures would have to be along lines of administration, management, and medical care.) Even when the standard is how much they are "learning," it is associated with discerning improvement and retrogression in various patients.

How do the nursing personnel discern such improvement and retrogression? Both in common sense and in quasi-psychiatric ways. By "common sense," we mean judgment that is essentially the same as judgment by a lay person. The nurses perceive similar kinds of signs and interpret them in lay terms: It is clear that the patient is improving, for his speech becomes more coherent, intelligible, and sensible; the formerly regressed patient, who could not control his bowel movements or feed himself, is again able to manage those bodily functions; the noisy, violent patient has calmed down and acts more decorously; the ritualistic patient no longer goes through his routine motions. Or patients may grow more confused, more incoherent, more regressed, more uncontrollable. The great preponderance of nurses' perceptions and evaluations of patients' psychiatric conditions are akin to those of laymen, but some judgments do rest upon more sophisticated psychiatric knowledge. Nurses do develop the ability to observe keenly patients' behavior and symptoms. Their interpretations of patients' actions can often pass muster with persons who have been more extensively trained in psychiatry.

Whether most of the nurses' judgments are minimally psychiatric or closer to common sense is much less important than that they disagree, with considerable frequency, from judgments made by the attending physicians. We shall attempt to explain why. The physicians whom we interviewed are characteristically skeptical about the possibility that hospitalization will bring any profound changes to patients, except for infrequent special cases. They settle for the minimal improvement that will permit a patient once again to function passably, at least for a time, outside the hospital. Because psychiatrists, especially the psychotherapeutically oriented, think in psychodynamic terms, they to not believe that daily or weekly changes during hospitalization necessarily represent genuine improvement or retrogression: At best these changes are only preparations for further treatment at the office. When a patient begins to improve in the limited sense that these physicians conceive of improvement, the special signs that they read may be overlooked by nurses, let alone by laymen, and may even be read by nurses as deterioration. (As one nurse commented, "The doctor says she's making progress. I don't know how these doctors sometimes can tell what's getting better anyhow.")

To understand the nurses' perceptions of patient "movement," one must consider the implications of their daily contacts with patients, since nurses' ward work, when combined with their less than systematic psychiatric orientation and education, often causes their views of movement to differ from physicians' views. On each ward, patients come and go as they get better or worse than is deemed appropriate for the given ward. Sometimes there is a rash of arrivals and departures; at other times, movement is reduced to a trickle. Sometimes almost all the patients seem to be getting better at once; at other times, everybody seems to be on a plateau, with no apparent movement. Sometimes patients get better swiftly, sometimes slowly. Sometimes patients improve, only to reverse themselves and become worse. Sometimes they get worse before they get better. Some patients pass through cycles, swinging from one extreme condition to another. Some patients enter the ward at a very low points, while some enter almost well enough to qualify for a more "advanced" ward. Sometimes patients enter the ward when all its patients are relatively well and sometimes when all are relatively deteriorated. At any rate, nurses perceive a given patient's improvement against a backdrop of other patients' movements. Any progression is perceived also in terms of the nurses' related conceptions of a current and an ideal "shape" of their ward. If they believe their ward is ordinarily successful with patients and if their ward is at the moment terribly "out of shape"—as, for instance, when it contains too many patients who require medical care or too many adolescents who require long hospitalization—then their morale can be low because work achieves little success. How the ward's shape and its complement of patients relate to judgments of success with patients is easily pictured in another way. One need only imagine that each new patient becomes better in a day or two, so that the ward has an almost daily turnover of patients: The nurses' sense of accomplishment can then easily be imagined.

At PPI nurses are accustomed to patients entering in various conditions of illness, to divergent rates of improvement, and to various kinds of forward and backward movement. The nurses are prepared for almost anything, so long as it does not too radically disturb their wards' shapes. Nurses definitely prefer not having too many deteriorated patients enter simultaneously, too long a period of time without progress among patients, too many patients whose movements swing unpredictably from better to worse and back again, and even too many patients who are improving—if improvement brings troublesome behavior. Under such conditions, nurses feel neither successful with their therapeutic work nor capable of doing their best work.

Of similar importance for their judgments of patients' improvement is a phenomenon that can conveniently be called "patients' reputations." Patients rather quickly, within perhaps two to four days, begin to gain reputations among the staff. The personnel talk among themselves about each new patient, describing his behavior, recounting interesting events that he has precipitated, and making judgments about his condition, his illness, and his behavior. The day-time personnel make log-book notations about each patient; this information is passed along to the evening and night staffs, abetted by the head nurse's report to the evening staff, which she often supplements with anecdotes. Each patient's reputation is composed partly of therapeutic judgment—whether he is getting better or worse and by how much—and partly of managerial judgment of how troublesome he is, for example.

Much of each ward's daily communication consists of phrases and stories passed among the staff about each patient, especially about those patients who are interesting, colorful, troublesome, or "moving." Each patient, unless he is remarkably unnewsworthy, is the subject of a continuing story: "He's the same today" or "You should have been here when he acted out again." Each day features episodes in the continuing stories of the more troublesome, loved, or colorful cast of characters. (We may term these episodes "focal events.") Each day is likely to have its single most salient event, although of course many days may be devoid of truly memorable incident. Some of the stories are success stories—"You should have been here when she first began to eat!"—and some are stories of failure. On some days, indeed for days on end, the staff may focus principally upon its struggle for success with a single patient. (We may term this phenomenon "focal attentiveness," and we may call the patient the "focal patient.") The staff becomes engrossed in the continuing story of the focal patient. The jubilation or gloom that may pervade the atmosphere at the nursing station need bear no relationship to any objective statistical assessment of the progress of patients as a whole. One or more focal patients can have more impact upon the staff's sense of therapeutic worth than would seem warranted by considerations of mere arithmetic.

[In this chapter] we are concerned only with how and why their [nurses'] views of patients' movements are unlike doctors' views. The doctors, at least those who are psychodynamically oriented, not only think more systematically about patients, but they scarcely can view patients within such a rich context of ward life. Even the ex-residents do not: They may understand the staff's perspective, having once operated within it themselves, but one has only to listen to the ward co-ordinators advising nursing personnel to recognize that memories are short and that a practitioner's view is very different from a nurse's.

One qualification must be made, however: The judgments of nurses and physicians are not always so disparate as we have described. Occasionally patients worsen enough to be sent to a state hospital; much more often they improve sufficiently to leave for home. Concurrence of physician and nursing personnel does not mean that the two agree exactly, but at least there is agreement on the direction of change.

Yet even then, there may be no agreement on the causes of change. This point again raises the question of how nurses weigh the respective contributions of themselves and physicians. It is not always an easy question for nurses to answer confidently. When physicians have "co-operated" and everyone has "worked together closely," then the question is unlikely even to arise, whether the patient has improved or deteriorated. At the other extreme, when the nurses have carried out their own therapeutic program for a given patient, because his psychiatrist either seemed to have none or was unwilling to communicate it, then the nursing personnel can easily believe that their claims to success or imputations of blame have been justified. These divisions of labor—with quite co-operative and quite unco-operative physicians—together undoubtedly involve a majority of patients, exclusive of those given EST. Success and failure are relatively easily judged for the latter: Either shock succeeds, or it fails. But if nurses step in, believing shock inappropriate or unsuccessful, then they credit their own programs with any apparent success. In the remaining cases there may be some question about who has been the more effective (or destructive) therapeutic agent.

We are not concerned with detailing how that question is answered but with two other issues. The first is that nurses may not find it easy to assign credit and blame. The causes of change in a patient's condition are difficult to ascertain, and nurses are aware of the difficulty, except when the credit or blame is exceptionally great. In addition, nurses face the knotty problem of vindicating their claims to success and their assignments of blame.

Actually, with most patients, this problem need not arise since open contests between physicians and nurses are unlikely. If there happens to be strong feeling among the nurses that a considerable share of the credit is theirs, they take it quietly through a variety of almost automatic tactics. They support one another as they talk about the patient and how he improved. They make assumptions about how the ward and their own action helped the patient. Most often they do not make a clear distinction between credit due themselves, credit due the ward itself, and credit due the psychiatrist's action and orders: All merge into an undifferentiated "helped the patient." As for the psychiatrist, he usually does not announce that credit is due to anyone, unless a particular nurse or aide has been particularly useful.

When a patient deteriorates, however, or is so troublesome that his treatment is called into question, then both physician and nurses are vulnerable to charges of error and blame. Then the central administration is most likely to enter the situation, sometimes acting as an interested mediator and sometimes as an interested participant. Other audiences also may enter or be pulled into the fray for at least two reasons. The patient's reputation may have traveled to far corners of the hospital, stories about him circulating among all levels of personnel. He and his treatment may have become something of a *cause célèbre*. Various persons will have expressed different opinions and taken sides in judging him and his physician. Outsiders may also enter into the affairs of a ward when its nurses pull them in. Nurses may illegitimately bombard other attending physicians with questions that bear upon the vindication of their own position. Some attending men must invoke their professional code to remain neutral. Some do not remain neutral but get caught up in the issues; or become involved because of their own opinions of the colleague whose treatment is being challenged by the nurses; or attempt to placate the nurses. In their search for vindication, the embattled nurses will speak to almost anybody who enters the station—including sociologists! We may call this general process the "scanning of potential vindicators."

For the nurse, it is a very important process precisely because she is a minor partner in the collaborative therapeutic enterprise. She is in a weaker position than the psychiatrist, weaker because her formal status allows less claim to psychiatric knowledge and judgment and because she has less confidence. She must seek sympathetic audiences and allies whenever she is accused by an attending man of error or incompetence. She must find people who will listen to her, to whom she can appeal, who will help her make her own claims and accusations "stick." If she can find such allies among the central administrators or among the colleagues of the offending psychiatrist, so much the better. When the nurses themselves are divided, the same processes occur—except that the atmosphere becomes more like that of a civil war. The entire search for vindication is of momentous consequence for nurses, for it pertains to perhaps the central question that they face: Where does therapeutic nursing fit into the total treatment of a patient? To this abiding question neither the central administration nor the attending men offer clear answers. The nursing profession has no single ideological position that will give her a clear answer either; although, as we have said earlier, if PPI's nurses were more firmly trained in one ideology, they might have less difficulty in coping with this crucial problem. We believe the problem would still exist, however, as long as the attending men themselves either possessed no clear answers or were willing to reveal their private beliefs only to colleagues or researchers.

ALIGNING MANAGERIAL AND THERAPEUTIC FUNCTIONS

At the outset of this chapter, we named two major problems confronting psychiatric nurses, especially those who work with psychotherapeutically oriented psychiatrists. One problem has been discussed: How does therapeutic nursing fit into the total treatment process? A second problem arises from the necessity for nurses to align their managerial and therapeutic functions. To this second problem there is no easy answer, but answer it each nurse must. Even a firm answer has potentially hazardous consequences for her, since it may work better on certain wards in certain hospitals.

Around each psychiatric nurse at hospitals like PPI, there is a field of institutional forces, which pull her sometimes in the direction of her managerial duties and sometimes toward her therapeutic obligations. She is not allowed to forget that she is a *psychiatric* nurse and that her major function is therapeutic. This philosophy is explicitly enunciated almost daily and is implicitly expressed in continual interaction with colleagues. Her head nurse, the nursing administration, and the central administration all expect appropriate therapeutic action from her, as do some attending men. Even the patients may have such expectations. There are also other expectations, however, pertaining to the nurse's managerial, adminis-trative, and custodial duties. The very same people who expect her to engage in competent therapeutic action also expect her to be a good ward manager. Even the attending psychiatrists may emphasize now one aspect of her work and now another, with respect to their patients' welfare, although differing in the weight placed on each aspect. All these expectations or requirements have the effect of catching each nurse in harrowing cross fire. They also intensify whatever internal struggles she herself may have over the proportional weights that ought to be given to therapy and management respectively. Her safest answer is to make a commitment that harmonizes the two kinds of demand. Yet even this answer is constantly brought into question.

There is, however, a supporting structure for combining managerial and therapeutic functions. We have suggested that the dominant philosophy of this hospital emphasizes that those functions naturally work together. The very division of the institution into five separate wards gives symbolic and actual support to nurses, in the sense that, when an improved patient is transferred, the personnel on his original ward can believe that they and their ward have helped him. Furthermore, those physicians whom nurses consider among the best and with whom they work most comfortably take pains not to disrupt unduly the ward's orderliness. In working with these co-operative men, a nurse is able to combine the frequently warring aspects of her dual job. This collaboration between physician and nurse allows the latter considerable freedom to manage therapeutic action. Ideally, the physician's orders and observations help the nurses to organize appropriate action toward and around the patient—action that can be *both* therapeutic and managerial. This action leads to results that the psychiatrist in turn can perceive and interpret. He then reports back to the personnel. Similarly, the nursing personnel can make observations about a patient that can be utilized by his physician. The physician's actual therapeutic sessions can also serve both managerial and therapeutic ends—when the physician is co-operative. Management and therapy can ideally be fused by the nurses provided they can act as the physician's delegated managers, performing certain acts that he himself cannot perform either because he is not there or is not trained to do them.

Another institutional support enables nurses to combine management and therapy. It consists of an effective terminology used throughout the hospital by every echelon. The terminology is sufficiently ambiguous to allow at least three possibilities: It can refer to therapeutic action, managerial action, or both. For instance, "giving contact" to a patient may be used to mean therapeutic action or that such action should be taken merely to prevent further troublesome behavior—or both meanings may be indicated. Virtually all the terminology used by and to nurses, except for certain strictly psychiatric terms like "hallucination," has dual meanings. A physician's orders to give contact, for instance, may be read in two ways by different personnel. His very diagnosis can be converted from therapeutic to managerial connotation, since certain diagnostic terms suggest how patients can be expected to behave. The physicians themselves play into this ubiquitous lingual system, because they use these very terms as a shorthand for giving both orders and managerial suggestions.

By accident or design, a nurse can find other supports within the hospital setting for softening the potentially sharp conflict between therapy and management. Especially if she is shrewd or creative, she can find opportunities for maximizing therapeutic at the expense of the managerial effort or *vice versa*. We shall cite a few examples. On $_3$EW, the head nurse is assisted by two younger women, each of whom has her own *forte:* One is good at and enjoys working with patients; the other is adept at the administrative work, which is principally performed at an enclosed station. Each nurse tends to function in accordance with her particular ability. Since $_3$EW is a large ward, its head nurse consciously tends to play along with her assistants' desires in the daily assignment of work. She herself is

93

exceedingly busy with ward administration and finds it useful to have both an administrative assistant and one who can supervise "work with patients." On PPI's most open ward, there are relatively minor problems connected with keeping order and less paper work than on other wards; the nursing personnel can spend much time working with patients. Indeed the head nurse runs into much less trouble with physicians over managerial problems than she does with the nursing administration, since the latter is more managerially minded than she. During the evening hours, on any ward, a floor nurse can better escape surveillance and feel freer to work with patients if she wishes, especially since she is less burdened with paper work and other administrative duties. A nurse who puts therapeutic action relatively low in her scale of values, however—a few PPI nurses do—may discover on the night shift a relative freedom *not* to work with patients. Here are two final examples: One nurse reluctantly allowed herself to be made a head nurse and then, caught in conflict of management and therapy, attempted repeatedly to be demoted in order to escape the extra stress engendered by her administrative position. One nursing supervisor grew restive with her wholly administrative duties and stepped down to replace a head nurse who had quit her job. In short, the hospital as constituted offers potentialities for working out various kinds of nursing commitment, whether they lean toward management or therapy or fall between the two.

The hospital also erects barriers to the implementation of nursing commitments. Beside those already discussed or suggested, others can be listed. The perennial transfer of nurses from one ward to another and from one shift to another allows some nurses to discover genuine satisfactions in working at the hospital; but this transfer system can also be immensely disrupting to nurses who have nicely managed their environments. Transfer not merely shatters routine and necessitates the learning of new routines, but it also means that new alliances must be made, new channels of negotiation found, new conditions of work be handled. To some degree at least, a new environment must be managed. Yet transfer and rotation of nurses are frequent in most hospitals, which are perennially "understaffed" according to administrative criteria.

It does not require much observation to see that some nurses fail to learn how to bend the hospital setting to their desires. Some quit the hospital. Some battle it out, looking for or stumbling into conditions that will allow them to do what they wish. Fortunately, too, some are abetted in their search by their superiors. Other nurses swing back and forth between the managerial and therapeutic poles, leaving themselves exceedingly vulnerable to attack and clearly restive about their unresolved positions. Lest we give the impression that all nurses are trapped, we hasten to repeat that many nurses find or create conditions that give them relative freedom for what they wish to do at the hospital.

Nevertheless, the implementation of any nurse's commitments is directly affected by her conditions of work. She needs relative control over those conditions, or she cannot carry out the dictates of her convictions. This control is hard to achieve in a hospital administered by physicians and used by a multitude of attending men. Even when nurses obtain relative control over their conditions of work, it must constantly be guarded and reconstituted when undermined. Some situations that lessen control are perennial and are therefore partly predictable. They can be prepared for to some degree. Other disruptions are difficult to foresee for many reasons: For instance, the hospital itself may be undergoing rapid changes; new physicians and new kinds of patients may be appearing; new kinds of therapy are being tried; and, of course, the views of attending physicians about nursing functions are neither consistent nor entirely understood by the nurses themselves. All these elements are crucial to an understanding of the world and the work of psychiatric nurses.

TRAINED VERSUS UNTRAINED PSYCHIATRIC NURSES

One outstanding feature of the PPI nurse is that she is not a "trained psychiatric nurse." Because she lacks the specialized training given in programs of psychiatric nursing at collegiate schools of nursing, she lacks the ideological staunchness so typical of many graduates of those programs, who often share the ideological fervor exhibited by the social workers and psychologists at Chicago State Hospital. In a certain sense, the PPI nurses' lack of formal training is useful at the hospital. Since such nurses have no firm and articulate commitment to a clear ideological position, they can work with somaticists and psychotherapists, without undue violation of their beliefs. Generally they can even work well with the individualistic psychotherapists, which might be more difficult if the nurses were self-consciously ideological.

At least one excellently trained psychiatric nurse has remarked, however, on hearing about this hospital and its nurses, that the situation would be quite different if PPI's nursing service were headed by a genuine specialist. There is some merit in this argument, for one might then imagine certain new consequences for the nurses' work. The nurses would be inducted by the nursing director—a militant professional—into some variant of psychotherapeutic ideology. They would receive solid personal support from her during moments of stress. She might also gain more purchase on the central administration in terms of therapy rather than merely management. The director might also leave her educational mark upon residents, if not upon attending men, conveying the truer work and functions of the psychiatric nurse.

Assuming that this hospital's central administration were to change its views about psychiatric nursing sufficiently to hire such a director, it would still be difficult for her to change the situation radically. The attending men are not easily concerted or even influenced. The residents would surely be affected while administering the wards, but by the time they had become attending men three years later, the director's influence would unquestionably have been counterbalanced and probably far outweighed by the combined influence of supervisors and personal career aspirations. Furthermore, a core of nurses with staunch psychotherapeutic ideology would undoubtedly precipitate certain new problems.   95

Somaticists would find it harder to deal with these nurses, whose contempt for somatic practices would be more explicit and certainly more pronounced. Perhaps more important, the greater claims of nurses to participation in therapy would surely make more explicit the currently masked opinions of most attending men about the minor contributions of nurses to the therapeutic process. As we have noted, even the most cooperative attending man rates that general contribution rather low. Unless this opinion were altered, it is not difficult to imagine the reactions of nurses. Meanwhile, central administration would bear an increased burden of mediation between the attending men and the nurses. That is, the director would be teaching her girls that management and therapy support each other and are not separable (or perhaps that management is subordinate to therapy), but the older attending men would hardly accept her views of therapy either in general or concerning specific patients. (She would sometimes be unable to convince all her nurses.) As long as the hospital's work is organized around the private patients of attending physicians, the director of nursing service would face, as sociologists are wont to say, a most difficult "structural" problem.

It is also important to understand that another of the current basic problems among the nurses would be difficult to solve: the proper assessment of the relative contributions of physicians and nurses to a specific patient's progress. This problem, it will be remembered, rests partly on the differential reading of signs: Nurses read more behaviorally, more like laymen. The introduction of trained psychiatric nurses would change this situation of course, for then nurses would read signs much more professionally. We would anticipate that this change would only make the content of their therapeutic claims more explicit. While both echelons might now more frequently agree, their fewer disagreements would be far less masked and covert.

In painting so skeptical a picture of the value of introducing specialized nurses into a setting like PPI, our intent has not been to argue that it should not be done. Our purpose has been primarily to underline briefly what problems confront the various nurses and psychiatrists at PPI as they work together. Secondarily, our purpose has been to suggest *some* of the possible consequences of introducing strongly psychotherapeutically oriented nurses into hospital settings comparable to PPI. As the trends toward both psychiatric sections in general hospitals and specialized psychiatric nursing continue, we can expect that the kinds of problem outlined here will figure prominently—because for many years the nurses who man our psychiatric hospitals will not be formally trained in psychiatric nursing.

SUGGESTED QUESTIONS FOR DISCUSSION AND ANALYSIS

For undergraduate students

1. How do the nurses go about keeping order on this kind (psychiatric) of ward? What resources do they have at their command? What are the special kinds of problems they face in maintaining order? Why is order so important to them?
2. When psychiatrists do not agree in their basic psychiatric philosophies, how does this affect the therapeutic efforts of the nurses? Do you think it would

have made a difference if all the psychiatrists at PPI had had basically the same philosophy?

3. How independent do you think psychiatric nurses can become in their work on hospital wards where the patients "belong" to private psychiatrists? Can an innovative nurse get *some* measure of independence or degree of control in her nursing care of patients?

For graduate students and teachers of nursing

1. What difference do you think it makes when nurses have been trained in psychiatric nursing, as compared with nurses who have not, in settings like PPI? Would some of the same problems occur for the nurses, or would they be entirely different?

2. If you were the head of nursing services at PPI, how would you organize the wards so as to minimize the problems discussed in the foregoing pages? Would you organize them differently if there were just one psychiatric ward, say in a large community hospital?

3. Is the problem of ideology (philsophy of etiology and treatment) characteristic only of psychiatry and psychiatric nursing? Do similar ideological conflicts appear on nonpsychiatric wards; If so, how do they affect nursing care?

5. Mental illness and the TB patient

Shizuko Yoshimura Fagerhaugh, RN, DNSc

Shizuko Fagerhaugh, while a research assistant for a study of tuberculosis patients in clinics and in an associated county hospital in San Francisco, did extensive observation and interviewing of tuberculosis patients and of the hospital staff. She was struck by the kinds of problems that certain patients set for the staff, by how the staff defined patients as difficult and even mentally ill, and by what happened when the bedeviled nurses called upon the hospital psychiatrists for help with their problem patients. Dr. Fagerhaugh had studied psychiatric nursing, so she was particularly attuned to the different perspectives of psychiatric and tuberculosis staffs. The result of her observations and analysis is the following perceptive paper. It has implications far wider than for merely tuberculosis nursing.

Managing the long-term care required by patients with tuberculosis is a challenge to health professionals in most institutional settings. When the patients' problems are compounded by mental illness, the professional staff finds this group the most difficult of all "recalcitrant" patients. Assistance from psychiatric services within the care system for either commitment or management of these patients has been found wanting. Yet from my observations and interviews with tuberculosis and psychiatric professionals in one large urban county hospital system, the problem seems to arise from the difference between the perceptions of mental illness of the two professions and their expectations of each other.

Much conflict existed between psychiatrists and tuberculosis professionals in the care system of the study undertaken. The two groups often disagreed whether or not a certain patient was mentally ill—some behaviors defined as mental illness by tuberculosis workers were not considered so by the psychiatrists. Both professions differed in assessing the status of mental illness and whether a patient required care in a psychiatric facility or could remain on the tuberculosis unit. The two groups differed widely in their expectations of each other in the management of these patients.

As in many public municipal systems of tuberculosis care, most of the patients were poor and represented the less favored sectors of society—the aged, the nonwhites, alcoholics, and new immigrants from underdeveloped countries. Most of the professional workers in the field were older physicians and nurses who had finished their professional education 20 to 30 years before; many had worked in the tuberculosis field ever since.

The psychiatric professionals on the other hand, were younger, reflecting a health trend in this country. As incidence of tuberculosis has decreased and interest in mental health grows, professional men have been attracted to psychiatry.

FAULTY COMMUNICATIONS

In the hospital under study, discourse between the psychiatric and tuberculosis services was infrequent. The psychiatrist under pressure in his department, did little more than examine the tuberculosis patient, make a diagnosis, and recommend treatment when necessary or commitment to a psychiatric unit that had a separate tuberculosis unit. Occasionally the psychiatrist made suggestions on management of emotionally disturbed tuberculosis patients left on the unit.

The different concepts of the two specialties of what constituted mental illness were largely the result of the different treatment approaches to each disease, the priority each discipline set for its assigned responsibility, and the ages and professional outlook within each group.

Tuberculosis and mental illness have some common properties or characteristics. In the acute phase of both illnesses the patient is incarcerated in a hospital on the grounds that his illness endangers his life or the lives of others, and he is legally committed if he resists. Both illnesses bear a certain stigma: in the acute stages, the patient is isolated and his movement regulated.

On the other hand, there are major differences between the diseases and very different treatment approaches. The most obvious distinction is the reason for isolation. Tuberculosis is a communicable disease, the reason the patient is in a hospital is different from that of the mentally ill. Patients with communicable tuberculosis who suffer mental illness cannot be transferred to a psychiatric unit because of the danger of infecting others. The most significant difference, however, is that tuberculosis deals primarily with physiological functioning, and mental illness with psychosocial functioning. As a result the precision with which each can be diagnosed, treated, assessed for the degree of dysfunction and future outcome, and the sensitivity of each to social and cultural variables are quite different.

99

CONTRAST IN TREATMENT

Tuberculosis is an infection of the body by a specific bacilli which acts in a specific way. By objective tests, the status of disease and response to treatment can be established with fair precision. Patients with tuberculosis are treated with specific antitubercular drugs, and the treatment is concrete, routine, and well codified.[1] The first priority is seeing that the patient continues drug therapy for two years.

Mental illness, by contrast, is quite ambiguous and includes an array of deviant behaviors and groups. These groups include people with psychotic conditions, learning difficulties, stress reactions, antisocial behaviors, sexual deviations, mental deficiencies, and drug addiction, as listed in the *Diagnostic and Statistical Manual of Mental Disorders*.[2] The etiology of mental disorder is believed to include a wide range of factors including the unresolved oedipus complex, biochemical changes, and unfavorable social conditions, poverty for one. Treatment may include physical measures, such as drug and electric shock therapy; psychological techniques, like psychoanalysis; relationship therapy; group therapy; and environmental approaches, such as milieu therapy.

Also, the traditional psychotherapeutic techniques are often unsuccessful for certain groups of people, particularly patients from lower socioeconomic classes.[3] Thus, a psychiatric diagnosis does not necessarily determine how a doctor will treat and manage a patient. In mental illness, therapy like its etiology, is nonspecific. It is difficult to identify one specific cause for the varieties of mental disorders, or one treatment to cope with the variety of behavior problems in an array of social situations within the diversity of social groups. All of these factors make it difficult for psychiatrists to agree on the disease status of a patient at any given time, or to predict his future behaviors in various social situations—at home, at work, or at social gatherings. Thus, although mentally ill patients can be legally committed in a psychiatric facility, as a danger to himself and others, it is often difficult to assess accurately the degree of danger, except in extreme psychotic conditions.

The patient-professional relationship is very different in the two forms of illness. Observations of patient-professional interactions, both in the tuberculosis wards and the clinic, indicate that, although warm relationships are philosophically important, operationally this is of secondary consideration. Since drug treatment is specific to tuberculosis control, persuading the patient to follow the concrete, routine drug treatment has primary importance. In psychiatry, the patient-professional relationship is crucial: a trusting relationship between the two is of great importance. Knowledge of the patient's social situation, his feelings, and his perceptions of his situation are important factors in treating the patient. Each patient exhibits his mental illness in different ways, depending on his personal experiences and perceptions. Of course, in a city system inundated with troubled and troublesome patients and a shortage of personnel, individualized care is not always possible. But psychiatry gives priority to warm patient-professional relations, even though operationally this may be difficult.

Psychiatric treatment is a slow process. By the use of various treatment modes, the patient slowly gains "insight," becomes "self-motivated," and eventually resolves his problems. For patients lacking insight or the social attributes of "treatability," such as an impoverished capacity to communicate, drug and milieu therapy may be the only approaches available. Forcing patients to undergo psychiatric treatment is not usual unless there is clear indication that they are in immediate danger to themselves or others.

MEDICAL MODEL OF DISEASE

Diagnosis of tuberculosis is by objective tests of sputum and x-ray examinations; but defining mental illness is much more complicated, since all behaviors occur within a group context, and the frames of reference of the evaluators or the names of illness are not always comparable. Since the definers of mentally ill behaviors are located in different foci of interaction with the patient, the behaviors they are concerned with may differ significantly, and vary in importance. What may be viewed as deviant in one group may be tolerated in another. The process by which persons are identified as "mentally ill" and acted upon, will depend upon how serious the consequences of the deviant behaviors are for the group.[4]

The tuberculosis staff's perceptions of mental illness and of psychiatry and their expectations of psychiatrists were shaped by their medical orientation, their commitment to tuberculosis control, and their professional training. Since the tuberculosis staff deals with a physical disorder, their understanding of mental illness is largely based on the medical model of illness. Furthermore, because of the long time interval since their medical training, and their limited contact with psychiatry since, a generation-information gap occurred. Managing mentally ill tuberculosis patients often meant to them incarcerating the patient in a psychiatric facility with a tuberculosis unit, if he could not be treated or managed in short-term therapy. This has been the practice until more recent changes evolved in psychiatric commitment procedures which coincided with other changes in the community health movement. There were, of course, varying degrees of sophistication within the staff about mental illness and psychiatry. However, many held the view that over the years psychiatry *must* have made progress and developed into a more exacting science.

DIFFICULTIES IN DIAGNOSIS

Because of the nature of mental illness and the difficulties in accurately assessing the status of the disease and future behavior of the patient, the psychiatrist sometimes considered not seriously ill patients who later proved to be so. Some troublesome patients in the hospital phase of care became quite manageable during out-patient care. Other emotionally disturbed patients were tractable while hospitalized, but became a problem during the clinic phase of care. When such discrepancies occurred, the tuberculosis staff tended to indict the psychiatric staff–criticize the caliber of the psychiatrists, charge them with wrong diagnosis, or dismiss them as "queer ducks," anyhow.

This misunderstanding of psychiatry seems rooted in the preciseness of diagnosis and treatment in tuberculosis which generates intolerance for the ambiguity attending mental illness and psychiatric treatment. As one tuberculosis specialist summarized the general feeling: "I simply can't understand the psychiatrist's criteria for 'committable' and 'noncommittable' [to a state mental hospital]. One would think the psychiatrist could be more exacting. After all, mental illness is a *disease*."

The kinds of behaviors defined as mentally ill and of particular concern to the tuberculosis staff were those that influenced tuberculosis treatment and ward operations. Interviews with hospital staff and examinations of charts of patients whom the tuberculosis staff defined as mentally ill or emotionally disturbed, revealed that the behaviors described were those that interfered with the treatment process or with the sentimental order of the ward–behaviors such as fighting with the staff or other patients, refusal to follow the proper barrier techniques to prevent the spread of infection, or unwillingness to abide by the rules of the unit. Poor cooperation in following the treatment regimen was often cited. Interestingly, when it came to those patients who exhibited bizarre behaviors, such as delusions or hallucinations, information was meager. Partly, this is due to the fact that the staff, who, unfamiliar with psychiatry and psychiatric techniques interacted less with such patients. For that matter, delusional patients were well tolerated by the staff as long as they cooperated with the tuberculosis treatment process and did not unduly upset the ward. Understandably, the most difficult patients were the paranoid patients who refused to cooperate in the drug regimen on the grounds that it was a conspiracy to poison them. Although many of the staff spoke of the need to interact with the withdrawn patients, as such behavior may indicate a deepseated emotional problem, relatively little attention was accorded them.

Because of the priority of drug therapy in tuberculosis treatment, patients who refused to cooperate in the drug regimen because of mental illness, or other reasons, were indeed a problem. A patient's refusal to cooperate after having received an ample and logical explanation, was interpreted by the staff as using "illogical thinking." Such thinking could only be attributed to some peculiar thought process–mental illness–and these patients were labeled "deniers." The psychiatrists, of course, are not likely to label such deniers as being mentally ill. To them denial of disease is a psychological mechanism, or a symptom of disease, but certainly not a disease in itself. Frequently, these patients were interpreted by the psychiatrists as acting out their frustrations against the confinement of hospitalization, or the behavior was attributed to some deep-seated personality defect for which there is no quick psychotherapeutic solution.

The tuberculosis house staff are responsible for the patient 24 hours a day for months at a time. Any patient who upsets the order of the ward becomes a major problem. For example, one patient in a four-week period, left the ward six times against medical advice. Each time he returned to the hospital, he was roaring drunk, disrupted the ward by abusive behavior, and ran around the open ward naked. To make matters worse, in his drunken state, he made sexual remarks to the nurses using foul language. This patient was seen by the psychiatrist who labeled him an alcoholic and depressive. The patient saw no need for psychiatric help as he perceived his problem as primarily stemming from personal problems at home and the confining hospital situation.

At times a disgruntled patient is able to organize the discontent and frustrations of the entire ward, creating a medication strike. In such situations, understandably, the hospital staff want help from the psychiatric staff in reinstating compliance to the drug regimen, as well as in maintaining control over the unit. Unfortunately, the psyciatric staff is unable to meet this request both in terms of personnel or in treatment approaches effective for these patients. Thus, consultation after consultation had the notation, "Patient has no insight into his problem. Psychiatric help offered, but patient refused. Patient not committable to psychiatric facility." And so the house tuberculosis staff is left with the conviction that they alone have an insoluble behavior problem and most often they are correct.

COMMUNICATION PROBLEM

Related to this difficulty between the two professional groups is the fact that each inhabits separate conceptual worlds with entirely different languages. The tuberculosis staff, generally unsophisticated about psychiatry and psychiatric language, were unable to describe adequately patient behaviors helpful to, or of concern to, the psychiatrists. Rather, as stated earlier, only those behaviors that had consequences to the treatment process or to their work were noted. Furthermore, the psychiatric diagnosis provided in the course of consultation had limited usefulness to the tuberculosis staff who were unable to put these diagnoses into operation to serve as sensible guidelines to manage the patient. Even the suggestions that consultants did make for patient management, such as "help the patient become part of the ward community," or "set limits for the patient," were too general. On the other hand, the psychiatrists, without further detailed information about a given patient, or knowledge of the social context of his behaviors, would not give the staff the much desired "how to" answers for patient management.

The psychiatrists viewed the situation from their discipline's framework, which is concerned with human behavior based on a psychological and interpersonal frame of reference. They believe that the barrier techniques used in tuberculosis and the staff's concern for ward order is evidence of the staff's compulsiveness and rigidity. They tended to make invidious judgments—that a compulsive and rigid person would be attracted to such work in the first place, and that they used the communicability of the disease as a rationalization for an underlying hostility and authoritarian nature. Further, they believed that the use of the masks and gowns created barriers in establishing warm patient-professional relationships. Several psychiatrists felt that the nature of tuberculosis, which requires extended isolation   **103** from the outside world, and the stigma associated with the disease, in addition to the coercive attitude of the tuberculosis staff, contributed to most of the patients' behavior problems. They felt very strongly that the tuberculosis staff created their own behavior problems because they lacked sophistication about the emotional needs of the patients and were inept in interpersonal skills. The psychiatrists believed minor personality disorders of some individuals became exaggerated in the tuberculosis ward situation. The fact that many of the patients perceived their problems as stemming from the extended hospital confinement helped confirm this view. It is understandable, then, why many of the patient's behaviors were viewed by the psychiatrists as situational anxiety.

A particular point of irritation to the psychiatrists was the tuberculosis staff's prevailing notions that psychiatrists possess some sort of magic by which the patient would become manageable after three or four sessions with the psychiatrist. From the psychiatrist's perspective, language, insight, and motivation are essential factors in psychotherapy, and most of the patients on the tuberculosis ward did not meet these criteria for treatability. Furthermore, a patient who created havoc on the ward might not meet the criteria for commitment to a psychiatric hospital on psychiatric grounds. He could only be committed if he showed evidence that he was "imminently dangerous to self and others."

At the time of the study, the psychiatric staff was concerned with major reorganizational problems related to changing concepts in community mental health. Additionally, since the psychiatrists are peripheral to the tuberculosis system, they did not feel a strong responsibility toward resolving the problems of another care system.

MEANINGFUL DIALOGUE

The outcome of the contrasting perceptions and expectations of the two groups could only result in accusations and counter-accusations with little room for engagement in a meaningful dialogue. Such interprofessional animosity results in inadequate care to the emotionally disturbed patients and prevents more constructive approaches in resolving the conflict. It would appear that both groups should objectively review the sources of conflict and seek solutions. These would include: inservice education programs for the tuberculosis staff; reduction of factors that contribute to patient anxiety in a long-term care facility; and more and better psychiatric consultation that is appropriate to the particular situation.

REFERENCES

1. Cohen, Archibald, *The Drug Treatment of Tuberculosis.* Springfield, Ill., Charles C Thomas Publisher, 1966.
2. American Psychiatric Association, Committee on Nomenclature and Statistics. *Diagnostic and Statistical Manual of Mental Disorders.* Washington, D.C., The Association, 1952.
3. Hollingshead, A. B., and Redlick, J. C. *Social Class and Mental Illness,* New York, John Wiley and Sons, 1958.
4. Lemert, E. Legal commitment and social control. *Sociol. Res.* 30:370-378, 1946.

SUGGESTED QUESTIONS FOR DISCUSSION AND ANALYSIS

For undergraduate students

1. What is the medical model of disease management? How does this model affect the social organization of the health care system and the work of various health team members? How is the medical disease model of social organization incongruent in meeting the physical and psychosocial needs of patients with chronic disorders?

2. The problem of managing emotionally disturbed tuberculous patients is a definitional problem of "mental illness" among the various health team members. Why is the problem maximized in the mental illness–tuberculosis combination? Do similar problems prevail in other mental illness–physical disease combinations? Why?

3. Describe the behaviors of an emotionally disturbed tuberculous patient (or a patient with another physical disorder) in your nursing experience. How did the patient's behavior disrupt the treatment process, work routines, or ward order? What factors in either the hospitalization process, treatment process, or hospital situation might tend to foster patient behaviors that can be defined as "mentally ill"? In what areas and to what degree are the various health team members (head nurse, staff nurse, aides, physicians, and students) accountable to treatment, patient management, and each other? How did the various team members define the same behaviors? To what degree are their areas and degrees of accountability related to their definitions of the patient's behaviors?

For graduate students and teachers of nursing

1. Identify the areas of incongruence in managing mentally ill and tuberculous patients. What kinds of patient management approaches in both tuberculosis and mental illness decrease the many incongruences?

2. How might clinical nurse specialists be utilized to remedy the situation described above? What kinds of educational experiences would the nurse specialist require? Keep in mind question 1.

3. What kinds of questions do you need to raise in developing training programs that would help the tuberculosis nurses described above to cope with the problems?

6. Nurses in the intensive care unit

Patricia Benner, RN, MS

The following series of observations by Patricia Benner were done as part of a larger research project on which she was a research assistant. They are useful from several perspectives. First, they describe the nature of the nurse's work in the intensive care unit (ICU). This awe-inspiring, machine-dominated, lifesaving setting is not infrequently off limits to many students. However, even when not physically off limits, the high crisis and highly technical orientation of the ICU generates a mystique to this setting that makes it figuratively off limits to students and uninitiated graduate nurses alike. In almost any social system, there is a frontstage reality shown to outsiders and a backstage reality reserved for and known only by the insiders. It is often very difficult to break through to the backstage reality.

Benner's expertise and experience in ICU nursing, and her knowledge of the backstage reality makes her observation of nurses and activities in this setting particularly useful. Having worked in several ICU's, including the one in which she was observing, Benner provides the reader with backstage insight, but she herself encounters some difficulty in moving from the participant to the observer role. There is also a possibility that perceptions, observations, and possible interpretations are more selective when the observer knows and is known by the personnel whom she is observing.

Another perspective to be gained from these field notes is the subtle, and sometimes not so subtle, sparring for control and autonomy between physicians at various levels and nurses. Here also, we see nurses whose work emphasizes more the cure and care aspects, rather than the coordination of either of these elements, although the latter is still evident to some degree.

Monday, August 16, 1971

I had called Jean Johnson, the assistant head nurse, and made arrangements to come and observe on Monday, because Jean would be working days on Monday. Jean was the only person I had worked with during the year who could give me both formal and informal sanction to come into the unit and observe. (Alice, the head nurse, was on vacation.)

Walking into the ICU, I recognized that it was quiet. The most striking impression was the absence of nurses. Usually I saw nurses first and then patients; this morning I saw only beds and patients. I was struck by the isolated unattended patients; there were no curtains drawn, no nurses standing around patients' beds. My heart sunk a bit; I felt that I had picked a bad morning—that there wouldn't be any activity going on. (I guess that really shows how crisis oriented I am—"nothing" is going on unless there is activity!)

A janitor was mopping the left side of the hall, which was the usual entrance. I had walked around the utility room "center island" in the center of the large, open ICU and approached the nurse's station from the right hall. I felt awkward about doing this. I am not sure that it is the design of the unit, but custom dictates that the entrance to this unit is on the left. Open-heart patients are kept on the right side of the room, and access to this side is much more guarded. There were no open-heart patients on the "open-heart side" this morning, and there was not even a prepared space (prepared by many IV bottles, CVP lines, waiting electrodes). In one bed there was a comatose 50- to 60-year-old man who was breathing very loudly, grunting and blowing with every exhalation. A young woman, a relative, was standing at the foot of his bed. I felt uncomfortable, since I did not see any nurses and I did not want to talk with her before making by presence known to the nurses, and yet I could tell she wanted to talk. I also knew that I could not even refer her to anyone at this point.

There was another man in the corner of the open-heart section; he was very alert. Around the corner at the end of the U shaped unit, was a white-haired man with a neck incision (I assumed, correctly, that he had had a carotid thrombo-endarterectomy) struggling with a urinal underneath his breakfast tray (still no nurses). I succumbed to his plight and took the urinal. (I had chosen to wear a nurse's uniform, thinking it would facilitate my entry, but more important, because I felt most comfortable wearing the nurse's uniform. It fit my own familiar, comfortable nurse image. I soon found that the uniform was evoking expectations not only from patients and families but from myself, too! It would have been hard for me to ignore this man's need for assistance had I not been in uniform, but in uniform I found it impossible. My plan was only to observe, and this could wreck my entry.) I was at a side sink where I had measured urine in the past, when Jean came up. I said, "Hello," and asked her if the urine needed to be saved. She said, "No, but we measure them all and do specific gravities." I replied, "I know." She took the urinal from me and said, "I'll just measure it back here and do the SG." She went back to the utility room. I felt really put down. I resented being treated as an outsider, one who does not know the ways (the sacred rituals) of an ICU. *One never discards urine in an ICU without at least measuring it and doing an SG!*

Trying to reestablish some identity as "one who knows," I said to Jean, "It's quiet." She said, "Yes, it's a good thing, because the new interns just came and the new residents start tomorrow." I said, "Oh, that's right, it is a good thing!" I found I was clinging to my identity as an ICU nurse, not because it might help me gather data, though I knew it might, but I thought I was latching onto a more familiar, comfortable role than that of "a research observer." Also, I didn't want to be cast into a role where I would not have an opportunity to demonstrate my hard-earned expertise. Such egotism!

I then looked around for a good place to sit and found none, so I leaned against the doctor's order-writing desk. Two other staff nurses appeared. One, a young tall blonde nurse named Amy was talking to the relative briefly, and then to the nurse aide. Amy was saying, "I never smoke." The aide replied, "You were smoking Friday night." Amy answered, "That's because I was drunk." They both laughed. Amy then went over to the comatose patient (just as the relative was making motions to leave) and withdrew about 30 cc of bloody drainage from his NG tube. She did not speak to the patient or to the young woman. Amy then came back over to where I was sitting (the doctor's order-writing desk) and said, "I've forgotten your name." I gave her my name, and she then said, "Maybe I can get some work out of you." (She had asked for my help in the past.)

She asked me what I was doing, and I explained that I was just observing. "I am learning how to do participant observations," I said. She smiled and said, "We'll get some work out of you." I smiled, knowing that she was not busy, and asked her if she needed some help. She said, "No." (When the ICU is busy, nurses don't ask for help, the need is usually very visible and simply demands it.)

An intern went over to the comatose patient's bed, Amy joined him, and they exchanged first name introductions. The intern then came over to the medicine station where the second young nurse, Carol, was drawing up meds. She asked him how his weekend was, and he replied that it was fine, just not long enough. He seemed a little nervous. He then asked how her weekend was, and she replied, "Nice," but then she moved into a conversation about all the bloody stools and Sustagen stools the patients had had all weekend. "Between Mrs. Smith and Mr. Jones, it was really bad," she said.

I decided to retreat to the head nurse's office (it is possible to duck in there unobtrusively) and jot down some notes. I was trying to capture my feelings, when I realized I really couldn't conjure up any awareness of feelings. Even though I was there to be an observer, I had assumed the ICU nurse role and had lost much of my observer "reactivity." It was as though hiding my feelings was a part of the demeanor and posture of the ICU; or was it that I was so busy emanating my ICU nurse image that I had no energy left to perceive my feelings? I was jotting these notes down when Jim (the intern) passed the office, saying, "I'll be back to see him, so make sure you don't let him sneak by before I get my liver biopsy." I assumed that he was talking about the comatose patient who, I had since discovered, was in a hepatic coma.

When I returned, Amy and the other young nurse, who seemed to be her friend (I was never introduced), were getting ready to go on their break. As she was leaving, Amy reported to a young bearded doctor about the bloody drainage and the fact that the comatose patient only put out 12 cc of urine in the past 2 hours. She then said, "I ordered a Gomco—his NG was draining on the bed." The doctor made no response; he just nodded his head and kept studying the chart. When Amy returned from her coffee break, she mentioned the urine again: "Did I tell you that Mr. Rolo only put out 12 cc of urine in the past 2 hours?" He shook his head and said, "No." She said, "Well, I mumbled it, but I didn't think you heard me, so I though I'd better tell you again." She had not really mumbled before. I was assuming that this, too, must be a new intern. The pattern of communication was not at all set up; he did not respond appropriately to information by asking further questions or by giving any indication of what he would do or what to watch for in the next 2 hours. (Maybe he couldn't sort out the depressed urinary output from all the other signs and symptoms he was reading about!)

Then the young nurse, Carol (I was feeling old), came out of the room of the patient who had been on Sustagen (the patient was a 57-year-old woman with generalized myasthenia gravis and an MI) and said to the ward clerk, "Mrs. Smith is being switched from Sustagen to a blenderized diet." (This was one of the patients who had had the Sustagen stools she had discussed earlier with the intern.) She had just "received" the order from the intern. (I thought, "Aha, the socialization of the interns is beginning—every year over and over—again. This one is quick; he picked up the nurse's message about the stools very rapidly!")

The very alert man in the corner of the open-heart section had asked Jean a question earlier that had made her respond that he was probably going to be transferred later in the day and that he looked much better. She had also explained that the only reason he had been moved back up to the ICU was because of his lungs and that they were primarily watching his lungs. When the anesthesiologist came up, she acted as a spokesman for this patient as she stood by the patient's bedside and said, "Mr. Blain asked me if they were only drawing blood gasses for practice." She said this with a smile in her voice. The anesthesiologist took the cue and explained to the patient that the reason so many different doctors had drawn the blood gasses was that different doctors were on call. Then he talked to the patient about his x-rays. (This was an unusually alert patient for the ICU, and he was really putting things together. This is a good example of the effect that changes in intern and resident rotations have on patient care.)

The only other nurses I had contact with were Sue and Elise. Sue poked her head out of the room of a 16-year-old boy with broken legs and internal injuries—he had been in an automobile accident. She looked around for help and then asked me to ask Elise whether she should change the dressings on the boy's leg. I peeked into the isolation room where Elise was and asked her; she said she did not know. "Have they been changed before? Probably the doctor should change them. I don't know; I have been off for 4 days. She will have to use her own judgment." I repeated the information and then introduced myself to Sue, explaining that I was just visiting and observing. I felt that I had to clarify that I would not be able to help either.

Upon returning from her break, Amy had noted that her favorite song was playing on the radio and had turned the radio up. A second favorite song came on, and she turned up the radio even louder, saying that she would just have to stay right there all day. (I felt a bit indignant—she was not fitting my image of an ICU nurse.) I had messages for her from her patients. The very alert man was requesting a breathing treatment, and he had used the commode while she was gone. She said, "Good, I asked him to wait two seconds after I left and then ring for you and ask to go to the bathroom." She refused to take me and my new role too seriously. (Ducking out for coffee immediately before you suspect a patient will be using a bedpan—or even better, right after giving an enema—is one of the "in" things that many nurses talk about but seldom try out on newcomers.)

I decided to leave the unit at this point—I had to go to a meeting. Some afterthoughts: The unit was completely different today than I had ever seen it before. Everything seemed to be in a state of flux. Jean mentioned that they were having the usual turnover of nurses. I noticed only four familiar faces out of the eight nurses on duty. I came away remembering the age, diagnosis, and general condition of every patient on the unit. I am not even sure when I made all these observations. I felt that things were so out of control today that I had to make some order for myself. I might even have taken charge if Jean had not been there! I had never come out of this unit with this much awareness of the total unit before. Usually Alice (the head nurse) was there, and she was controlling and monitoring every activity in a very formal, quiet, and controlled manner. It was as though the unit had been completely stripped of its formal side, and the informal structure left wasn't working too smoothly. There were many new nurses and new doctors, and the formal leader was away.

Thursday, August 26, 9:30 AM

I was struck by the quietness and control in the unit today—there was soothing music playing, and there no sounds other than respirators and soft human voices. Loud talking would have seemed out of place to me in here today.

I had the feeling that everyone had to really stay on his toes in order to keep on top of everything today. My first impression was that they had a lot of complex patients and that the nurses and doctors were really busy.

At the entry way (the division between the right and left side of the unit) there was a large polygraphy machine, which graphs EKG, blood gasses, and respiration. I noticed that Dr. Murphy, the medical director of the unit, was there making rounds. Alice, the head nurse, was talking to a new RN. I didn't see one familiar RN other than Alice.

110   Alice didn't interrupt her conversation with the other nurse to greet me at first,

but finally (I felt that I had to wait to be acknowledged), she asked me if I needed any help. I said no, that I just wanted to look around, and she said, "Fine."

At the end of the desk a new nurse was being instructed by the ward clerk. She was giving the nurse a new IV order and explaining to her that the nurse would have to start the IV herself, because the "IV nurse" had been called up the day before and had complained because she (the IV nurse) did not consider it her job to start IV's in the ICU. The new nurse said, "Okay, but I'm not too red hot at starting IV's." Then she had difficulty because she didn't have the right-sized bottle and the day's supply had not come up yet. She checked with Alice to see if it would be okay to use two smaller bottles. (I thought that if she had been working there longer, she would have known a way of getting the solution some other way, either from another floor or by checking to see when the supplies would arrive. She would probably learn to save herself some time by these tactics.) Fortunately, the fluids did come up before she had her meds mixed in the IV; she was slow in getting her equipment together. She was even slower in starting (I mean even beginning to start) the IV. I had sympathy for her when I noticed that her patient needing the IV was rather obese. This meant that it was probably going to be even more difficult for the beginner.

I remarked to the ward clerk that all the nurses looked new, and she said, "Yes, part of the reason is that all the older nurses have to take duty on evenings and nights so that the new nurses can be oriented on days. Sometimes I don't even get to know their names. It would be nice if they could stay longer." I agreed with that. Then I noticed that the urine was overflowing out of a large urine collection bag in the corner. I pointed out that the urine was spilling and asked if there was someone to empty it. (I felt really dippy—that is, strange—and out of character to ask if there was someone else to empty it instead of doing it myself, as any self-respecting nurse would do. To ask for another nurse to do this made me feel that I was really breaking the norms. I was still wearing the nurse's uniform and still battling my expectations as well as the expectation of others.) The ward clerk said, "No, his nurse is at coffee. Could you take care of it for her?" And I took care of it. (Here I was going again! I wondered if a non-ICU observer would have even seen or mentioned this overflowing bag.) When the patient's nurse came back I introduced myself to her and then explained the problem and gave her my guess on how much urine was lost. I explained that I was observing in the unit for a little while. She smiled and thanked me. Alice was busy mixing up a medication, and then she was at a patient's bedside. (I was always impressed at how much direct patient care she did, and it occurs to me now, some weeks later, transcribing my tape-recorded notes, that one of the reasons that she could be so free of paper work was that she delegated much of her paper work to the night nurse in charge.) I said to her, while she was preparing the medication, that the unit was pretty busy, and she answered in a very controlled, almost monotone voice, "Yes, it changes overnight."

I went to coffee with Alice, who had made arrangements to go to coffee with an   **111** "old timer." (I had seen the old timer around, but I had not met her, and I didn't know if she was an RN or a technician. I didn't know her name.) The old timer had the elevators waiting for us. Alice asked her about her health and whether she was feeling better. She said, "Yes, I made myself sick because I didn't get enough sleep." Alice said that it was perfectly okay to take mental health days; "We all need them." In fact that is what she (Alice) had taken the day before; she was just so tired that she knew that it was just no use to come to work. Alice made quite a point to legitimate mental health days, saying that some people felt guilty about taking them, but that they shouldn't.

Alice explained the morning report situation to the old timer. She had only four nurses plus one (the "plus one" was herself), which meant that besides herself there were only four nurses, and there were twelve patients. Also, they were getting a "heart" back that afternoon. She had called Mr. Jackson (the supervisor), and he had said that there was no way that he could send anyone. Alice said that she had sat through the report and had realized that there was no way that she could possibly get through the day without another nurse. So she had called Mr. Jackson back. He hadn't had the information that someone had requested a special day off, so then he had sent a "little student" down from the nursery.

In the cafeteria line the old timer asked me if we had met and I said no, that I had been an instructor on the unit earlier in the year. I gave her my name, but she did not reciprocate, and I did not push the issue. I got the feeling that she was not as interested in my name as in "who" I was.

During the course of our conversation, I was talking too much rather than eliciting information. I was so busy trying to integrate myself into the group—not at all a research stance—that I felt a need to be accepted by the group. I said that I was very interested in the career patterns of ICU nurses because we had found that there was a 6% higher drop-out rate in the ICU than in other regular hospital units. (People in the coffee conversation that was not monopolized by the "researcher" were Alice, the old timer, and a newcomer, a very pretty young nurse.) The old timer nurse responded to my high ICU dropout statement by saying, "That's because not all of them can take the pace, and yet, after working in intensive care, they can't go back to any other kind of nursing. It's like it's just too boring." I got the idea that her opinion was that doing any other kind of nursing would be "stepping down." (I'd heard this expressed before from other nurses.) Alice clarified that all the dropouts were not for marriage, travel, moving away, or having babies, and I said, "No, none of the nurses are counted as dropouts if they leave for any of those reasons."

The conversation drifted to other topics. Alice told the old timer about the psych conference the day before. She explained that they now had a liaison psychiatric resident working with the ICU staff for a 6-month period and that it really helped to have the residents longer, because they built up a rapport. They mainly worked with nurse-patient, nurse-doctor, and nurse-nurse interpersonal problems. "Sometimes you don't say what you feel because you think you are the

112

only one who feels that way, and actually, many others feel the same way." (She really seemed to approve of the psych conference.)

Then Alice asked the old timer if the "Big Monster" was working. (The Big Monster is the polygraph machine I mentioned earlier.) The old timer nodded affirmatively. Then Alice said, "By the way, I heard that they tried to use it on Mr. [X]. We're supposed to be giving only minimal care to him. The fact that we were asked to give only minimal care to Mr.[X] is an example of one of the conflicts we have in ICU–the girls brought that up in the psych conference yesterday. We can't just give minimal care. Our whole mind is set to give intensive care; we just aren't geared to give minimal care." Then the old timer spoke up. "Well, it's discouraging to take care of such a big, heavy, and difficult patient and then find that it's to no avail and doesn't make any difference." (Wow! The silence and exchange of looks at that point! Again, I was very aware that I was both "in" and "out." As an insider, I knew that the old timer had broken a taboo–one never says that any life is not worth saving–but I felt like an outsider in that Alice apparently felt the need to raise the curtain and give a frontstage performance, which she did by her next statement.) Alice said, "Well, the problem *is* that there are patients who really need intensive care, and yet, all your time and the unit's resources are taken up with a patient who really can't respond to intensive care." That seemed to be a more "acceptable" comment, and the old timer nodded in agreement. Then they went through the history of the patient's becoming comatose. The patient had a strange neurological disease. The evening nurse said that the patient was doing fine, and then the night nurse came on and found that he wasn't breathing. He had never regained consciousness.

Friday, September 17, 8:00 AM

The unit was really full today. There were pairs of nurses at almost all the bedsides and in the corridor just outside the three rooms. (This is the typical report procedure after the large report, which is given to all the oncoming nurses by the night charge nurse.) The sounds were also familiar. One patient was coughing loudly, a rather distressing congested, moist cough. I was most uncomfortable coming in at this time because everything was in limbo–it was that time when all the nurses were tied up and I would feel the most internal pressure to "care for the patients." I spoke to Jean (the assistant head nurse) at the desk. She was very intently filling out some kind of paper–it looked like some kind of schedule. She asked about my vacation, and I asked about hers. She said that it had been a year since she had had a vacation and that she really needed one, and so on. She ended the exchange by working very hard on her paper, as if she had to finish it. I positioned myself by a post, actually the back wall to the nurse's station. May, a night nurse (whom I recognized as a former Brighton ICU nurse), was giving a report to a new day nurse. The report was involved; they were going over a number of things on the Kardex, line by line, and at 8:10 AM May and the nurse to whom she was giving the report moved over to the bedside of a young girl. She explained to the nurse about the CVP line, the 10% dextrose, and the special precautions   **113** necessary in taking this young patient's CVP. The patient was unconscious, was on a respirator, had chest tubes, was on peritoneal dialysis, and had three IV's going. Her heart pattern and respirations were displayed on the oscilloscope above her bed. (Such a young patient. I wondered if she had had open-heart surgery and had gone into renal failure due to poor perfusion.) At this point I decided to take a few notes.

The unit was overwhelming to look at "as a whole" today. (I was focusing on one or two beds; I thought I just couldn't process all the information and stimuli coming in if I looked at the whole.) My attention was particularly drawn to a young, attractive Oriental lady in the second bed. She was an open-heart patient and looked very alert, despite the fact that she was still intubated (endotracheal tube) and was on a respirator. (This indicated to me that her surgery or progress after surgery must have been somewhat complicated; otherwise, she would have been extubated by now.)

There were three house officers and a nurse standing around the bedside of this patient; she looked at each of them intermittently, but no one said a word to her. As I mentioned before, she was hyperalert. (An alert patient really stands out in this kind of unit.) One doctor asked for a skin suture set; he remarked to the bed and unit in general that he would have to stitch the CVP line in place a little. He opened the tray up on the bed; at this point another doctor walked up and asked him, "What did Mr. [Y]'s autopsy show?" The doctor working with the suture tray said, "Really inflamed lungs . . . " and then something about the tissue in the lungs being really bad. He then described in detail the appearance of the tissue. The nurse was standing there handing the doctor things he needed; she didn't say anything. On the opposite side of the bed, the other doctor, who was now working with this patient's pacemaker and looking at the scope, interrupted the doctor who was suturing by frowning and saying, "It's up to 2 milliamps now." The patient was looking in both directions with wide open eyes. Was she looking for reassurance? For answers? For someone to say something to her? The doctor working with the pacemaker said, "Her pattern looks good this morning." The doctor working with the skin suture tray nodded and then continued talking to the inquisitive doctor about something else that had showed up on the autopsy. (I cringed every time the word "autopsy" was mentioned. I wondered what the patient was thinking. I would like to have interviewed this patient after her ICU experience to see what she remembered. I left to jot down some notes.)

As I returned, I saw May, who by now had put her sweater on and was getting ready to go home (8:35 AM). I asked her if she had worked nights at Brighton. She replied, "Yes," and stated that she had been wondering where she remembered me from. She then asked what I was doing, and I told her that I was interested in the time and task demands on nurses in the ICU. (I didn't feel comfortable using the work "research" with her, so I didn't.)

"I could tell you a lot," was her response. I said, "I'd like to talk with you." I then invited her to go to coffee. She declined. (I had heard her refuse to go to breakfast with some night nurses earlier.) She explained that she had gone over to one of the girls' places for breakfast the day before and had not been able to get to sleep until later in the afternoon. Her pattern was to sleep in the morning, and if she interrupted that, she had trouble sleeping.

I asked her how she liked working here. She said, "I like it." "Better than Brighton?" I asked. "Well, Brighton is better. I left there because I had had several patients die and I was depressed and getting into a rut. I felt like I needed a change. I wanted to get away from intensive care nursing. I went to a doctor's office, which was really a change . . . I didn't like it . . . the doctor or the work. Then I worked for a registry for awhile, and then I worked for a hospital in the East Bay, and for a hospital in San Francisco, and then I came to work here."

"How long have you worked here?"

"Nine months. Brighton has much better staffing. Like last night, the little girl on dialysis should have had a nurse all to herself. I had one other patient. Sure, my other patient only had q. 4-hour signs, but she had to have three tube feedings, and when she rang her bell, I felt that I should answer her. Sure, other girls could answer, but she was my patient and I felt responsible. The little girl had had VT [ventricular tachycardia] the day before, and I had to watch her. Wednesday night, I had three patients in the first three rooms. [These are set up to be isolation rooms and may be used for isolation or very sick, complex patients.] The man in Room 2 had a nurse all to himself last night, and he should have had one the night before. He was on the Ohio respirator and had a lot going on with him. The woman in the first room has an abdomen full of fistulas, and the one in the third room was pretty sick, too. It makes you feel bad—you might as well be on the floor . . . that's the reason for working in here. You can do so much more for patients in here. But, if you have too many—you might as well be on the floor. I am going with a fellow who is doing his internship now. If we should get married (we have been going together for a year), he may do his residency at Brighton. That would be nice because I could go back and work in that ICU."

She then left the head nurse's office, where we had had this conversation, and went to find Jean to give her a time-off request. I, too, looked for Jean to explain that I was leaving.

Some afterthoughts: I was beginning to realize that my presence in the ICU today had, at most, a very dilute effect, because the nurses were so busy and preoccupied with their work demands that they had no time or energy to do image-management for me. (As an observer, this was good, and I should have been happy about it. But as a person, it just told me that they screened me out as one "who did not know or understand," and that deflated me!)

Monday, October 4, 7:05 PM

I arrived and asked for the charge nurse. I was told that she was out to dinner and would return in 15 minutes. The secretary (who was young) would have let the conversation drop at that, but an older nurse's aide had stepped up and was listening. "Can someone else help you?" she asked with some authority. I then introduced myself and explained what I wanted to do. (I had switched to wearing a lab coat over street clothes. I thought that this would make my entry more difficult, but I could maintain distance and an observer role better than when I was wearing a white uniform. I was becoming more intrigued with and receptive to my observer role. I was also becoming more acclimated to "doing nothing" in this place of institutionalized activity.)

The unit had only seven patients this evening. A renal transplant patient and an open-heart double-valve patient had returned. There were eight people standing around the bed of the open-heart patient (man or woman? I wondered). I had noticed two distraught, anxious-appearing family members standing in the hall and peering in the door. I wondered to whom they belonged.

One of the doctors requested mannitol. (Was the patient in renal failure secondary to poor pump action?) Someone asked if the patient had responded at all yet. The answer was, "No." (I have only recorded this one clinical inference on my part, simply because it would take several pages to note more! I was immediately clinically involved in the meaning of the activity around the bed: the empty urimeter, the lack of response, the two hanging emergency medications, the Isuprel drip, and the crowd of doctors. All this brought to mind many inferences and questions. What kind of valves? How much space were they occupying? How much blood? What about vascular overload with the mannitol? I was in terrible conflict. I was trying to relinquish my right to be integrated into the group because of my previous "ICU citizenship," but problem situations like this really turn me on.) Approximately 3 to 5 minutes had passed since my entry. I left to wait for the returning charge nurse. Being very careful of protocol increases my respectability and trustworthiness, I think.

When I came back, there were still eight people around the heart patient's bed. One of the doctors said, "he raised his knees—a little volume helps." Then a doctor asked the patient to wave his arms or to do something if he could hear. He called the patient by his first name. Apparently there was no response. Then there was some talk about anesthesia—some humor and laughter about "biting on a bullet and lying still." Then the conversation moved to a sport events that had occurred the day before.

Lucy, the charge nurse for the evening shift, was back. The unit secretary pointed her out to me. She was putting electrodes on the renal transplant patient. I had noticed that he didn't have electrodes earlier and had thought this strange. I later found that he did not want them; nor did he want his O_2 nasal prongs. His doctor was insisting on both.

As soon as Lucy finished, I introduced myself as a research aassistant who was being trained to do observation. I was learning to objectively describe events. Lucy said "Sure, you can observe." (Lucy seemed very accustomed to having visitors and did not seem uptight or concerned about my presence.)

The mother had returned to visit the young unconscious girl in the last bed on the acute side. "Susy can you hear me? It's your mother. Susy, I love you." There were only seven patients, and I was really aware of the amount of human tragedy and drama in the unit. This line of thinking was triggered by the mother's plea to her daughter. Then I heard two RN's talking. "The baby is doing well, and the father got to hold it today." I asked, "Is there a mother in here?" and they explained, "Yes, Susy. She was in an accident and was 7 months pregnant. She was transferred here from San Anselmo for burr holes; she had a subdural. When they did the burr holes, she went into labor. The baby is doing well." "How is the mother doing?" I asked. "Not too well—she's not responding like she should," one of them said. The other RN interjected, "You see, she was in another hospital for a week or two before they brought her here." "Was she conscious there?" I asked, completely caught up in the tragedy. "Yes." "Oh," I responded, "she's never been conscious here?" They said, "No." Then I could hear the husband standing at her bedside saying, "Susy, we have a beautiful baby girl." The two RN's were very matter-of-fact and unemotional as they talked. They emphasized that the baby was doing well and that the father had held the baby today.

The seven patient stories told only in age and diagnosis are:

Bill, a 48-year-old man who had open-heart surgery a month ago and had been in the ICU 34 days. He was transferred out of the isolation room tonight.

A 50-year-old man with a pulmonary embolus. He seemed a little out of his head. His hands were tied down.

A young man with a kidney transplant; "gone bad."

A 54-year-old man with a double-valve replacement.

A middle-aged man—diabetic with a new below-the-knee amputation. He was in heart failure and was confused this evening.

Susy, the 19-year-old mother of a premature infant. She remained unconscious despite burr holes.

Only Bill was talked about as a person with a personality. The nurse taking care of him was the only one who talked about him as a person. For example, when he was transferred out of Isolation, much attention was called to him. "Hey, Bill is bagging himself [with an Ambu bag]. He doesn't need any help; he can handle it by himself." Later, Linda said to Cindy, the nurse caring for Bill, "You look happy tonight." (Cindy was dancing to the music on the radio.) "I *am* happy; I am out of Isolation." In a minute she explained to me that they had had a wave of infections with the heart patients and said, "It's really a drag to be the nurse for the patients in Isolation." "Why is that?" I asked. "The extra work—you really have to be organized," she said. "Tonight, it's not so bad. It's not as busy as some nights. Some nights, you can stand at the door 30 minutes waiting for someone to bring you something. Finally, you just find that it is easier to wash your hands, take off the gown and come out and get it yourself. Bill's really glad to be out, too. He says, 'Now people will come to see me.' He bagged himself during his transfer! He is really a nice man. I used to think he was kind of kooky or weird, but I guess I would be, too, if I were in there that long. He had a lot of complications; a lot of infections after heart surgery. He's been in here for 34 days."

The renal transplant patient (sorry, but that was his only identity to me—I hadn't heard anyone call him by name) was angry. He wanted to be **transferred**; he did not want the nasal O_2. His doctor's response to his complaints was to order Valium. The patient said that he knew that the Valium wouldn't do any good and that he wouldn't get any rest. His nurse had called the doctor and explained that he really should be transferred since he was so upset. The doctor said, "Absolutely not," that there was a potential for a dangerous arrhythmia and that the patient should be monitored. Two of the nurses related this problem to the resident on duty. The resident said, "Well, he is going to cause an arrhythmia just by being so upset. Call Dr. H. and I'll talk to him." The nurse thanked him, and I didn't see or hear a follow-up conversation. The renal patient was dozing in the ICU when I left at 11:00 PM.

The open-heart patient now had five doctors standing around his bedside; they had been there for 45 minutes. The patient had six IV's and one unit of blood going. The nurse caring for him was very quiet and deliberate. She moved slowly but didn't seem to waste any motion. She worked quietly weaving in and out around the doctors, to care for the patient. The doctors were talking about internships and residencies. Then they announced that it was time to start rounds. They had stood glued to the bedside for an hour. A very formal presentation of "the case" had been made by one of the doctors. There had been discussion about his mannitol therapy as compared with a lecture they had all heard. As they were ready to move on, the nurse caring for the patient asked about the Isuprel. She had timed it and noted that it was turned off; the doctors had been adjusting the Isuprel flow rate—increasing and decreasing it—and it was important for the nurse to clarify the status of the Isuprel rate before they left. (Usually it's "off-limits" for the doctors to adjust the Isuprel flow rate without telling the nurse.)

8:15 PM

The family of the heart patient came in—the man's wife and daughter. They were alone with the patient at first. (The patient was blinking his eyes and turning his head now.) They asked if his brother could come in. The wife went and got him. The daughter stood by the bedside alone. When the brother and wife returned the nurse went over to the bedside and explained, pointing to the respirator tubing, that the patient could breathe without the machine now but that the machine was to help him—make it easier for him. She then said, "He's doing pretty well; his blood pressure is good; it's stable now and has been for the last hour." The brother heard and pointed out an irregular beat on the monitor and asked, "What about that?" The nurse said, "Well, that's his only problem. We're giving him medicine for that. The next 12 hours are really important, and we'll watch him really closely."

The nurse got out a wash basin set and put it at the foot of the bed. The family left. (I don't think it was because of the nurse's behavior; they were already making motions to leave.) I reacted internally upon seeing the wash basin. Not here, too!

118

All the patients had to have a bath the night they returned from surgery. The lack of individualization and thinking–rationale–bugged me. This patient was still cold, and the bath would only make him colder. This typified some of the "nurse thought" tangents I was prone to while observing. I had to consciously avoid getting bogged down or "tripping out" (as in mind wandering) with all the "shoulds," perfectionisms, and beliefs of my own ICU practice.

The nurse, Gail, working with Mr. [Z] (A diabetic amputee with heart failure) came over to the nurse's station and said to two other nurses, "Mr. [Z] says 'I am not going to tell you about that woman I saw.' I asked him, 'What woman?' and he said the woman he saw over here. I asked him if he knew where he was, and he said, 'I told you I am not going to tell you anything about her.' " Gail then said, "He's always been weird, but tonight he is really cranked out of his head." She then returned to his bedside. She just seemed to be repeating what was to her a funny incident. She didn't wait or indicate by her tone of voice that she wanted any feedback from the other nurses. Later on in the evening, about 10 PM, she asked the nurses if anyone other than Mr. [Z]'s wife had been in to visit him; she said that he continued to talk about a woman who had made derogatory statements. The nurses said, no, but that maybe it was his wife. Gail said, "I just wondered if there was anything I had missed out on–he knows where he is–I am just trying to figure out if he is confused or not." By this time I was wondering about Mr. [Z]'s blood sugar, but no one mentioned this, and I turned off those clinical thoughts.

9:15 PM

The heart patient was now having frequent PVC's. I noticed that his nurses, Jane and Gail, were at his bedside. Jane had phoned the doctors, who were to come right up. At 9:30, the patient had an episode of VT (ventricular tachycardia), and Jane quickly and quietly gave a bolus dose of Xylocaine. The VT subsided. The nurses brought over the defibrillator, and the doctors arrived, were shown the VT on the rhythm strip printout, and were told about the Xylocaine. "Well, you're doing a good job, Jane. Keep up the work. We have to document this for the day crew, mark it, and put your name on it." Another doctor said, "They'll just throw it out." They then talked about the patient's low potassium level (3.7 mg %) and decided to give him intravenous potassium over the next hour. They gave Jane the order, and one of them said, "I'll write an order to cover it later." She nodded and immediately started the potassium in the volutrol. The doctors stood at the bedside, and Jane said that she had lost $60 over the weekend in LA, at a party. There was laughter and joking.

Jane asked if the doctor wanted the patient to have a continuous Xylocaine drip, and the doctor said, "No, Jane, you're doing a fine job. The thing I am worried about with the Xylocaine is the renal failure." Jane said, "But who's going to hold my hand?" They laughed. They then rolled the patient's bed down to take arterial pressure readings. The patient became nauseated and had a coughing spasm. Cindy explained to me that there was water in the respirator tubing, which traveled down the tubing when the bed was rolled down and that this made the patient   **119** cough. I said, "Oh," and nodded, delighted with myself that I didn't show that I knew this, and appreciative of my new role. When the nausea began, Jane pulled the bed covers down, palpated the patient's stomach, and reached for the sump tube, which the doctor immediately inserted.

A few minutes later, Gail brought over a Gomco, which caused the doctor who was sitting at the desk with the chart to ask, "Why are you using a Gomco with a sump tube?" Gail explained, "We always use intermittent pressure with a stomach tube." The resident said, "But that's the idea of the sump tube; you use it so you won't have to use intermittent pressure, then the tube doesn't get stopped up. We use regular wall suction on day shift." (I could have warned this resident not to identify with the day shift.) Lucy said, "They do not; we never use wall suction with an NG, and besides, the large wall suction doesn't work anyway." The resident laughed and said, "You go to hell." Lucy laughed and said, "You're out of your mind. I have been here for 2½ years and I've never seen them use a wall suction for an NG." The resident explained, "You can turn them down (meaning wall suction used for chest tubes and ET suction), you know." (He really had his back to the wall now.) Lucy returned, "Yes, I know, but we always use intermittent pressure with an NG." The resident jumped at this statement. "I'll bet you a six pack," he said. Lucy said, "Ok, I'll bet you a six pack; I'll call Alice, [the head nurse] and ask her. No, she's not home." The resident persisted, "But the tube gets blocked; remember the patient with the Maalox running back out the tube." Gail, remembering, said "Yeah, but that doesn't happen if you keep the tube patent." (There was much derision and disbelief of his "gall" and lack of knowledge. This was expressed in the nurses' laughter, nonverbal signs, gestures, and clicks of the tongue. I really felt the social power of the nurses. I was sure that the doctor was *absolutely* right, but I took sides only mentally and didn't get emotionally involved. Probably because of the triviality, I felt amused. At any rate, the girls made it clear that they would hook up a Gomco and a Gomco only.) The resident's voice sounded more authoritative now. "Well, the impasse is at the use of the sump tube," he said, "The whole reason for using a sump tube is that they have an air outlet making the intermittent pressure unnecessary. That's why we use them. They are expensive; if we use intermittent pressure, then there's no use for a sump tube." Lucy responded (I think her voice sounded conciliatory at first), "Well, that makes sense, but the wall suction, the larger ones, are broken, and there's no way I am going to hook a sump to the ET suction bottle." The resident replied, "No." (At this point he had given up; earlier, he had pointed out that the other high suction outlets could be turned down and used. The stand-off was over for now, but the issue remained unresolved. We had all gathered in this discussion group. I participated by listening and sometimes smiling as the "point" was tossed back and forth.) The nurse, Jane, who was caring for the critical open-heart patient, cocked her head toward the group and came over (a distance of about 2 to 3 feet) to lend support to the evening nurses position. Now there was a lull in the conversation, and Jane came over to Gail talking softly to her. The rest of us could not hear what she was saying. The resident asked, "What's Jane telling you?" Gail said, "She was telling me to watch the monitor while she gets a cup of coffee and a cigarette. What's the matter? Are you getting paranoid, Dr. Sims?" The resident said, "No." (He *had* sounded as if he thought they were talking about him.) Then the conversation turned to drinking after work and partying.

I had introduced myself earlier (same spiel as outlined before) in the evening to Jane, and she said with a smile, "Yeah, you're checking on me." I said, "No, far from it." Then she was busy. I followed her into the coffee room a few minutes after she had started her smoke and coffee and charting break. I asked her to tell me what had gone on.

She explained, "The patient went into a serious arrhythmia, and the doctors had left me an order for Xylocaine in case of such arrhythmia, and I gave it."

"Do they always leave an order for Xylocaine?" I asked.

"No, he had been having an arrhythmia that led up to that episode."

"So they were expecting it?" (I continued to check out my assumptions; I must admit that I felt proud of myself. I was beginning to really get into the role of a "systematic," if not scientific observer.)

"Yes, in spite of the fact that we are all acting pretty casual, the patient isn't doing well at all."

"What happened when you decided to give the Xylocaine?"

Jane's response was to digress a bit. "If this would have happened 6 months ago, I wouldn't have been able to take it this well. You take care of just one patient and you get used to it. You are a nurse aren't you?" she asked.

I said, "Yes," and asked, "What were *your* main concerns with this patient?"

"Well, there are five IV lines and he can have no more than 250 cc all evening. You see, patients come off the pump wet, and you really have to watch their input to get them dry. Both Keflin and potassium have to be given in (IV) fluid. You can't let the Keflin go in too fast, or the patient could get into trouble."

"It's like juggling," I said with respect.

"Yeah, we go out drinking afterwards." She smiled as she said this.

"That's probably the most therapeutic thing of the evening," I noted, hoping to show some understanding of the stress she had experienced.

"Yeah," she replied.

"So the main things *you* do first," I paused and waited for her to explain more.

"First we take vital signs every 15 minutes, then every 30 minutes. There are arterial lines, and there are really potent meds—a lot of really potent meds. The doctors wanted me to start up Isuprel, and I refused unless they were up here. He went into VT *without* Isuprel. It's really strong and can cause an arrhythmia."

There was a pause, and then she said thoughtfully, "You really have to depend on the doctors to make a decision; if they are indecisive, you can't do anything more."

"Do you feel that they have been indecisive?" I asked.

"Yes," she answered.

"What would you have them do? Do you have something in mind?" I felt that she did have some other approach in mind.

"Yes, give a continuous Xylocaine drip." Her voice sounded convinced.

"Why do you think they didn't?" I asked.

She answered quickly, "Denial. Dr. Sims is concerned about the patient's renal failure, but I've taken care of other patients with that problem, and no one seemed to worry about it. I think it's just denial on their part. They looked at the bigeminy and trigeminy on the monitor and said, 'It's not that bad; you just have to really watch the monitor.' "

This made me remember the omnipresent collection of doctors around the bedside during the evening, and I asked, "Earlier in the evening there were six to eight doctors standing around the bed; did that bug you?"

"Oh, at first they were talking about the patient, then they forgot to move away. It didn't bother me too much. You just have to tell them to move when you want to do something. Sometimes it's worse, and you really have to tell them. It's just one of the things you have to put up with in a teaching hospital." With this, Jane looked at her watch and began to chart on the "intake and output" sheet. I took the cue, thanked her, and excused myself.

Tuesday, November 9, 4:10 PM to 5:30 PM

The unit seemed to be in a hubbub. The noise level was fairly high with lots of talking among nursing staff and doctors. I noticed on my way into the unit that Alice (the head nurse) was in her office. Alice came back and gave Marcia a piece of paper and said, "Hi, Pat." I saw one other day nurse still on duty and the staff development person.

Things seemed to be in flux. I walked to the end of the nurse's desk and caught the attention of the afore-labelled "old timer." (I still did not know her position or name.) She wanted to know what I was doing, if I needed any help. I seemed to be disturbing her work. She apparently did not recognize me. I went through my spiel about learning how to describe, and she very nervously said with a bit of a laughter, "You best not observe or write down what I do." I put my hand on her arm, smiled, and said, "No, I'm just trying to describe all the work you guys do in here; trying to make some order out of it." (I was saying more than I wanted to—I wanted to reassure her, but I wasn't making any headway.) She laughed and said, "If you make any order out of it, would you let us know?" She seemed satisfied. At no time was there any feeling of a need to tell this person my name or for her to tell me hers. She went back and continued her conversation with the doctors.

(I had heard that they were expecting someone up from the emergency room. I wondered what type of emergency.) Marcia was busy assigning dinner times to everyone along with the person to relieve the nurse going down for dinner. She was constantly being interrupted by questions. Trish, a rather new nurse, came over with a BP cuff with the bulb, pump portion detached and asked how to get it connected. Instead of telling her (as I would have done), Marcia took the cuff and put it together. Trish watched and then thanked her and took the cuff back over to the area where she was preparing for the new heart patient. I realize that all this sounds rather disjointed—an apt description of the activity in the unit at this point. A lot of unordered, though not unusual, random stimuli kept coming into the desk area where I stood. Marcia was handling all this randomness and directing it. Another nurse came up and said that she was caught up with her work and that she could circulate (meaning that she could go around and help others.) Was there anything in particular that Marcia wanted her to do? A phone call had just come in that the heart patient was on his way and would be there in 10 minutes. Marcia immediately directed this nurse to help with the new heart when *it* arrived. Then there was some discussion about how old the child coming down was: Marcia said a 12-year-old; Trish, the nurse assigned, had understood that the child was to be a 5-year-old. (I was thinking how little history these patients have when they come into the ICU, unconscious from heart surgery.) About 7 minutes had passed since I entered the unit; questions were buzzing in my head, and I felt the need to order some incoming of stimuli. I asked Liz, the nurse's aide, who seemed to be the only unpressured one in the unit, the following questions: "You have a patient coming up from the emergency room? What's wrong with him?"

Liz answered, "It's an MI from the emergency room."

"Oh, is CCU full?" I asked.

"Yes. We have another MI patient, a real nice patient."

"It's good to have a quiet MI patient for a change?" I wanted to know why she considered this patient "nice."

"No, he's not quiet, he's just cute. They say he's disoriented, but he's not really; he just speaks Russian." (I had followed Liz into the utility room now, and she was nodding her head, pointing out a little old man with nasal O_2 prongs in his nose. He looked disheveled and sunk down in bed. There were brown paper bags at the end of his bed.) I asked Liz how she knew that he knew what was going on, also making a comment that it must be awful to be in this strange place and not have the benefit of speaking the language. She smiled and said, "Yes," and related with pleasure and pride, I thought, her unique exchanges with this man that no one else had understood. She had found out that he did not like coffee; he preferred tea. She asked if he could drink Sanka. He grunted and gave signs that he could, but only as a last resort. She then went out and got some plain hot water for him. (An MI patient is not allowed caffeine, because it increases myocardial irritability.) Liz explained that she had had trouble procuring the hot water from the girl outside (dietary, I assume). I could tell that she was irritated (maybe incredulous that she should have any problem) with the trouble involved in getting the hotwater. But I also felt that she was pleased that she had gone to all this trouble for this patient and that that was her point in telling me all this. Liz smiled and said, as if to finally prove her point that this man could communicate, "And he prefers two sugars!"

We were now standing out in the hall. Again I had followed Liz. She excused herself rather abruptly and went behind a closed curtain in the corner. It had been pulled ever since I came in 30 minutes ago. I looked around, and there was an orderly who had just come in with a cart with a shiny metal dish-like tray about 6 feet long. It completely covered the cart—there was a metal handle at each end. I looked at the cart, wondering, "What on earth? Is it to collect instruments?" Then it dawned on me that this was a morgue tray and that the person in the corner behind the curtain must have died. (The dish-like tray sent shivers up and down my spine—it reminded me of the time that I, as head nurse, had had to go down to a postmortem to see the blisters a cooling blanket had caused on a patient's back. The coldness of the metal and the dish-like shape gave me the mental image that the body no longer had integrity and that the fluids coming from the body were now looked at differently and treated differently.) Liz excused herself and explained, "I didn't mean to ignore you—I have to go down to the morgue with this orderly." I heard a nurse say, "Get him out of here." She was referring to an older man standing, holding his wife's hand, at the bed just across from the bed where the body was. Another nurse quickly and without explanation deftly pulled the curtains in front of the man and his wife. No explanation was asked for or offered. The body was quickly removed.

I was concerned about the Russian man, who seemed to be the only one who might view the morgue cart on its way out. But he had become interested in what was in the brown paper bags at the end of his bed and was too distracted by looking through these bags, which contained his belongings and medicines, to notice the cart. The cart really looked more like a heap of linen now than a body. The body was completely shrouded in a sheet. I was caught up in this game of protection. Once it started there seems to be no choice. I wondered if the man standing by his wife knew about the death, anyway. If he had been there very long, he could have been in the waiting room when the family was told. I knew nothing about the person who had died. I had heard no one mention anything about the death.

I was pleased and surprised to notice that the man had been allowed to stay with his wife for over a half hour now. This kind of extended visiting privilege is unusual on the unit. His wife seemed very ill and fearful. She looked very pale and had very bloody urine. The nurse and husband had been ministering to her with a cool wash-cloth and reassuring phrases.

The MI patient was then brought into the unit from the emergency room. She was accompanied by a nurse and an orderly. She looked to be in her late 40's or early 50's. She was sitting upright in her bed, supported by an elevated back rest. She was smiling, looking around. Her face was a bit flushed. She had oxygen and IV running. Carol, an ICU staff nurse who had approached the patient, completely ignored the patient. She did not greet her with either eye contact or verbal greeting, but zeroed in immediately on two small transistorized monitors located at the foot of the woman's bed. Carol's response was, "Look at these—how neat!" (What incredible selective perception to notice and acknowledge the portable monitors first!) Then the nurse assigned to this patient came over to help with the bed. Still no one had greeted this woman, who was still smiling and looking around expectantly. There was a bit more talk about the portable small monitors. Beds were moved, and the patient was placed in location Number 8. After the patient was in her bed, Judy, her nurse, was getting ready to attach new electrodes to the patient. The first formal greeting or acknowledgment was given by Judy. "I'm Judy; I'll be your nurse, so if you have any complaints, I am the person to talk to." The woman was still smiling (She didn't seem to believe what was happening to her, and she could only respond with smiles—she looked amused, actually. I was thinking that this woman was a low priority patient in this unit because of the relatively few curative, procedural demands of her illness. How different her greeting and her importance, in terms of priority, would have been in the CCU. Since she was a relatively young woman with an MI, this would have given her a high priority in the CCU. In the CCU she would have gotten much more attention and introduction to the unit, the monitoring, the nurses, and so on. Here, the greeting and introduction were limited to, "I'm Judy, I'll be your nurse, so if you have any complaints . . . " What a negative set!)

I noted that Marcia had posted the dinner list. She had also made out a list of missing supplies. There were about eight precise items, such as "two 12-inch long French catheters." I wondered when she had had time to make out this list. She had had so many interruptions. A nurse had come in from the adjoining unit and asked to borrow something, and communication had to be straightened out regarding the transfer of a patient. The Russian patient was to be transferred to the eleventh floor and not to her floor.

I was standing at the end of the nurse's desk now, and Marcia was inside the nurse's station talking to an anesthesiology resident. He asked about the patients that were going to be transferred in. Marcia explained that Dr. Murphy (medical head of the unit) had made the final decision on the four patients who were to be admitted. (I inferred that there were more than four patients vying to get in. Otherwise, Dr. Murphy would not have had to make a decision.) But he had not informed anyone of his decision yet. The anesthesiologist explained that he was not really on call yet and that he had been doing research in the pulmonary function lab all day. He asked who was on first call.

Marcia then said that there had been some trouble changing the endotracheal tube on Sally Jones and that she had expired. The resident looked stricken and said, "No, I don't believe it." Trish was standing at the desk, waiting for her heart patient to come, and said twice, "Dr. Murphy was here." "Dr. Murphy was here then, huh?" the resident asked. He was reassured again by Trish and Marcia that Dr. Murphy had been here. The resident was looking for the deceased patient's chart. (This was the first time I had heard anything about the patient who had died.)

The resident was studying Sally Jones' chart when the anesthesiology resident on days, Dr. Boyd, came up and stood beside him. The new resident asked him, "What happened with Sally Jones—were you here? How come they couldn't get her intubated?" Dr. Boyd explained, "Well, they did have trouble with the intubation, but that wasn't the cause of her death. She was breathing on her own for awhile. And then they did get her intubated. Her blood gasses were okay. Jim [Dr.

125

Murphy] was here." Then he went into a brief neurological description and explanation that I could not follow. (I picked up on the phrase, "Dr. Murphy was here." I interpreted this to mean that, "The expert, Dr. Murphy, who is well respected, was here, so everything that was possible to do was done.")

Marcia and Trish were still standing at the desk. Dr. Boyd was explaining that Bill Webber and he were still unsure of their roles in the ICU. The other new anesthesiologist chimed in, "That's three anesthesiologists who are unsure of their roles in the ICU." (Apparently they were on a new rotation.) Marcia smiled and wrote the appropriate names of the doctors on call.

Then the heart patient returned from surgery. His name was Jimmie—the anesthesiologist accompanying him from surgery was calling to him, "Jimmie, wake up. You're okay. Your surgery is over." There were eight people around the bed; the anesthesiologist, Marcia, Trish, two doctors on the heart team, an orderly, and the two new anesthesiologists.

Trish and Marcia were busy rearranging arterial and venous lines—hooking up the chest drainage to the wall suction and connecting the patient to the monitor. They were also noting the amount of blood and fluid in the IV's and connecting the CVP, which had become dislodged during transport from the OR. Trish got down on all fours—forearms and knees on the floor—to look at the chest drainage unit. (This made me shudder since I was so rigorously instructed, and have come to believe, that the floor is the dirtiest of all places in a hospital. I wondered if Trish would wash her forearm.)

Two more heart team members arrived. One female resident asked the doctor attending the boy how he (meaning the surgeon) was doing. "I'm doing great. I am happiest when I am cutting and sewing. If I never had to go out and see or talk to a patient and could just do surgery, I'd be in my element." This young surgeon really looked elated; he was smiling, his face was flushed, his eyes looked very alert.

The surgical anesthesiologist had ordered blood gasses, a chest x-ray, and an EKG. All three were accomplished within 10 minutes. (There was very little time lag between the doctor's orders and the doing—communication and action were very streamlined. In fact, I did not even know who called for these tests after the doctor verbally requested them, probably the unit secretary. This streamlined communication and action is typical of the ICU's I have worked in.)

The initial care of the new heart patient was well under way. All the vital reconnections of tubings and monitoring were made. The x-ray technician came, and Marcia directed him down the right side of the unit. Marcia then noticed at 5:20 PM that the two girls assigned for the 5:15 PM dinner time had not yet left and rounded them up, receiving very brief reports from them, based mainly on her specific questions. She really had to take over and prod these girls to get them off to dinner on time.

My thoughts at this point were: It had really been a chaotic evening. Marcia had been running, coordinating, doing, overseeing, and clarifying ever since I had

126

arrived at 4:10 PM, and still there was one more patient to transfer out (the Russian man with the MI) and four more patients waiting to get in. It was likely to continue to be a very disconnected, changing unit this evening since the four new admissions represented unknowns.

It was from this frame of reference that I said to Marcia in way of leave taking, "It is really hectic tonight—there's so much going on." She answered me as she would answer an outsider. "It just seems busy because it's strange to you. All of this is very familiar to us."

To an outsider this was an accurate statement. I would ask Marcia later if she considered this evening to be unstable and rather unpredictable, which was what I was referring to. I think a backstage reply to an insider might have been quite different—something like, "Yeah, everything is really up in the air—more like days." As I left, I was impressed with the continued hubbub of much talking and conferring throughout the unit. For the most part, the talk was between and among the doctors and nurses.

SUGGESTED QUESTIONS FOR DISCUSSION AND ANALYSIS

For undergraduate students
1. Cite an example of a "role message" being given by the following: a nurse to a doctor, a nurse to another nurse, a nurse to a patient, a patient to a nurse or a doctor.
2. Cite instances in this narrative where a nurse might feel instrumental and expressive role conflict. (See Skipper, James K., Jr., "The Role of the Hospital Nurse: Is It Instrumental or Expressive?" In Skipper, James K., Jr., and Leonard, Robert C. (Eds.): *Social Interaction and Patient Care*, Philadelphia, J. B. Lippincott, 1965, pp. 40-48.) How do you think nurses might handle these conflicting role demands?
3. Who are the central figures in Benner's descriptions of the ICU? Based on this description and your inferences about this description, what would you say are the major goals or objectives being carried out in this unit?
4. Have you ever been requested to give minimal care to a terminally ill patient? If so, did the patient's setting influence or affect your feelings about giving minimal care?
5. Which patients do you think might be high priority in the ICU? Why?
6. What are the major role behaviors of the charge nurses described in these observations?
7. Have you seen or participated in "protecting" patients or family members from seeing a corpse removed from a hospital unit? What do you think are the benefits of this protection? What do you think are the negative effects of this protection?

For graduate students and teachers of nursing
1. Give some examples of ways in which the nurses in this description made their world more manageable. What are some of the ways a head nurse or director of such a unit might facilitate the nurses' handling of the stresses such as (1) instrumental and expressive role conflict (see Skipper and Leonard), (2) high death rate, (3) high personnel turnover, and (4) close working conditions and other stresses?

2. Does the ICU nurse's social power differ from that of the regular hospital nurse? If so, what differences in the social systems of the regular unit and ICU might account for this difference in social power?
3. How would you help students understand the seeming incongruity of loud music and dancing in a high life-death crisis area?
4. Do you agree with the old timer's assessment that ICU nurses might consider any other type of nursing a step down?
5. How can you evaluate and reward expressive nursing care? Can expressive nursing skills be taught?
6. Do you think that it is possible for ICU nurse to give both expressive and instrumental nursing care?

7. Work in the premature nursery

Anselm L. Strauss, PhD

While doing field observations and interviews of residents and interns at the University of Kansas medical center, Dr. Strauss, a sociologist, observed some of the interaction on the premature baby service. He had the opportunity also to talk extensively with the nursing staff. This kind of ward presents some very special challenges and problems to the nurses, but above all, the work that they do is special because of the nature of their patients and the clinical problems that they present.

LOOSELY AND TIGHTLY GOVERNED SERVICES: PERMANENT NURSE AND ROTATING RESIDENTS

As the housestaff physicians rotate around the services, they are brought into contact with nurses who are permanent members of each service. This sets problems of diplomacy and control for the young physicians; but the nurses, especially the head nurses, have comparable problems with the housestaff. The head nurse can rather naturally be expected to believe that her longer stay on the service has given her greater knowledge of how it works and ought to work. In this hospital, as elsewhere, the doughty head nurse is a problem to the resident who officially is her superior.

When the service is unquestionably a "resident's service," then his official authority is maximized. At the other extreme, we might visualize a service that is almost completely given over by the senior staff to the head nurse, whatever the formal ranking of authority. Listen first to the head nurse on the former kind of service, and note what the rotation of housestaff means to her.

Reprinted from Strauss, Anselm L.: *Professions, Work and Careers,* San Francisco, The Sociology Press, 1971.

I asked whether the interne was important to her. He is, because the students are supposed to draw the bloods, and sometimes they do not do it on time or so readily; and the interne is important to her because he is responsible for getting on them. She said you have to keep on the interne to do these kinds of jobs. She said the interne that she had before the present one was not so good in this respect. He did not keep up to snuff. She had to keep on him. This fouls up things for the nurse; because if she does not get the IVs done, this means she has to delay on breakfasts, and then she gets behind generally. She said the interne is likely to change every month; meaning that it is about half over before he knows the ropes entirely. When I pressed her on this she said it only takes two or three days for him to kind of know his place, but I think the first statement more accurately represents her viewpoint. As for the residents: she spoke of idiosyncracies. Recently one resident when he first came on wanted short needles for IV's (she said with kind of a snort). So she got him short needles. In this way she gets on his right side. It is, as she said, a matter of sizing up what they want and pretty much giving in to it. But in return, of course, she gets certain concessions. "You order them short needles, and they write you the orders when you want them." For if she does not have the orders when she wants them, it upsets her whole scheduling. The idea is to get orders written ahead of time in case they have to be used when the residents are not around. This nurse, however, has an arrangement with other services, who bed some of their patients with her: then she finds things need to be done with their patients, rather than calling them up and having them come down to write orders, she is allowed to go ahead and do what she wishes, and then later when the resident appears he will write the orders. On these particular services the residents are much more stationary; on the resident's service they rotate, of course.

The major difference between a service run by a resident and one run by a staff man seems to be that on the former service the nurse depends more upon whatever relationship she can build with each new resident. Her control over him probably is less firm, more unstable.

Be that as it may be, observe now a nurse who has a very great deal of control over her residents. Hers is an unusual position and an unusual service. She is in charge of the premature baby service. She has no assisting internes, and only one resident (and one student) at a time. The care of premature babies apparently calls for considerable skill, for the margin between death and life is very slight. Whether or not the faculty men have given this nurse de facto authority over residents on this service, it is clear that she believes they have.

The sociologist first came across her domain when a pediatrics resident told him about Miss Geer:

He said she had been there for fifteen years and she knows a very great deal about new born babies, that she is quite good just out of sheer experience. As a consequence she practically writes the orders. She will say to the residents, "Here are the orders." If you cross her and give her other orders, she simply will end up not doing most of them. You can complain about her and she'll be alright for perhaps a month and then you are back again in the same position. Also she will withhold information so that it will embarrass you. For instance, there was a jaundiced child, and you come into the room with the staff man and discover it, and she says she had told you the day before—but she had not. So I said to this resident that in other words she pretty much runs the nursery and he said that was right; but it was not proper she should do this. On the other hand the residents, it would seem, have very little defense against this. He was cheerful about this, but displayed a strong air of resentment.

The sociologist, when he went to visit Miss Geer, was much less interested in the amount of her control over the nursery than he was in her attitude toward that control. By now he was well aware of rotational consequences, and wished to know how her perspective influenced the life of the resident while he was assigned to the nursery.

I let her know from the very first what I thought her problems with residents were: saying I realized she has been here for some time, whereas the residents were constantly rotating. How in the world did she ever handle the situation? Within five or six minutes she was talking freely, talked for thirty minutes without much of a break, and ended up at my request enthusiastically showing me the nursery. Her whole demeanor and style of speaking indicates that she thinks this is her own terrain, at least as far as anything but research on these babies is concerned; and research is done by the staff itself. Right now she has a "good resident." "We work together." Some residents do not work with her. But on the whole "we cooperate and get along." She stressed experience as important in handling premature babies, for it takes a good deal of experience to handle them and to know just what is going on. There are frequent emergencies, when one has to act very quickly to save the baby's life. Now the point here is that, as she noted, you supposedly have to get hold of a resident, and he is not very often around, but you have to act quickly. It was quite clear from the way she said this, that she does act on her own accord. I asked, what if she gets a resident who will not cooperate and will not write orders quickly and so on? She said that she can—if she has to—call on the faculty man. I got the impression that he is a great source of authoritative strength in such show-downs. "It makes a big difference that he is behind me."

She went on to describe the difficulties that residents sometimes made for her, as when they are not tactful to parents of the babies. She made a point of remarking that some residents regard the babies as cases rather than as patients. She spoke of a resident who had ordered three times too much drug for a baby. She said something to him about it and he asked whether they should give more. She disgustedly imitated his question, and said "you have to know your babies."

It is evident that if the resident can get on good working terms with Miss Geer—mainly her terms, of course—then he can learn a good deal both from her and from the greater freedom of movement within the nursery that he will enjoy. But what of the students? Presumably they too can learn something from this specialist—providing that they will forget she is a nurse and regard her as a clinical teacher; and providing they play the game according to her rules.

I asked if she had much contact with students. She spoke, her voice one big exclamation: "One every week!" Some do not even know enough to wash their hands to put on their gowns. She added, "I sometimes wonder why they are here." They do the physicals and then the residents are supposed to check them. I asked whether she got any benefit out of these physicals, suspecting not from her tone of voice. She said "no," and with a kind of weary patience added that physicals got done three times: once by the student, once by the resident, and once by the private pediatrician. Then I asked whether students ever asked questions of her about the babies. She said "no, they don't ever ask anything of us, except occasionally they may say that this is a nice baby."

Her remarks do not tell us about the amount of learning—and teaching—that may go on but they do suggest something of the consequences of rotation when an established nurse is given considerable authority. Even an outsider like the field worker, can sense quickly that this is a ward where medical service is paramount, and teaching and learning is quite secondary. Since the babies are important subjects for research also, we may guess that research also takes precedence over teaching functions.

131

SUGGESTED QUESTIONS FOR DISCUSSION AND ANALYSIS

For undergraduate students

1. If you have worked on premature baby services, what has been your experience? Has the service been operated much as described in the foregoing pages? Or did you find differences? Or did you not see the kinds of things described because of your purely student role?

2. The sociologist who wrote the above selection would tend to say that student nurses work in a bit of a vacuum because they tend to be students rather than "regular staff," and so are not so subject to some of the usual pressures of the regulars—especially with regard to relations with staff and visiting physicians. Do you agree or disagree with him, wholly or in part, and why?

3. Are there any implications for student nurses' learning in this account of the young physicians rotating around the services? What are they?

For graduate students and teachers of nursing

1. The assignments given student nurses are much like the rotation of residents and internes around the hospital. Think through some of the implications of that kind of rotation for the student nurse and her learning. Could we do it better than we do it now—with more rotation or less; with slower rotation or quicker rotation; with more carefully chosen services or just a more realistic sampling of all kinds of services and agencies?

2. What kinds of experiences have you had working on or with services where nurses had more "say" or less "say" in the running of the ward?

3. Think through some of the implications of the fact that head nurses on *any* service must negotiate with the chief resident or interne in order to give good nursing care—and that sometimes the young physicians are "good" and sometimes "not so good," sometimes "cooperative" and sometimes "uncooperative."

8. Children on the pediatric ward

Marlene Kramer, RN, PhD

How do differences in ages of patients affect the nature of the nurse's work? For the most part, children express their needs differently than do adults, with more nonverbal and diffuse communication, such as crying, rather than with explicit verbal communication. The differing needs of children and the rapidity with which their health status changes for better or worse leads to environmental, structural, and functional differences in the work of the nurse. For example, are there fewer or more constraints on the pediatric nurse's autonomy than are found in observations of nurses working with adult patients?

Another factor markedly affecting the nature of the nurse's work in the pediatric setting is the high potential social loss generally associated with the death or prolonged disability of children. This factor introduces a stress, strain, and emotional current that becomes very obvious in observations on this unit. A parallel factor here is also the association with the role of mother, which is often a source of conflict, particularly for young married nurses who work in a pediatric setting. Such are the foci of the field notes describing the observations made by a nursing professor on a pediatric ward. They were done specifically for entry into this book.

Friday, 8:00 AM

As I walked through the adult units to get to the pediatric unit, I particularly noticed the somber quietness of these units. The carpeted floors muffled the steps of the nurses scurrying around. Voices were controlled and hushed. When I hit the pediatric ward, I was bombarded with stimuli—light, color, noise, and activity. The contrast to the somberness of the units I had just come through was overwhelming.

The pediatric unit was bright, noisy, cluttered, and active! There were a lot of

133

bright colors, drawings on the walls, and papier-mâché things tacked up all over the place. One of the windows behind the nurse's station had an entire glass panel filled with pictures of children who had been patients on the unit. The noise level was something else again. There were children crying in the background as well as close up to the nurse's desk as I approached it. There was a steady hub of noise from conversations going on all over the place. Added to this was the periodic calling out of the children or nurses. Each could observe one another through the large glass windows, so communication was by yelling. "Nurse, nurse, bring me some water." "I gotta go peepee, nurse." "Sit down in your chair, Timmy, you'll fall." "Okay, Marc, I'll be right there."

The pace of activity on this unit was startling. Everyone was moving. The nurses walked and moved very rapidly. Seemingly in one flowing, unencumbered motion, one child was picked up and another deposited. This one was moved off of a lap or moved over to make place for another. The ward secretary was busily working with one child on her lap and another at her feet. There was an aliveness about the atmosphere here, even with the sound of crying and pain in the background.

The hallway was filled with paraphernalia—a scale, wheelchairs, potty chair, laundry hamper—and there were children under foot everywhere—sitting on the floor, in laps, in the hall, in a wheelchair. They were toddling back and forth, and one was immediately on guard to be careful and not stumble or run down the children as he walked up and down the corridor. (I wonder how all this noise, clutter, and activity must seem to a 3-year-old—like a constant loud buzz and kaleidoscope of color and changing figures?)

I approached the nurse's station. There were six physicians (of various kinds) in animated conversation in the middle of the station. (How typical!) The ward secretary wove in and out among them as she needed to get various forms, and so on. There were a couple of other people around in varying colors of blue, pink, and yellow uniforms. I assumed that these were the nursing personnel. It was impossible on this unit to distinguish the difference between RN's, LVN's and aides by uniform; everyone wore quite short, stylish, colored uniforms. It was even difficult to pick out the parents from the nurses because some parents had on the same style of dress.

I identified the head nurse. She had on a white uniform and a "head nurse" name tag. I wanted to introduce myself, but she was deep in conversation with the night nurse. I identified her as the night nurse for several reasons; she looked very tired, very harried and harassed. It was about 8:15 in the morning and the night nurse, I knew, was supposed to be off duty at 7:30. As I waited to introduce myself to the head nurse, I overheard part of their conversation. (It wasn't difficult since it was taking place right out in the middle of the corridor in easily heard voices.) It was obvious that something had happened last night or early this morning that had caused a great deal of confusion and apparently had caused the night nurse to become disorganized and get behind in her work. (I found out later that a child had died.) The morning report had apparently been quite jumbled, disorganized, and very difficult to follow. The head nurse was saying how difficult this made it for the day staff when they didn't get a good, clear report. The head nurse asked the night nurse, "Did something happen in the early part of last night that you got so far behind in your work?" The night nurse stated, "Well, yes, I had to go to a meeting from 1:30 until 4:00." The head nurse said, "Well, you don't have to go to the inservice meetings if you are not caught up in your work." The night nurse said, "Well, I was caught up at that time. While I was gone, this and this and this happened, so I got way behind."

At this point the head nurse picked up (it was more a grab, because she had to push the night nurse's sweater away to get at it) the night nurse's clipboard and said, "Well, let me see if I can help you with your organization. You always seem to get far behind in your work and don't seem to be too well organized." Then she said, in tones that reminded me of a mother talking to a small child, "If it is too much responsibility for you, I'll relieve you." The night nurse countered defensively, "Well, no, I don't think it is too much responsibility. This is one of the first times this has happened, and I really enjoy being in charge. I really like to try it and see if I can do it." At about this time the night nurse looked like she was starting to cry, and perhaps, at this same time also, the head nurse noticed I was standing there, because she said to the night nurse, "Well come on, let's go into my office and talk about it some more."

I had some mixed reactions to this episode. First of all, it was very obvious that the night nurse was very, very tired and that she had had a bad night. She was also at least an hour late getting off duty, and I really wondered about the timing of this kind of counselling conference with the night nurse. The head nurse's approach and technique were also rather aggressive, but I was identifying with the night nurse, and in situations like this, the "top dog" always seems to be meaner than what she perhaps actually is. On the other hand, when would have been the appropriate time for the head nurse to discuss this matter with the night nurse? Early morning was probably the only time that the head nurse saw the night nurse. But in terms of any criteria for an effective counselling session, I wondered if this session had any positive effect at all.

One of the other things I overheard the night nurse saying was that this was her first night back after having been off duty for 5 days. She used this as one of her reasons for being somewhat disorganized last night, but this was "put down" by the head nurse.

Since I wasn't able to talk with the head nurse, I introduced myself to the other nurses on the unit and to the ward clerk and explained what I was doing, and so on. They were very friendly but also very busy, so they more or less told me to go about and do my own thing and leave them alone.

I walked down the hall and again was struck by the activity on this unit. The nurses walked very rapidly, with long, striding steps and a great deal of free motion and twisting of arms and body. A child was lifted into the air, another one was placed back in bed, a third one was patted on his rump, while a fourth was chucked under the chin—all in a single nurse's sortie down the hall.

There were about four nurses that I could identify at this point on this 24-bed **135** pediatric unit. There were four large wards and one private room, all with large glass windows in the walls and doors. In the first room I walked into, the nurse, Joan, was caring for the three children in the room; two girls, aged 13 and 16 months, and a boy of 4 years. She was feeding, or helping to feed, the two girls and at the same time was supervising the feeding of the boy. The infants were in high chairs; the older boy was sitting at the table. Joan was interacting with all three children almost simultaneously and almost in a continuous running fashion—first cooing to one baby, then saying something to the boy, smiling at the other infant, and spooning food into the mouth of the first baby. (It was funny to watch, especially since I know I do this myself, but with every spoonful of cereal Joan brought up to the infant's mouth, she also opened her own, as if to receive a spoonful.)

In the next room the children were alone; they, too, were all set up and were eating breakfast, as were the three older children in the last room on the right side. I crossed over to the other large ward on the left, Ward A. Here there was much activity.

I observed in this room for quite a while, so I will take the time to describe it in more detail. There were five beds in the room—two on the left-hand side and three on the right. In the center of the room there was a low round table. Seated around this table were three children, about 3 to 5 years old, and a woman. The woman was feeding one of the children, who I later found out was her own. In the corner station on the right-hand side there were a man and woman dressed in hippie style. A student nurse was making up a bed—the first bed on the right as you entered the room. Another nurse was bathing the child in the second bed on the left. This was an infant about a year old, who was marasmic, dehydrated, pale, and whining. An IV was running; the child looked very, very ill.

I first took in the room as a whole. There was absolutely no interaction between any of the five adults in the room. The mother who was feeding her child was crooning and talking softly to the child. The two hippie parents were looking off into space or out the window. The student nurse was *absolutely* silent; even her manner and way of movement was mouselike. The staff nurse talked frequently to the baby she was caring for, as well as to the infant in the first bed on the left. The content of her remarks were, I am sure, completely meaningless to the infant. (She was talking about things she had to get at the grocery store, what she was doing, and so on.) The level and tone of her voice, however, had an obvious soothing effect on the baby. She used a great deal of hand contact—rubbing, patting, and stroking of the infant.

The infant in the first bed on the left side was a very appealing baby—blonde, blue eyes, and on the chubby side—there didn't seem to be anything obviously wrong with the infant. The thing I particularly noticed was the sporadic and frequent interaction of the staff nurse with this baby, named Joey. Every now and then she would look over, smile at the infant, say something, and then go back to the baby she was caring for. There was no particular stimuli from the infant (such as a cry) that I could see that provoked these interactions.

During the 30-minute period I observed continuously in this room, at least six nurses entered (not six different ones; some came in twice). As I observed their interactions and approaches, I began to see a pattern. The person entering would stop first at Joey's crib (first bed on the left), coo at or pat him, receive a smile, and then approach Carol, the staff nurse bathing the very ill year-old baby. A question would be asked of or a message delivered to Carol (all of the entrants apparently had their business with Carol), and then a "coo-pat" interaction would be begun with the baby Carol was caring for. Often, this was begun while Carol was responding. On the way out there was some variation in the pattern. People frequently interacted with the two children seated at the table who were feeding themselves. If the mother looked up (she was seated on a low chair) at the nurse, a greeting was exchanged, and the nurse would comment on how the child looked, how much she was eating, and so on. Two of the nurses commented to this mother that she herself looked more rested today. After this interaction, there was another "coo-pat" interaction of the nurse and Joey, and then the nurse left. None of the six nurses interacted at any time with the student nurse, the hippie parents, or the small child being fed by her mother. None of these people, however, gave any observable cues that they desired interaction. But then, neither did Joey, Carol's baby, or the two children at the table. Did Joey have higher social worth than the other infants?

I left Ward A and walked down the hall. I noticed now that there were a variety of signs, toys, pictures, and playthings all around the unit. The clutter in the hall again seemed quite hazardous, but everyone deftly stepped around and over children, tricycles, wheelchairs, and so on. This unit would have driven anyone of a neat nature up a wall. The equipment seemed to be necessary and seemed to be used at periodic intervals; the nurses said they liked to keep things within easy reach.

I must comment again on the physical movements of the nurses on this unit. They had very free, open strides with arms swinging; I am sure that some of this was due to the great deal of lifting on the unit. The patients, being small, were frequently lifted and handled from one nurse to the other, moved bodily around the beds, into the wheelchairs, and so on, so that the movements of the nurses were very energetic and wide sweeping.

I went back into the first room, where I had earlier observed Joan feeding the two infants, and observed here for a while. Joan had finished feeding the children and was now saying to the older boy, "Ricky, I am going down to coffee now; would you watch the two girls for me until I come back? Or would you like to take your bath while I'm gone, and I'll have someone else watch the children?" Ricky said, "No, I'll watch Susie and Marie until you come back." Joan said, "Okay, if you watch them while I am gone, then when I come back, you can take your bath while I bathe Susie." Ricky said, "Okay." (I had observed this practice of asking older children to look after the younger ones earlier, but this was my first observation of deliberative, participative planning of care between a child and a   **137** nurse.) Joan then moved Susie into a wheelchair and Marie in a high chair out into the corridor outside of the room and said to Ricky, "I appreciate you watching them for me." Ricky said, "Okay," and looked up at her with a grin. As Joan was walking out to go to coffee, she called loudly to another nurse and to the ward secretary (so Ricky could hear it?) "I am going down to coffee now. Susie and Marie are out in the hall, and Ricky is watching them. He'll do a good job watching them." (What tremendous positive reinforcement this must have been for little Ricky!) Ricky stood by his two charges the entire time Joan was gone. Every now and then, if one of the babies started to cry or fuss, he would go over and pat the baby or pick up the rattle or the toy that the infant had dropped. He really seemed to take his charge very seriously. As I watched, I had the impression that it was a rather common practice for Ricky to do this. I asked the ward secretary why Ricky was there. She said he was recuperating from open-heart surgery and had been there for quite some time. "He's one of the pets of the ward." (I had noticed before that patients who have had open-heart surgery seem to have high social value—maybe because of the staff investment to "bring them back to life.") When Joan came back, she thanked Ricky for watching Susie and Marie while she was gone and then proceeded with the bathing as planned.

The other thing that I particularly noted was the frequency of brief, fleeting interactions between nurses and infants. Much of this interaction was nonverbal, with a lot of touching and patting. For the toddler group, some differences were noted. They seemed to be in their own world, and the nurses were in their own world. Every now and then, the two would meet. The interaction was very seldom sustained, but it seemed to be characterized by a continuing theme. It was almost as if the nurse had a continuing dialogue with a floating object who streamed in and out of her sea of consciousness. The nature of the interaction was ongoing, rather than discrete.

I will illustrate the nature of this sporadic interchange with a continuing theme, by a conversation (if you could call it that) that took place over a 4-hour period between patient Ricky and nurse Joan. It started at breakfast, during which Ricky wasn't eating too well. He was a very thin and emaciated-looking child, and he really looked as though he could use some good nutritional intake. Joan said to him, "You know, Ricky, you really have to eat better than that, so you can build up your body, and so you'll be able to get well and go home and go outside to play." Ricky nodded, and a period of 10 minutes elapsed before, seemingly out of the clear blue moon if you hadn't heard the previous remark, Ricky said, "I'd like to ride my bike; I like Frosted Flakes." Joan responded, "Bikes are fun to ride. I'll get you some." When Joan came back from coffee, she said to Ricky, "What color is your bike?" Ricky said, "Blue." After a pause he said, "I'll drink some chocolate milk." A while later, Joan asked, "Ricky, what would you like for lunch?" Ricky didn't say anything. A full 15 to 20 minutes later, the head nurse came into the ward, smiled, and said "Hello" to Ricky. Ricky looked at Joan and said, "Peanut butter." So Joan said, "Would you like a peanut butter and jelly sandwich for

138

lunch?" and Ricky said, "Yes, I like peanut butter." Around 11:00 o'clock or so, the head nurse came in and said to Ricky, "Here's a peanut butter cookie, Ricky." Ricky smiled, took the cookie, and began to eat it. (Keeping up an ongoing dialogue like this with several children, all on different subjects, would seem to produce quite a cognitive overload for the nurses, but they seemed quite comfortable.)

In addition to the yelling and calling between rooms of the nurses and children, there was also more yelling on this unit between nurses and nurses, and doctors and nurses. The head nurse or ward clerk sat at the desk and called across the corridor or down the hall, "Dr. So and So has changed the pencillin order on Ricky," or "Be sure to feed Lynn slowly; the night nurse said she upchucks if she takes it in too fast." When I asked the nurses about this, they explained that the communication on peds could be open and free because the children didn't understand, and it didn't matter to them if they heard what was going on. (They had an intercom system, but I observed that it was used only for one child in isolation.)

Later the same day

Since the head nurse and night nurse had not come out of the little back room for quite a while this morning, I had never introduced myself to the head nurse. When I arrived on the unit this time, the head nurse was standing at the desk in conversation with Dr. Simpson, a woman pediatrician. They were discussing the amount of analgesia that children who are postthoracotomy or post–open-heart surgery might have. The gist of the conversation was that both Miss Hatch, the head nurse, and Dr. Simpson really felt very strongly that these children need some morphine in very small doses for pain medication after this chest surgery. The nurse related that these children splint the left side and walk droop-shouldered after surgery, that they do have pain, and that she felt very strongly that they need some pain medication. She was telling Dr. Simpson that she had gotten into some big battle with Dr. Rode, the surgeon, because his whole idea was that these children don't need any analgesia, that it's bad for them, and so on. Dr. Simpson went on to say that Dr. Rode read an article once that said that children did not have pain and should not be given analgesia. She said the trouble was that the article compared giving nothing for pain with giving too much medication—there was no middle ground or middle of the road. The thing that impressed me about this conversation was that there was a mutual sharing. There seemed to be a collegial relationship between the head nurse and the doctor, in which the nurse gave some detailed description and observations of a particular child, how much morphine he had received, and how he did as contrasted with another child who had gotten more or less analgesia. (Was this because Dr. Simpson is a woman? Because children are the patients? Or was this a common occurrence?)

When the head nurse had finished this conversation with the physician, I stepped up, introduced myself, apologized to her for not having introduced myself earlier, and explained I had not wanted to interrupt her, and so on. She was very warm and gracious, saying, "Oh, go right ahead. In a teaching hospital anything goes; the girls are used to being watched." She then asked me if there was anything specific I wanted. I said, "No," and I went on about my way.

I walked down the corridor, and again, even though it had only been a couple hours since I was here before, I was struck by the absolute clutter in the hall, the swift walking of the nurses, the light, the color, the noise, and the steady stimulation on this unit. I walked into Ward A, the same room I had observed at length before. This time, all of the children were in their beds. In the middle bed on the right-hand side, two of the nurses were catheterizing Michelle. Michelle was about 3½ to 4 years old. One of the nurses was holding her in a spread-eagle fashion. There was a great big light over the child's head; she was sweating profusely and was yelling "bloody murder." The other nurse had on sterile gloves and was lubricating and inserting the catheter. It must have been extremely terrifying to the child to have that bright light shining right down on her and to be restrained like that, although Roberta, the nurse who was holding her, periodically talked to Michelle and tried to sooth her. "It's almost over with now, Michelle." She kept up a running prattle of talk to Michelle in a very soothing voice. The child screamed and yelled throughout most of the procedure. Technically, the procedure was accomplished very efficiently and very effectively. (It would be so easy to castigate these nurses for inflicting pain and discomfort on a terrified child, but what else could they have done?)

This entire procedure was carried out in the ward—no screening, and so on. It was completely ignored by the infants and other toddlers in the room, but parents and other nurses frequently stopped by or looked in to see what was happening. (I wonder if this made the nurses uncomfortable, parading their technical skills and capabilities in front of everyone. This was quite different from an adult ward, where frequently a skill is performed only in front of a patient, who may or may not be in a position to judge the competency. In this instance, the nurse had to perform a difficult technical procedure on a squirming 3-year-old who was loudly proclaiming to anyone who would listen that she objected. Furthermore, this procedure was performed under the judgmental eyes of three staff nurses, a student nurse, four parents, a cleaning woman, a lab technician, and two physicians.)

The behavior of the student nurse was in marked contrast to that of the staff nurses. I had now observed for about 4 hours. The student nurse had yet to say a word to any child or person in my hearing; nor had I seen or heard anyone else speak to her. This was in such a contrast to the four staff nurses and the head nurse on the unit, who were constantly not only receiving communication but also giving out information either to parents or to each other, and who maintained a constant running prattle with the children. The nurses addressed all the children by name; the student nurse seemd to communicate solely by gesture or movement. The other thing that was so noticeable with the student nurse was the difference in posture, manner, and bearing. As I noted earlier, the staff and head nurses walked with an authoritative, swinging, confident walk. Their manner and bearing exuded a confidence that was almost overwhelming in contrast to the student nurse, who sort of slunk and slithered up and down the hall. She must have been terrified and overwhelmed by this absolutely overwhelmingly confident posture of the other nurses. I'd tried to catch the student's eyes a couple of times to explain to her who I was, what I was doing, and to just talk to her. But she absolutely averted my gaze. It was like she was shrunk into a shell. The staff nurses on the other hand, although they asked for no explanation and seemed to have accepted my presence like a piece of furniture, would look me straight in the eye if I smiled at them. They would smile at me, they would engage in any conversation that I initiated, and they would very readily answer my questions, although no one asked me for an explanation of who I was or what I was doing.

It's getting close to lunch, and the smell of food reminds me how hungry I am. Before I leave, some thoughts and reflections:

I thought at first that the ongoing, continuous sporadic interaction that I described earlier took place only between the nurses and the children. But I was now seeing that this also took place between nurses and parents, and nurses and physicians. There were at this time about ten different parents on the unit, cruising in and out, in many of the wards with many of the children not necessarily their own. There was a constant prattle with the toddlers, and there was a constant "coo-pat" interaction with the infants. It was apparent that the nurses here must have been able to tune in and out very rapidly from one conversation to another. This kind of rapid tuning in and out was also noted with the physicians. They would come on the unit and say, "Hey, did that kiddie void yet?" Or a nurse would ask, "Can Dickie have water now?" And very quickly each would have to tune in to exactly who or what the other was talking about. They usually responded by saying, "You mean Pam," or "you mean the open-heart patient?" (The physicians didn't seem to know the children quite as well by names; they referred to them more by diagnosis.)

Another example of ongoing sporadic interaction that was observed—Joan was walking down the hall with a washbasin and some dirty linen. Will's mother was pushing him, and the nurse asked, "How is he today?" The mother said, "Oh, he is not so good." They then discussed the mood of Will, who was about 2½ years old—that Will wasn't in a good mood, although he had been in a better mood this morning until they had started working on him. (I had observed earlier that another nurse had changed Will's dressings.) Joan then asked Will's mother how her rash was (location not specified). They discussed this for a bit, and then Joan said, "Will your husband be coming in this afternoon?" Will's mother said, "No, he is still on the road. He won't be coming back until tomorrow." Then Joan said, "I guess you'll be glad when he gets back. He must be a big help to you in terms of taking care of Will and the other children." They continued this dialogue and discussed who was caring for the other children at home and that sort of thing. Again, I was noticing that there was evidence of ongoing relationships between nurses, parents, children, and physicians.

It was particularly evident on this unit that all the nurses seemed to want to

141

know about all the children. Even though they might have been assigned to another room, they seemed to be knowledgeable about all the children and seemed to interact with all of them. This was undoubtedly because the children were wandering all up and down the halls, so that it was very necessary for the nurse to at least have a working knowledge of all the children and their present state of illness or health; whether they were NPO or not NPO, and whether they could be out of bed or not out of bed.

SUGGESTED QUESTIONS FOR DISCUSSION AND ANALYSIS

For undergraduate students

1. Describe some of the uncertainties and bases for insecurity that a new student nurse might have on a pediatric unit as opposed to an adult unit. What are the most striking differences in specific role behaviors of a "new pediatric nurse" as opposed to a "new nurse" on an adult care unit?

2. Place yourself in the role of the head nurse. What do you think her concerns and priorities were in talking with the night nurse? How else could the head nurse have helped the staff nurse to fulfill her role expectations on the job?

3. Place yourself in the position of the staff nurse. What do you think were her major concerns and needs? How else could she have responded to this situation in order to meet her needs?

For graduate students and teachers of nursing

1. What are some possible consequences of open-awareness context on the pediatric unit? What are the teaching potentials of the open-awareness context—for the children and parents? For other professionals?

2. From the observations described, what are some of the "unplanned" learnings for students on a pediatric ward? Do you think the student nurse described in this observation was having a meaningful experience? How might you have assisted her to make this a more meaningful experience?

3. Compare and contrast anticipated student and teacher learning goals in relation to clinical experience on this pediatric unit.

section D

The emergency room

9. The health care system of the emergency room

Ruth Fleshman, RN, MS

Written while the author was a graduate student in a research program, these field notes of a series of observations in the emergency ward of a large county hospital in a metropolitan area are rich with descriptions of the impact of social system constraints and cultural attitudes on health care. Also seen very vividly are details of the nurse's work in this kind of free-floating, labile, high stress-oriented environment. These observations provide an opportunity for the reader to assess the impact of acuity of illness and cultural differences in patients as variables affecting the nature of the nurse's work.

December 5, 1962, 12:30 PM

I arrived per my appointment with the Assistant Nursing Director. I was in a lab coat with an improvised name tag: "Mrs. R. Fleshman, RN, School of Nursing." I gained approval by looking very businesslike, and we discussed the total invisibility of lab-coated personnel. We walked over to the emergency ward, I was introduced to the head nurse, Miss M., and my purpose was briefly explained. Miss M. then took me around the unit, explaining the functions of the various areas, the routines, and the flow of traffic through as far as the patient route went.

For the first half hour or so, my only perception was of total chaos; people were rushing around in various uniforms, phones were ringing and being used to call all over, and references were being made to incomprehensible ward numbers as the destination of current patients. During most of the early period, I simply followed the head nurse, clipboard in hand. When she would return to the nurse's station and seem at ease, I asked questions regarding staffing. She replied by telling me the number of nurses per shift and the physician-staffing pattern. Shortly after that, I became aware of many more types of personnel belonging to the ward and was then able to learn that the service also had LVN's and orderlies, male and female.

The first patient of whom I became fully aware, after the quick tour and foot-of-bed summaries of patient conditions, was a woman holding her fussing baby in the pediatric ward and trying to control her other child, an active, curious boy about 8 years old. Through the glass walls I could see her flaring at the doctors and nurses, showing more and more signs of impatience as time passed and the baby fussed more and more. At last, about 1:00 PM, she stood in the doorway and in heavily sarcastic tones demanded to know if they intended to admit the baby or not, since it was, after all, an hour past his feeding time, anyway, and she wasn't about to keep him starving much longer. The head nurse turned to her and blithely assured her that the admission process was going along apace and that the only thing needed was for the pediatrician to finally get down to examine the child. The tone had nothing of apology, soothing, anxiety, and so forth, in it but was quite matter of fact without being curt. Contributing to the mother's tension was the fact that her other child was also getting bored and had begun exploring further afield. Although none of the staff had remonstrated with him, the mother kept calling to him to get out of the way, come back in here, don't go in there, and so on. I learned that the baby was a referral from the pediatric clinic to be admitted to the hospital for a routine circumcision.

The function of the admitting unit was also handled within the same area as the emergency service and by the same staff. The area and staff served as a funnel through which patients were poured and sorted into several categories. Except for a few OB patients, a few psych patients, and one other service I can't now recall, all other admissions to both the acute and rehabilitation hospitals must also have come through here to be seen by the appropriate physician from the prospective service and then to be shuttled off. Next to them may have been a patient brought in from the outside as an emergency case. The process here was that any patient who had to be given a body examination (as opposed to a cut finger, and so forth) was directed to the appropriate ward room and told to undress and get into bed. During my first period of observations, an old regular came shuffling in with the complaint that his penis was raw. Told the routine procedure, he objected since, "All I have to do is drop my pants!" But the procedure had to be followed. He managed to evade part of this by eventually undressing but never getting into the bed; he sat on the bedside chair while waiting.

Within the nurse's station were kept the drugs and supplies that were often dispensed to the patients when they were discharged, as well as during their stay. Near the intercom were two telephones that were generally indistinguishable when ringing, causing whoever answered to get the right one more by chance than by anything else. The head nurse answered my query about it by saying that there had never been a clerk or secretary in the station. In fact, she told me, it had been only recently that she had been able to have a clerk, instead of one of her LVN's, put out at the central "booking" desk to start the paper work. One of the head nurse's jobs was phoning—for old charts, for social service work-ups, to check which floors the patients were to be admitted to, and so on.

There were many more people around the area then simply the medical staff and patients. Other hospital employees included the ER orderlies, pink-coated orderlies returning patients from x-ray, male and female social workers from the adjacent area, occasional student nurses (from a 3-year Catholic school in the same city), and physicians—some in hospital attire as consultants from other services and some in street clothes. The latter were usually older men, status unknown but always addressed by title by the other MD's. There were also a great number of men in police-type uniforms, and I gradually became able to distinguish men from the sheriff's office, city policemen, and badged-and-uniformed city ambulance stewards. The first two groups were usually in pairs, attending a male prisoner from one of the respective jails who had been brought in for treatment—usually of injuries sustained during the course of their violations, most often connected with drunkenness.

I gradually became aware of the bantering conversations that went on between the nurses and the various staff members—the nurses and the police types (stewards), and the nurses and the physicians. The first of the two combinations seemed almost a parity relation with a familiar, sardonic tone, with first names being used both ways. My feeling was that there was a sense of work division here where each made his own contribution without any infringement on the other's territory and each sharing a commonly accepted goal. The banter with the physicians was of much the same nature but less familiar. Although the MD's called the nurses (except the head nurse who was "Miss Mac") by their first names, they in turn were addressed by title, even during the coffee break.

During her tour of the patients, the head nurse spoke to me about the condition of each patient as we came to him in a tone that was not meant to exclude his listening and included several friendly phrases, such as referring to a florid-faced man in his 60's as "this young man." However, after a while I began to hear the exact same tone used with every patient, drunk or sober, freeman or prisoner, male or female. It may be that this was a device she had arrived at to use in patient situations. The other nurses, being younger and newer, were not quite so consistent, and their tone tended to be more casual, even flippant.

Unless it was an actual critical emergency, patients brought in through the double-glass doors were directed to the booking desk where an older man in a white hospital smock and police star began to get the data for the chart sheet that followed them through the process. This was usually only name, address, age, and so on, and not any medical information beyond any obvious clues he could gather (a possible fracture was only designated by its site). The patient was then directed by him to the appropriate way station. If the patient was ambulatory and needed no body physical, he was sent to sit "on the benches"—one bench and two short rows of folding chairs against the wall at the first part of the emergency hallway. There was always a nurse assigned to this area, which also consisted of two minor-surgery-type rooms separated from each other by a lab and from the hall by doorways that could either be curtained off or actually closed with a sliding door.

These three areas actually comprised one large room with partial walls so that traffic (and sound) could flow inside or out to the hall. Across from one of the doors was the entrance to a small cluster of treatment cubicles that I saw being used for ENT procedures and certain storage tasks. On the same side as the treatment rooms was the pediatric ward with several cribs and one full-sized bed. Opposite this was the bend of the corridor occupied by the nurse's station. On the outside of the bend on the other side was the women's ward with a dozen or so beds that could be separated by curtains on an overhead rod. Immediately south of this was the linen closet, well stocked. Down at the end of the hall were a series of small rooms—one on each side was a "holding room," formerly referred to as a cell, that contained only a mattress and bedspread. The window was easily 10 feet off the floor. The heavy door with a peephole was propped open unless actually in use by an unmanageable psych patient, or, in one case, by a physician doing a casual physical when the men's ward became jammed. Also along this wall were the men's toilet, a tub room and a kitchen. At the end was the men's ward, containing 13 beds with the same curtain arrangement. I was interested to note that bed No. 13 was used only for a "station" for the orderlies and LVN's who never came into the nurse's station except on business. This bed was covered with little pieces of busywork—gauze, wrappers, file folders, and so on, and was surrounded by chairs. The intercom unit, which was over each bed, was the method by which the head nurse communicated with attendants when they were in this "station." I later asked her why no patients were ever put in bed No. 13, even when they were spilling out into the corridors, and she told me that it was set up too close to the closet where patients' clothes had to be stored to be convenient to use and said it had nothing to do with its number.

Although patients came in fairly steadily, there were intervals when the previously deserted nurse's station had most of the MD's and RN's in its vicinity, and there was casual chitchat, interspersed with comments about various current patients, requests for x-rays, charts, and so on. Then they would gradually disperse until only the head nurse and I were left, and I would sit again in the No. 2 chair.

Just prior to 3:15 the head nurse was headed with a chart toward the booking desk and I was following close behind. Coming into the lobby, one could hear a siren winding down outside. The head nurse dropped off the paper and swung around toward the door, saying, "I'll just take a look and see what we have here." At this point the doors burst open as a gurney was pushed through them on which was a young child over whose face a worried-looking steward was holding an oxygen mask while the other steward carried the tank and helped push the gurney. In one rush, the gurney sailed into the second treatment room and by the time I had changed direction, it had jumped back from the rush of people—three to four MD's were there, one cutting off the boy's clothes, another trying to introduce an endotracheal catheter, and another with his ear to the boy's chest, trying to listen for a heartbeat. At his request the others quieted momentarily until he decided he could hear one. Near me the mask-holding steward said to no one in particular,

147

(unless me), "I had a hard time keeping him going until we got here!" In answer to someone's question, he said, "Fuller and Washington—yeah, a city bus." In the central group around the table I saw three nurses; two were at the table and one was seated next to it keeping notes of the procedures as they were being done. An IV had already been set up, and a fourth MD was trying to start it in the left arm. On the periphery of this group were one or two LVN's handing over equipment, and so on. Along the edges were the bystanders—myself and the stewards from this and perhaps one other ambulance, since there seemed to be a fair number of people. I observed that the boy was a rather bad shade of green.

I decided to check what was happening outside on the rest of the ward while this crisis was occurring. One of the internes was continuing a physical in the men's ward. The orderlies and LVN's continued their routines. The head nurse was sitting at her station. By this time, the mask-holding steward had brought in the boy's book bag to give her the boy's phone number and address. She was filling out the report form and said to him in a serious, semisoft tone, "He doesn't look like he's more than 7, does he?" in such a way that suggested, to me, at least, a sort of "poor little thing" feeling. At the door of the pediatric ward, the mother, with the to-be-circumcised baby was standing holding him and said, "Oh dear, I have one 7 years old myself." Her expression was such that I figured she had not gotten the nature of the emergency since she had almost a smile, although sympathetic, on her face. The head nurse dialed the boy's phone number. The mother apparently answered, and the nurse identified herself and said, "Your boy was injured and has been brought in to the Brent Emergency just now. Is there someone you can get to bring you out?" The mother must have asked the nature of his injuries, since the nurse replied, quite honestly, that she didn't know yet, since the doctor had just gone in to see him. After she hung up, the surgical resident came into the station and asked if the call had been made. The nurse said it had, and he asked what she had said. She answered, "I only said that he had been injured, and she said she could have someone bring her out. She's on her way now. Was he DOA?" (It was apparently obvious, or I had missed the word, that the boy was dead.) The surgeon rather tentatively decided he had been and added, "I'm afraid big city buses kind of wipe out little kids." I noticed the time was now 3:23; only 8 minutes had passed. I went back into the treatment room. Now there were only two staff members—a nurse removing the IV tubing, tape, and so on, and a physician palpating the boy's body, apparently to determine the extent of injuries. As I slipped back out into the hall through the curtains, I noticed a black woman who had been waiting for treatment on the bench outside; her face was distorted, and she was quietly sobbing. One of the other nurses came over to her, put her arms about the woman's shoulders in a comforting gesture and led her into the other treatment room. Whether she had observed any of the events or not, this was the only visible sign of disturbance in the whole area during the crisis. All the other staff members had dispersed to their various routine tasks. While filling out forms, the head nurse happened to mention to someone that the boy had been DOA and was contradicted by this person, who said the surgeon had just decided he had expired in the ER. There was heated discussion about this, but she finally checked and found he had almost immediately changed his mind after leaving her and had changed the time of death to 3:22.

While she was still completing the necessary forms, the head nurse looked up at another nurse and said in a "routine" voice, "Call the priest, will you?" She turned to me and amplified on this by saying, "Of course, we don't know yet if he was Catholic, but sometimes it helps to tell the parents about it, if he was." At this point, the surgeon came through again, and she reminded him that the mother was on her way and that she would be in the "family room" for him to talk to. I asked her about this, and she explained that this room had been set aside for family use, that it had been nicely furnished by the hospital volunteers, but that so many things had been stolen out of the room by visitors and patients and they had to keep it locked at all times when it was not actually being used for such dire circumstances as this.

A few minutes later, I heard her say to the surgeon that both parents had arrived and were waiting for him in the family room. Without any change in his already sober expression, he turned and started to walk down the hall in that direction. (To my eyes, he seemed to be walking very much alone through a passage full of people along its fringes.) After the doctor turned the corner, the Catholic priest came out of the cubicle where the boy's body had been stored. He was a stocky, florid-faced man, and he had rather a strange expression: his head was bent forward, and as he turned to face the approaching head nurse, his glance seemed almost shamed (?), bullied (?), defensive (?). She told him both parents had arrived and were in the family room now. He said, "Of course, we don't know their religion." I added that the surgeon had just gone in to speak with them.

At 3:30 two student nurses came on duty, and as they walked by the nurses' station, one said to the other, "Oh, that poor little boy they brought in; he didn't make it!" The other matched her distressed look, and I became aware of the fact that these were the only two people who had actually expressed any regret in words. Several of the other staff members had discussed the incident further, though in terms of how often this sort of accident has been happening recently, and they had tried to recall just how few months ago it had been that another child had died as a result of tangling with a city bus.

At 3:35 the evening shift nurses had all gathered. The evening treatment-room nurse went off with the one from the day shift to get a rundown on patients waiting. The day head nurse took the evening staff and students around on another bed tour as she had done for me. I noted that while this was going on, one of the students was peering closely at my name tag, but no questions were asked of me. The head nurse had introduced me to the evening charge nurse directly, and I had given her my explanation also, but no one else had been able to hear it. During the tour, the head nurse was writing up a census sheet of those patients still in the wards at the end of her shift. Occasionally one of the patients would try to ask her

149

questions about what was being done to them, but she would turn them aside with reassurances that the doctors were working on it, that they were just waiting for reports, and so on. The statements used were almost in the nature of asides from the running commentary she was making to the oncoming nurses.

At one point in the afternoon, I was leaning against the outside of the nurse's station while two MD's were seated inside discussing a patient one of them had examined. He seemed to be trying to convince the other and himself that this patient should be admitted despite inconclusive findings. (In the decision to admit or not, the greater weight was given to trying to keep patients out of the hospital.) The examiner listed all his findings, points of the history, and the conflicts he had noted; he felt there was enough material to justify further studies. The second MD asked if there were a chance that this guy only wanted a place to stay, "a soft bed for the weekend," and if he had "hospitalitis." The first thought not. The second then asked, "Well, is he a good solid citizen?" The first replied, "He's more solid than most of our citizens. He came all the way in from Watsonville, where he had a job. He told me about the local MD saying he won't treat his symptoms without his record, so he figured this was the logical way to get *to* his record. And then, he came in without smelling of alcohol—so, generally, I'd say he came in like a human being." (I smiled sardonically to myself and wondered if he was now being treated as a human being.)

By 4:45 I had decided to leave for the day. Inventory to this point included awareness that I had begun to be accepted by the staff; the bantering that went on among them was extended to include me, not directly, but by a wink or teasing smile. Although no one had asked my function yet, they seemed to presume that it was removed from a work function, since once or twice someone would start to ask me for something and then recognize me as nonstaff and turn away. One of the reasons I had stayed to this hour was to be introduced to the evening staff so that later observations during their shift would not have to be prefaced by lengthy explanations.

One forgotten item: Just before the day head nurse left, she asked pleasantly if I were going to come again tomorrow. I said I planned to and thought I would be there in the morning. "Oh," she said, "come by 9:30, and we can have coffee together." I thanked her with some surprise and gratitude, mentally vowing to strive to be there, since this would provide an opportunity to see the off-ward nurse.

December 6, 1962, 9:30 AM

Made it! As I arrived on the floor, the nurse's station was swarming with chattering personnel, so I kept to the background. When there was a pause in the activity, I said good morning to the head nurse, and she said, "Ah, you're just in time! Let's go off to coffee." She turned to one of the other nurses and said, "You have the keys, don't you? I'll be over for coffee, then." She led me around the corner beyond the family room to the next door, which opened into a locker room cum lavatory, in which was a huge round table and side table with a coffee urn, cups, and a torn-open bag of doughnuts. Two nurses in smocks were already there, and she introduced me to them as a graduate student from UC and also as a nurse doing research. They, it seemed, were from the recovery room, and it was apparent from the tone and informality of conversation that a close rapport existed among the three. They were discussing an inservice program that had been held 2 days before, which only the ER nurse of the three had attended. She said, "Ordinarily, these talks on rehabilitation bore me stiff, but this one was absolutely fascinating! Of course, the two speakers were great, but this was the first time I've ever heard it so well discussed." One of the RR nurses said, "Well, that's probably all right for some places, but that sort of thing wouldn't work on a service like ours." With elaborate sarcasm the ER nurse said, "Why, what do you mean? We do rehab all the time—we give the patients a bath!" During this conversation, the medical resident from the ER had come in, poured coffee for himself, and sat down with us. The conversation turned to the interesting phenomenon the ER nurses had observed that giving baths to weak little old drunks brought in off the street often killed them. The MD explained the mechanism by which this could occur (borderline shock aggravated by the vasodilating effect of hot water) and advised cool baths. The RR nurse told of her experience in the past of turning little old ladies on their left sides for preprocto enemas and having them die also. This seemed to puzzle everyone, so the topic was dropped.

During our several cups of coffee, two other MD's and two of the ER nurses joined the group. When the surgical resident came in, one of the nurses commented, "Well, I see our little boy made the front page today." Someone else replied, "Oh, really? I haven't seen a paper yet today; what did they have to say?" The fact that this was a minister's son had been given stress in the newspaper and the whole incident was discussed by the group. The general response was to the effect that "these dammed city buses keep doing this sort of thing" and "something really needs to be done about that city bus system." Someone commented that they had heard that the city had to pay out $2,000 every day for injuries done by the city buses. One of the doctors replied that he wouldn't be the least bit surprised and, in fact, would wonder that it wasn't more.

After coffee was finished, we returned to the ER. I became aware of a lot of joking going on between the nursing staff and a middle-aged black man in street clothes lounging around the hall opposite the nurse's station. It soon became obvious that he had been an employee in the ER sometime in the past and had had some illness during which he had lost a great deal of excess weight, the resultant slimness being the center of the banter. I was unable to account for his presence until a black woman was wheeled out into the hall near him, awaiting discharge home by ambulance. This was his wife, also a hospital employee in another department, who had injured her back on duty. Even though she was also a patient, the staff attitude toward her was predominantly that she was part of the ingroup. The nurse quite openly gave her the prescribed drugs from the ER supply in an amount sufficient to save her from having to buy any. Although this was   **151** occasionally done for some particularly sympathy-arousing "ordinary" patient, it was clearly contrary to rules, and when it was done it was always in a surreptitious manner.

December 7, 1962, 6:00 PM

Friday evening had been predicted by the day head nurse to be violently active, "because that's when they all get paid out here." The physician staff was now comprised of the evening shift, who had to work from 5:30 PM until 7:30 AM the next morning. By contrast with the previous 2 days, it was now the pediatric area that was busiest and the adult areas that were quiet. The evening head nurse explained sardonically that this was due to the fact that these were the patients who were too lazy to come in to the clinic during the day, and now that it was closed, they would jam the ER until bedtime. I soon became aware of the pediatric interne, a short chubby young man, who was rushing around between the ward and the nurse's station making cheerful, noisy comments. His boisterousness must have often bothered the head nurse, since she would frequently suggest he keep his voice down, hush, and so on. He appeared not to hear her.

At 7:00 PM two adult women and one man came in carrying a boy, about 5, and a girl, about 3. The boy was screaming and kicking, apparently from fright. The girl was placid but wide eyed. Their skins were dark and their hair black; I made the assumption that they were American Indians. As per the routine, the children were placed in separate cribs in the pediatric ward and undressed. The physician came to them in their turn and learned that, between the two of them, they had ingested 45 baby aspirin. He was preparing to start the stomach-pumping routine, when he chanced to ask them what time this had occurred. When he was told it had happened 5 hours previously, at 2:00 PM, he nearly exploded. "Five hours ago? Where have you been all this time? Why did you wait so long?" He came stomping out to the station to tell us this latest bit of information, adding venomously, "Such stupid people—the kids could have died by now for all they care—stupid!" The charge nurse began to pick up these phrases and repeat them. She added to me, "Boy, we sure get 'em here!" The doctor had whipped back into the pediatrics ward and then came out again still frothing about such stupid parents, and I had had more than enough. With a bland look, I asked "Why necessarily 'stupid'? Maybe, 'ignorant'? After all, they *are* Indians." The head nurse looked up and jeered, "Yeah, *Texas* Indians." I asked, "What does that mean?" She said, "Oh, that's what we call Mexicans around here." Although the doctor had taken no part in the conversation, he had been within range. Although he may only have finally vented his spleen, when he returned to the ward, he stopped the "stupid" business and proceeded to treat them with the same manner he used on all the others—though I wonder if there was any relation to the fact that these were the last patients to be completed before he left for the night.

During the early evening, adult patients were being brought in fairly steadily by the stewards, and many were labelled "transfer from Central Emergency." This got to be a nearly standard joke between the nurses and stewards, one of whom finally said, "When Dr. [X] came on duty, he really cleared 'em out!" The head nurse told me this was one of the constant fights. "They have just about as many beds up there as we do, but they keep shipping them all down here. I don't see why they can't take care of them just as well there," she said. (The thought apparently never occurred that these might be the patients Dr. [X] thought would have to be admitted.)

About 9:00 PM the pediatric interne had just been telling me how many parents come in to the ER rather than make the effort to come in earlier to the clinic, when two black women and one man came in with a child. Since he was standing up by the counter, the pediatric interne asked cheerily what was wrong with the baby, and the mother said something about his not having eaten because he had lumps on his tongue. The doctor asked how long this had been going on, and she said all day. At this point he started asking sarcastically why they hadn't come to the clinic, and the man answered rather tartly with some excuse. The doctor turned on him and started haranguing that this was an emergency service, and so on, and so on. The man rather sassily commented, "How would you like it if you hadn't been able to eat all day?" The doctor stiffened (I could only see his back but he was communicating anger as if he had taken a deep breath and held it.) With a funny grin the man ducked behind one of the women. In a controlled, deeper voice the doctor directed them to put the child in one of the cribs.

After finishing one more task, which left only the Mexican family and this new one in the ward, he decided to take the coffee break he had been demanding for the last hour or so. I trailed him in and kept the conversation going. He told me of various episodes he had had of parents assaulting him and that his standard response was to simply freeze and stare at them angrily. He then went on, "These California patients simply expect and demand too much in the way of medical services. They've gotten spoiled! Now I really like to practice medicine; I really do. I don't expect to be fawned over or anything, but I do think I could expect some thanks or at least a nice smile. But these people come in here *demanding* service. They say they're taxpayers and have a right to it. *I* say to them that if they pay taxes, they can afford to get private care. I come from Bellevue, and the patients never acted that way there!" I couldn't stand much more, so I asked, "Have you ever seen the patients at X [another medical center hospital]?

"I haven't worked there, but I've passively observed them."

"Well, are they better patients?"

"If you want to get into socioeconomic factors . . ."

"No, strictly on a behavioral basis."

"Well, yes, they are. That's more like it ought to be."

"Are they as good as at Bellevue?"

"Oh, I'd say maybe better—more like the private wing at Bellevue, the university wing."

I couldn't help grinning at this, since I have my own opinions on the comparative behavior of "demanding" and "docile" patients, but he didn't notice   **153** or ask about my expression—which was probably good, since I'm afraid I would have told him!

After we finished coffee, I returned to the treatment room area and found that a man had been brought in after having been slashed in some kind of fight. The surgery resident was inspecting the gaping wounds on his right chest and behind his right ear and said to the patient in a jocular tone, "Looks like you kind of lost *that* argument." The patient slowly and softly, but distinctly, said, "No, I haven't, yet." The MD did a little double take and laughed, saying, "Oh ho, no?" The man continued, "No, and the reason I haven't lost yet is because my mother always said . . . " The doctor broke in with another laugh and said, "That's all right, Tiger. We'll have you fixed up pretty soon now," and walked off about his business. Later on, the doctor was chatting with another doctor and the head nurse, when this patient came into sight being wheeled down the corridor by the friend who had brought him in. They stopped in front of the men's toilet room and the patient started to swing off the gurney. The doctors and nurse stared, amazed, and she tried to stop him. "Aw, gee," he said, "I gotta go, and I just can't go in one of those little jars." The surgical resident grinned and said, "Okay, Tiger, but let your friend go in with you so you don't get in any trouble." And the mission was accomplished without complications.

About 11:00 PM the night shift nurses began drifting in, and the evening nurse began writing in a little book the pertinent data on all the patients. I had not seen this used by the day shift and asked about it. The nurse told me that she always put down any elevated temps or blood pressures so there wouldn't be any chance that they could say she hadn't told them about it. The tone suggested that there was little love lost between the evening and night shifts. There had been a phone message that the night nurse would be late, and the evening nurse said, rather bitterly, "You'd think she could get organized enough by this time of night to at least get here on time." She had not yet arrived by 11:30 PM, at which time I found myself far too sleepy to stay a minute longer.

December 18, 1962, afternoon

I came on the ward to notice and be told repeatedly that things were very quiet, but that there had been all kinds of excitement this morning—a young woman had been run over by a truck; another poor woman who had had her defective gas heater on all night had been brought in comatose this morning. But now "nothing" was happening. After the initial friendly chitchat with the nurses and residents, I asked Dr. B., the surgical resident, if I could talk with him a few minutes, and he led me off to look for a quiet room. The coffee room had an LVN in it addressing her Christmas cards, so we went across the hall to the MD's sleeping-room and sat on the unmade bed to talk. I explained that I was a graduate student and that I was interested in his comments about the previous day and about the problems of telling families about a death. Dr. B. said, "In the ER it's traumatic, sudden, and inevitable, so it's not as hard as it is on the ward or after surgery. If a patient actually dies here, it's obvious that they were real sick. They're pretty much out of it, and as a doctor, it doesn't really bother me. I've found that the best way to deal with the families is to go in and tell them right out that so and so has died. I don't pull any punches; I don't say they've passed away or gone to Heaven, I just say they're dead. Then I just sit back and wait for the first stage of disbelief, and I give them 15 minutes to work it out however they will. I find the Latins will start screaming and moaning around, the blacks will get hysterical, the Chinese will just take it, and the Anglo-Saxons will take it with some quiet tears. Generally, you get just about those four reactions, though with some shading in-between.

"With the little boy, what had happened was already done before he got here; it was so serious, so irreversible once it had happened that there was just no other possibility. It was hard to have to go in and tell the parents that their fine 7-year-old son was dead. It was all right, though, because the father was a minister, and he was really held up by his faith, so they took it very well. And when it happens like that, at least the surgeon knows that everything possible that could be done was done. But when a patient dies up in the hospital, especially after surgery, it's because of the failure of your own technique or because what you selected to treat him with didn't do the job. It's especially bad with a patient who has had a lot of intensive physician care. I've seen internes get really attached to patients that way so that when they die, the interne just falls apart. Of course, sometimes it's hard not to, but by the time you've gotten as far as I have, you learn not to get attached. Actually, it's not such a problem on a surgery service—not so many patients die as on the medical service. This was a much bigger problem when I was a medical resident, where you have people who are sick for a longer period of time with much worse things.

"The types of patients we have here, though, are sometimes pretty hard to take. Like this morning, we had a pretty, young girl who'd been run over by a milk truck—that was pretty rough. That sort of thing kind of bothers me—I really feel their grief—of course, not as much as they feel it, but it gets to me. But I can't get very upset about the stabbings and gunshot cases. [I asked if he could weigh the separate factors in the cases—say, if the city bus had killed a 60-year-old?] Oh, that wouldn't be as bad as a kid. [Or if the woman had been drunk and run out in front of the truck?] Now that's one thing—I never make judgments—that's one thing I insist upon. I always teach that to the interne—we're not here to make judgments about people. Sometimes I can't feel too badly when some of these old bums die, and I can't get much of a reward from making some of them well. But that mustn't make any difference in what's being done or the way they're handled. Sometimes I heard medical students making real sneering comments—a gal comes in pregnant, and he asks, 'You married?' 'No,' she answers in a low voice. 'How many kids you got?' he asks. 'Four,' 'Four and not married?' he asks. That kind of guy I flunk right off, and I'll tell their professor just exactly why. Of course, we all have our own personal prejudices: I was raised in the South, went to school in the North, went to med school in the East, and now I've come West. But we're not in the business to make judgments against anybody—I don't know—do you have any

155

specific questions to keep me from getting off the track and rambling on?"

"Oh, this is fine," I said, "But how about the different kinds of families you have to deal with? What are the worst ones?" "Well, people like the boy's parents are the worst, because I really feel their grief—though not as keenly as they do. But you get these excitable kinds, like the Mexicans; they feel they have to scream and roll around, tearing their hair and clothes. They're the real problem. I find, though, that if I get the responsible relative, or two at the most, and take them off from the rest to tell them—that's a cardinal rule in dealing with them that I always teach my internes. And then I always take them off somewhere and don't tell them in front of a bunch of other people. Another cardinal rule I always observe is never to tell people over the phone that their relative has died; I just say they're very sick, and they'd better come in to see them. Otherwise they may crack up on the way in, or have a heart attack themselves on the other end—that's happened too many times!"

"What kinds of families are easier or harder to deal with?"

"Well, that just depends on individuals—some Latins are real bad and some are real good; some blacks are real rough and some are real good; I just hate to generalize about that. But the thing we have to realize is that many of these people have entirely differents sets of beliefs and morals than what we're used to. You'd really be amazed at some of the things they do without the least bit of concern. But the internes and medical students have to learn to keep their own feelings under control."

"You've spoken about teaching your internes. I've often wondered how it is that doctors learn about dealing with this. I know from being around nurses that they aren't taught to handle it personally, so they just avoid the whole thing."

"Well, it isn't actually taught anywhere. There are just several examples around, and the med student has to decide which one to select for imitation. But the nurses just don't have the responsibility the doctor does for this sort of thing. Here the nurses are more to serve, to follow the orders, give care and ministrations. [His word, I swear!] So, the burden just doesn't fall on them. They don't have to bear the onus of responsibility like the surgical resident does. I'm responsible for everything that goes on in the whole ward, even in pedi—if a kid goes home and dies there, I'm responsible, even if I never saw him. So I make a practice of checking every single patient. This makes it really rough," he said in an awed tone.

"How long are you stuck with this?"

"Three months, and it's a tough time. "

Shortly after we had talked, Dr. B. was called to the phone to talk with some doctor he had apparently left word to have call him. Later, I overheard an interne tell Dr. B. about a man with negative x-rays who still claimed his hip was too bad to walk on and who wanted to be admitted. Dr. B. asked a few pertinent questions, then grinned slyly and asked, "He wants a place to stay? He has hospitalitis? Well, I'll fix his wagon in short order!" He strode purposefully down the hall to the treatment room. I followed and listened as he most sympathetically questioned the man, examined his hip, and regretfully told him of the negative x-rays. I went off to ponder this shift in tone from a public hard cynicism to a private gentleness. But then I recalled that this was the man who the nurses had said at coffee was far too nice to be a surgeon; they had said that he was a real gentleman, and that although they kept expecting him to bite someday, he never did. A bit later, he came back into the station with a bottle of ethyl chloride, saying he had just cured the patient, and grinning wickedly, he started plaguing the nurses by spraying them with it. There was a whole flight of play over this, with girlish squeals and giggles, before he finally put it away and returned to business.

At some point in the afternoon, the booking orderly came back to the station and said to Miss Mac, "I see our little one from this morning didn't make it." Miss Mac said, "Who?" "Archer," he answered. "The gas inhalation one? She didn't?" she asked. "Nope—died at 1:10," he answered. Turning away with a distressed look on her face, she said, "Oh, oh—I'm sorry! I thought she would." The expression on her face seemed truly pained, but the subject was closed. I meant to ask for more details as to age, and so on, to try to establish the social loss factor but forgot it eventually. Later another nurse mentioned this to Miss Mac, and she said, "Yes, I heard. Pat told me." The tone was more matter of fact but still serious.

There was a slight stir of orderlies looking for two gurneys in the hall. Someone muttered, "Auto accidents, a pair." Looking out in the hall, I saw a blond, with her hair up in rollers, sitting in a wheelchair, writhing and moaning. At first I thought she was an OB patient in labor until I noted she was flat; then I noticed two dirty abrasions on her shins. She sat there moaning and crying, "Why doesn't someone do something right away?" I noted that I made a tart comment internally, and the immediate assumption was that anyone who could fuss that much couldn't be very badly hurt. I finally noticed a young man sitting near her with signs of similar injury, but he was making no comment at all. A bit later I went into the room where the surgeon was cleaning her legs, and an accident-investigation officer was interviewing her for her perception of the accident. He was asking if they were going fast at the time, and she replied in a heavy accent, "No, no, we were going slow—I had told him to go very slow because my hair was wet, and it made a terrible draft through the rollers." The surgeon grinned to himself and went on cleaning vigorously. She admitted that the assaulting car was not going fast, either. "If she had been, we would not have come out alive at all!" she said. But the driver was looking the other way and simply did not see them on their scooter. "I went all the way to Spain on a scooter, and such a thing did not happen there. It is these drivers here." At this point the surgeon had had enough and said, "Oh, yes, it's all America's fault. Perhaps you should go back to Greece, Lisa?" She replied crisply but without appropriate anger, "I just may!" At this point the policeman engaged me in conversation about what I was doing and left. I returned to the station.

The surgeon later came out giggling about Lisa. "She says she may go swimming with me in the Aegean if I ever come to Greece," he said. There was a bit of banter about this. He went on, "You know, I like her—she's 42, but she still thinks young. You gotta give her credit for that!"

157

Although I stayed on to 5:00 PM, I began to realize that there was little value left in staying. Having just written up the prior day's observations, I had come in prepared to view the staff as a bunch of ogres but had found, on arrival, that I had succumbed to their friendliness toward me and had begun to adopt their perspective, at least to the point that I found many more signs of tenderness, kindness, and concern toward patients than I had seen before.

I was seeing divisions among the staff a bit more clearly. At one point, the medical resident directed an evening orderly to take an urgent patient up to the wards rather than the chronic one he was wheeling. The orderly sulked and asked if there weren't someone else and went right on out. The resident said, "Oh yes," sighed, and went back to his writing. Apparently there was no point in making an authority issue out of it.

COMMENTARY

After 3 days of observing I feel I can make the following statements. The staff consisted of a tightly knit ingroup whose territory was this emergency-admitting area. The hierarchical ranking placed the residents on top, with the internes just below. Slightly below both were the nurses. Apparently equal, but perhaps a bit below, were the ambulance stewards and those police and sheriff's men who were regularly in attendance at Brent Emergency. Farther below but still in friendly contact with the nurses (though perhaps not with the MD's) were the LVN's, aides, and orderlies. (Concerning the aide position: a grimy little old man was brought in injured from the skid row area, and as she walked by him, the head nurse got a whiff of him. She turned casually to a bystanding orderly and said, "See if you can sponge him off a bit. Nobody will be able to get near him with a smell like that." I wondered what was her differential of "nobody," since it obviously did not mean the orderly.) Employees from other departments were recognized as privileged but not "in"; the janitor swept industriously but was unnoticed.

Far below them all, and perhaps even lower than in a general hospital, were the patients, with whom no contact at all was made. (The older nurses seemed to have arrived at a "friendly" tone for speaking to patients that they automatically and universally applied to all. The younger ones approached them as diagnoses. The MD's varied between using first names or nicknames and referring to them geographically. "Give Bicillin to the kiddie in bed 3," "No, the one in *that* bed." "What's the matter with the baby, Mama?" I did not observe aide-orderly interaction with patients.)

Family and friends represented a definite complication, especially when they were tipsy. (One evening episode of two drunken black friends who kept trying to wander back to check on their friend's progress occurred where the head nurse tried to tease them into behaving. "You have to kid them along because they can really get ugly if they get mad. And then you have to call the cops, and that always gets so messy. It's just easier to keep 'em happy and out of the way.")

The two predominant tones here were efficient business and sarcastic banter.

Geographically, I observed more of the latter in the area of the nurse's station than anywhere else. Even the coffee room conversations had a slightly different tone—more personal, friendly, serious. During my sojourns there, I noted only RN's and MD's in there, which may have made the difference.

I did overhear bantering conversations between nurses and LVN's out in the wards, but the general tone there was efficiency. This efficiency reached its peak in the treatment rooms, especially during moderate emergencies (the slashing, a hit-and-run case, and so on) and was maximal during the city bus–7-year-old boy episode, when I heard no banter anywhere.

I would hypothesize that these modes had been learned by succeeding generations of employees as the acceptable way of masking themselves from whatever emotional involvement they may have had. Because attention was prompt, I would imagine that the adult patients were directed into their particular wards too fast to become aware of the sharp break in modes of communication. This must have been more apparent to the parents of pediatric patients, however, since they were within sight and sound of the station. Because so much of the activity was open to view (even though curtains may have been drawn around the adults), the sense of business was communicated to all the patients. This may have led them to interpret delays as due to the general pressure rather than to any overt callousness on the part of the staff.

By the end of the third day, I realized with great clarity that in dealing with the patients, the staff members were making certain assumptions about them, and many of these assumptions were dead wrong. Immersed in the practice of municipal medicine, the staff members had become so familiar with the local procedures that they seemed to assume patients had this knowledge, also, as well as a familiarity with the general rules of hospital medicine. Thus, I found them impatient when questioned, "How long?" or "What is this for?" As best shown in the Mexican children episode, their only explanation for patients not following the rules was stupidity.

From experience, they had rapidly learned that their clientele was drawn from the lower class. The associated attributes they cited were dirtiness, stupidity, a certain canny slyness in getting things they didn't deserve, dishonesty, a certain callousness to obvious dangerous symptoms (a woman had come in 8½ months pregnant with her third child and had not been to an OB clinic since she saw no need; she had needed no care with the previous two), impertinence, a disinclination for following directions, and so on. These and other attributes may well have existed, though it is obvious that the staff members defined them by contrast with their own middle-class standards. Perhaps because it was easier, they also reacted to them as they would to such behavior in a middle-class person—a child and a not too bright one, at that. In attempting to accomplish their medical ends, the staff members would invoke a condescending tone of authority, backed with threats (the booking orderly wore a police badge, as did the ambulance stewards). They were not terribly optimistic that the patients would follow through, but they seemed **159** resigned to having done the best they could, all things considered. For those patients who seemed most in danger of harming themselves irremediably, hospital admission may have been seriously considered. Otherwise, they were discharged with the feeling that they would be back soon enough in worse shape still.

SUGGESTED QUESTIONS FOR DISCUSSION AND ANALYSIS

For undergraduate students

1. Put yourself in the place of one of the patients observed by Fleshman in the emergency room:

    The woman with the fussing baby and 7-year-old boy

    The man with the raw penis

    The parents of the 5 and 3-year-old Mexican children

    Lisa from Greece

    What do you think was the primary purpose of the emergency room? Physician or staff education? Rapid channeling of patients? Staff convenience? Or what?

2. What changes in the physical setup and functioning of the unit would you suggest if comprehensiveness and continuity of patient care were your major goal? Who would pay for the services described?

3. What is the nature of the nurse's work in the emergency room? How extensive are the hotel-type functions there?

4. What were some of the coping mechanisms used by doctors and nurses in this setting? Were they successful? By what criteria are you judging?

For graduate students and teachers of nursing

1. What are some of the necessary knowledges, skills, attitudes, and modes of working needed by individuals in the nurse role in the emergency room?

2. Is the ER nurse role as described here the desired work role for the nurse? Is it the role for which nurses are currently being prepared?

3. Is there any evidence that health care consumers are dissatisfied with the care received in emergency rooms?

4. If the consumer is not dissatisfied with his care, then the issue is one of preparing practitioners to fit the present role in the system. How is this currently being done?

5. If the consumer is dissatisfied with his care, then the system of care and the work roles of professional practitioners must change. What are your ideas for more viable changes? What corresponding curriculum changes would be needed?

6. In what kind of educational setting should nurse practitioners for the emergency room setting be prepared? On-the-job training? Technical nursing programs? Professional nurse programs?

7. What are the parameters of the work of the ER nurse? Is it routine or nonroutine work? Are the tasks to be done active or inert? Is the degree of resistance to the major tasks predictable or nonpredictable?

10. "Baby, baby, where did our love go?"

Karen Scholer, RN, BS

The following observations by a student nurse were part of a term paper written for a course in leadership theory and practice. Miss Scholer, a senior nursing student at the time, was having her clinical experience in the same emergency room ward in which the preceding observations by Fleshman had been made 8 years earlier.

It is suggested that the work of the nurse as described by Fleshman be compared with this student's perception of emergency ward care. Note in particular the structural and cultural restraints (or excuses) suggested by the student as reasons for the inadequate functioning of the health care system. Is the nurse, or in fact the entire health care system, impotent rather than autonomous in solving this problem?

Unskilled and unsophisticated as this student's observations may be, she calls them as she sees them. Many readers might say that the way in which this student sees the emergency ward is overdramatized, her observations overly influenced by her feelings, and that it isn't a true picture. This kind of protestation is reminiscent of the three umpires defending their integrity. One said, "I call 'em as I see 'em." The second replied, "I call 'em as they are." The third clinched the argument with, "What I call 'em makes 'em what they are."

"Brent Emergency is just a damn hotel to these drunks!" yelled one irate medical resident one recent evening while in the heat of the nightly Yellow-Bottle-Disposition-Problem argument. It might also be called the Brent Emergency Garbage Disposal Problem. At Brent is the strange conglomerate of (1) a patient population composed largely of "social undesirables" (ethnic minorities, drug addicts, alcoholics, homosexuals, prostitutes, juvenile delinquents, robbers, hippies, racial minorities, and just plain poor folks); (2) a well-educated, medically

161

competent, white middle and upper-class, crises-oriented medical staff (including a disproportionate number of attractive, vital, healthy, active young men and women); and (3) an institution that reflects and functions as the social conscience of the city of Greenbriar. In this role, the institution is satisfied that it has 'done its best' when it pours oxygen into a dying man. That he has first been degraded to the level of social junk is none of its affair. The social conscience hypocritically asserts at conventions and coffees the medical truisms of the day, such as "Alcoholism is a disease," and "Health care is a right," while the Brent ER maintains soup-line medical care. These elements—the patient population, the personnel, and the institution as a social conscience—confront each other nightly in the Battle of the Bottles. War strategy is as follows:

Battle of the Bottles

Combatants: *The Bottles*—representing all that is evil and decadent in human society. Also known as junk, garbage, persons of low social value; persons who look for in bottles, what they cannot find in society or in themselves.

The Reluctant Garbagemen—formerly trained as practitioners of medicine, now degraded to this loathesome station in which they have neither skill nor interest.

The Soup Line—otherwise known as Brent Emergency Hospital, serving its own particular variety of thin soup—much of it through impersonal, vitamin-filled IV bottles—a Christian mission, truly.

THE BOTTLES

There are multitudinous theories of causation proposed for humans in our society who do not adopt the mainstream style of life, norms, and values. The explanations may be as diverse as the individuals involved. Labels are many—deviant, social misfit, hippie, bum—but solutions for giving the disaffiliated a stake in society are few and costly. The problem is chronic; it strikes at the very ideology of our society and, many say, is insoluble. Alcoholics are only the highly visible representatives of this group. Standard treatment (if they are treated) for alcoholics at Brent Emergency is to start an IV infusion of vitamins. The bright yellow bottles encompass diagnosis, history, and treatment in one symbolic color. Only slightly less visible are the heroin addict's needle tracks and abscesses or the attempted suicide's multiple thin white scars along the forearm. The black person is highly visible; the Chicano's lack of English is a little less so. The poor are Bottles also, for as Jules Henry asserts, "In our culture, personality exists to the extent of ability to pay, and in terms of performance of the culturally necessary tasks of production, reproduction, and consumption."

The Bottles say, "I have nowhere else to go—I need help. A hospital is supposed to help people." They are also saying, "Society has rejected me—I have rejected myself."

THE RELUCTANT GARBAGEMEN

"You start hating the patients, and then you hate yourself for hating them." So said one of the medical residents at Brent Emergency. "I know working here has changed me, and I don't like the person I've become. I should have left a long time ago," a young, attractive nurse reflected on her callousness toward the patients.

Henry's Law of Distortion and Withdrawal states, "The tendency of sound people to withdraw from distorted ones is determined by the extent and nature of the distortion, by the degree of degradation of the sound individuals and their fear of distorted people, and by the distorted person's own resources, e.g. human warmth, property, etc."*

The Bottles are truly distorted people. Old, infirm, dirty, powerless, sick, and uneducated, they form quite a contrast to the predominantly well-educated, young, vital, healthy, attractive, powerful doctors and nurses who are charged with caring for them. Furthermore, the staff has been trained (and especially the emergency room staff) for and is psychologically in tune with acute, life-threatening medical emergencies. This is where the staff is rewarded, in the last-minute, last-ditch effort against death itself. The living dead, the Bottles, present the staff with chronic psycho-social problems of unfathomable and untreatable magnitude. The Brent Emergency staff ends up with the disagreeable, unrewarding job of tidying up the human junk long ago rejected by society. A garbage metamorphosis occurs, whereby the patients are transformed into garbage by many of the staff. "Wear gloves and you won't get your hands dirty." "Avoid personal involvement and maybe you won't be sucked into the human mire."

Not all staff members are able to make the garbage metamorphosis, however. "Unless a person feels degraded himself, he will not be able to degrade others," states Henry. Some staff members side with the powerless Bottle, others with the powerful Soup Line. Thus the lines are drawn each night, and positions are taken when the question arises: "Do we admit the Bottle or do we discharge him?"

THE SOUP LINE

Overriding the human drama played out in Brent Emergency wards is the medical Soup Line of the city of Greensbriar. This Soup Line, established as the social conscience of an affluent society, is content in providing the "essentials" of life—food, housing, medical care—for its indigent without concern for their psyche or quality of life.

The absence of death is not necessarily life. One is reminded that the Society for the Prevention of Cruelty to Animals was founded before the Society for the Prevention of Cruelty to Children. The staff at Brent Emergency is in the position of doling out the thin soup society has allocated to the poor; it is just enough to maintain an infirm existence. Thousands of dollars are spent by the city for esophageal repairs and then the "cured" patient is sent back to his poor housing (or no housing) and inadequate diet. The staff members are agents of the hypocrisy and

*Henry, Jules: *Culture against Man,* New York, Vintage Books, 1965, pp. 391-474.

purposelessness of the social conscience. The Christian spirit of love thinly veils the old-time hellfire and damnation for those who have sinned. An alcoholic can be admitted to Brent Emergency for the night at a cost of $144 to the city or sent back to sleep it off under a bridge or on the sidewalk from whence he came. These are the choices the staff can make.

DISCUSSION

From the brief sketches of the combatants involved in the Battle of the Bottles, let us now examine the "healthy organization" as outlined by James Clark.* The healthy organization, he states, incorporates the optimal resolution of tendencies toward equilibrium and capacities for growth. Growth is defined as a behavioral system that involves greater complexity of relations with its environment, an "open-ended" proactive system. Equilibrium is based on the pleasure principle that the main principle of life is to reduce tension. It is a homeostatic, defensive, "closed" reacting system. The need for proactive and reactive behavior occurs at all levels of organization.

It is striking to observe at Brent, among the pathetic and tragic patients and the filthy and disorganized physical facility, the great deal of socializing, pleasure-seeking, reactive behavior among the staff. One senses a polarization of groups, the "us" and "them" of staff and patients, with the staff group increasing its internal solidarity by increasing its external combativeness to the antithetical group—the patients. The proactive behavioral contrast would be a breakdown of group barriers and an establishment of give-and-take relations between the two groups. The discussion on distortion and withdrawal points out why this proactive behavior would not be likely to occur.

Proactive behavior appears to thrive more in an atmosphere of freedom and free communication. At Brent Emergency, authority positions (such as RN's and MD's) are rewarded with status and money, whereas true leadership based on proficiency and knowledge (many LVN's and orderlies) is not officially sanctioned or rewarded. Thus Joe, an orderly with a vast knowledge in orthopedics, is often consulted by the MD's on diagnosis. Joe, with a working knowledge of the social system of Brent Emergency, tried instituting changes in the system with the head nurse and the director of nursing. The director of nursing, the final authority, has not the slightest idea of the needs of the facility, yet she rejected Joe's proposals on sight.

Brent Emergency cannot grow, cannot increase transactions with its environment because of the social conscience ethic. It cannot grow in and of itself because of the authority ethic. The staff members cannot grow, because they are not doing what they were trained for and desire to do; and they are hostile to the patient group, where they could grow. The patients cannot grow, because their needs are not being met.

• • •

*Clark, James: "A Healthy Organization." In Bennis, Warren (Ed.): *The Planning of Change*, ed. 2, New York, Holt, Rinehart and Winston, Inc., 1969, pp. 282-297.

"I think we should admit him. He's sick."

"He's a bum. I don't want to waste my taxpayers' money on a bum."

"If he's in DT's or near death, the hospital says we can admit him to the Detox ward. Let's wait until the next time he comes in—he may be sicker."

And, from behind a yellow bottle, a slurred voice . . . "It's a disease."

SUGGESTED QUESTIONS FOR DISCUSSION AND ANALYSIS

For undergraduate students

1. Identify the attitudes and values of the health care personnel in the emergency room as described by Fleshman and Scholer.
2. In what ways are they different? In what ways are they the same?
3. Were there any changes or movements in society during the years 1962 to 1970 that might account for these changes in values and attitudes?

For graduate students and teachers of nursing

1. Discuss the statement: "Equilibrium is based on the pleasure principle that the main principle of life is to reduce tension." Do you agree? How does this apply to Scholer's perception of emergency room activity?
2. From your own experiences, have you observed some parallels to the Battle of the Bottles?
3. Could one nurse be instrumental in instituting a proactive behavior change in this emergency room setting? Describe possible ways in which this might be done.
4. If you were Miss Scholer's instructor, or if you were a staff nurse in Brent Emergency and Miss Scholer came and discussed her observations and conclusions with you, what would you do? What would you say? How would you advise her? What would your rationale be for each of your activities?

11. Process and persistence of value transmission

Patricia Benner, RN, MS

Who are the socializing agents for student nurses? The instructors? The nurses in the work setting? Both? Or neither? The reader can be his own judge of who is the dominant and most persistent socializing agent, and what the possible effects are of being influenced by one socializing agent more than another. The observations detailed here are of a series of conversations and conferences. The setting is the same Brent Emergency Room described in the two previous chapters of this section. The time is May 1971. The actors are Susan Schmidt and Martha Hopkins, both senior nursing students in a baccalaureate program; Ann, the evening charge nurse in the emergency room; and Pat, the nursing instructor.

This description was written by the faculty member who was responsible for the clinical nursing course in which both Susan and Martha were enrolled. She recorded it concurrently as the events were unfolding. In this description, the instructor attempted to view and describe both her own actions and reactions, as well as those of the students. The instructor's thoughts and reflections are inserted throughout and enclosed in brackets.

The senior year in this baccalaureate nursing program is called "the real world of work." Susan and Martha decided to make their senior leadership experience as "real" as possible and chose to work the 3 to 11 PM shift in the emergency room of a large general hospital. Besides their motivation to "learn how to nurse in emergency situations," their decision was also prompted by their interest in health care in poverty areas.

To get this clinical assignment, the students had to negotiate a special contract both with the school and with the hospital. Their clinical assignment was finalized when I agreed to be their clinical instructor. Two things prompted my interest: I was an experienced emergency room nurse and liked this type of nursing, and I was interested in observing and assisting students through the "reality shock" anticipated by such a challenging environment.*

Even while this experience was happening, I was aware of being both an observer and an actor. It turned out to be a clear confrontation of differing value systems and made me look at my own values, as well as those of the charge nurse and students.

My goal in this teaching-learning interaction was to assist Martha and Susan in assessing the role values of the emergency room staff and to put into operation their own role values in their everyday work. At times my friendship for Martha and Susan and my concern for Martha's survival both in school and in the ward setting overshadowed my preplanned goals and caused me to abandon them.

Martha called me after work one day (at 11:00 PM!) and gave the following description of what had happened Tuesday evening in the emergency room. (Martha was quite upset.)

Martha: Ann, the evening charge nurse, found an empty chart while making her rounds and said, "Hasn't anyone done anything for this patient since 3:00 PM? Martha, you do this all the time ... where are the vital signs? Ann's voice was getting louder, and I knew that I was in for it. So I asked her if she would like to talk to me in the side room. All activity in the male ward (a large, open, 12-bed ward) had come to a screeching halt, and all eyes were on me. I was in charge of the ward, and Jim, an orderly, Sue, an LVN, and Bob, a former medical corpsman, were also assigned to the ward and were present for the accusation. Jim, who had not taken vital signs all evening, began to take blood pressures. I managed to get Ann out of the ward. In the doctor's room, Ann said to me, "You'll never make an emergency room nurse! You talk to patients too much. If you want to talk to patients, you should become a psych nurse. Emergency room nursing is just not for you." [Martha's voice broke as she was telling me this and I remembered a similar devastating experience that happened to me as a student nurse. I wonder if such an experience is a necessary ingredient of nursing school.]

After sympathizing with Martha and listening to some other feelings, I shared my similar experience with her. I thought it might help her put Ann's comments into perspective; being called a "failure" by a head nurse does not ipso facto make it so.

Pat: When I was a student, I had been told that I would never make it, because I became "too involved with patients." [A head nurse had found me with tears in my eyes at the death of a patient.] Being told that you will "never make it" may be one of the initiation rites all students and young nurses have to go through. What happened after this total castigation of you?

Martha: Well, I tried to think fast. What was the reason for the empty chart? What had been my priorities for the evening? But I never defend myself very well

*See Kramer, Marlene: *Reality Shock: Why Nurses Leave Nursing*, St. Louis, The C. V. Mosby Co., 1974.

under pressure. It was an hour later before I remembered that the patient with the empty chart had been up in x-ray since 3:00 PM.

Pat: That's understandable. [I was thinking how involved and turned on to learning Martha had been in the ER. She had studied harder than she had at any time since starting nursing school. She considered this her best experience so far; the others had not been too pleasant. She is very individualistic and favors a hip life style, which had caused resistance from the faculty and staff alike throughout school. Her file was filled with such complaints as: "Martha continues to refuse to wear her name pin, though she had been repeatedly reminded." Her history, I thought, made this castigation even more devastating. I also felt disappointed because I had been so pleased with Martha's growth and interest in her clinical experience. I wanted her last clinical experience to be a good one for her. Besides, I really like Martha, and I didn't like the idea of her being attacked for what I consider to be a positive quality.]

Martha: I told Ann that I thought I had been doing a good job. That's what made this hurt so much. I haven't been goofing off; I think I have really been doing well. For example, I told her that tonight I had run a urine sugar on one of the incoherent patients and had had the doctor follow it up with a blood sugar. And it was a good thing we checked, because his blood sugar was really high. I also got Lactated Ringers started on a patient who came in with a pulse pressure of about 10. He was really hypovolemic, and I checked with the doctor and got the Lactated Ringers started. But Ann wasn't impressed. She was really mad. She said, "Hell, any nurse should know enough to get help for a low blood pressure!" [I think it would have been impossible for Martha to do anything clinically that Ann would have considered impressive. Ann had worked at Brent Emergency for 3 years and was very proficient technically. I thought that what Martha said would impress an instructor, but Ann is not an instructor. I wondered if Martha's defenses only spurred Ann's anger.]

Martha: I asked Ann to tell me why she thinks that I will never make it in the emergency room. She was very impatient and said, "It's not just one thing, it's many things; this has been building up for a long time." Then I asked her to give me some examples, which she did: "Well, for example, Martha, tonight you didn't take the 8 o'clock vital signs on two patients. You spent half the evening in the hall talking to patients. You can't be all over the place—in the lab, in the hall talking to patients, and running around trying to figure out what the doctors are doing all the time."

Martha: Then I asked her if we could have a joint conference with you and stated that I did not want to continue to work without settling or figuring out why my opinion and her opinion of my performance differed so greatly.

Pat: [I interrupted Martha at this point.] Martha, I wish that you hadn't come on so strong. It's more of a problem for you than it is for Ann if you don't finish your senior experience. [I was struck with the possible outcome of Martha getting an incomplete if she could not find another clinical placement: I had lost all objectivity. What a typical "instructorish" thing to say—"Don't come on strong. I wish you'd look at this and this."] What did Ann say?

Martha: She did not see any need to have the joint conference. She did not think it was necessary and said she did not have time for such a conference. [I was relieved. At least, Ann apparently was not going to raise a big formal complaint against Martha.] When I explained that it [the conference] was important for my clinical grade, Ann conceded. I think she's sadistic and wanted to see that I would not get a good grade.

Our phone conversation lasted quite a while and took the form of mutual reassurance. Martha agreed that she had been rash in her threat to stop working until the differences were settled. She also stated that she wanted to finish her clinical experience at Brent and graduate on time. She had not realized that she had jeopardized her time of graduation. I reassured her that I was pleased with my observation of her clinical performance and that she had done the right thing by insisting on the conference and validation of the accusations. Ann's response to my phone request for a joint conference was much like Martha had forecasted. (This I *know* about Martha, from repeated validation: she is painfully honest! She will never try to make things sound better or different from the way she perceives them. This is one of the qualities in Martha that I find most attractive.)

SELLING THE CONFERENCE TO ANN

Ann: I don't see any need for a conference. It's been building up for a long time, and I just blew off, and that was the end of it. I don't hold grudges. If something is on my chest, I just get it off, and that is the end of it. I told Martha exactly what I thought, and that was the end of it. [I was thinking that if Ann was that angry and just "blew off," that she probably was not even aware of half of the things that made her so angry. I was hoping that she could be more explicit and later on define or at least describe some of the behaviors that were making her so angry.]

Pat: Ann, I think there must be some things that Martha is not picking up on, some things that you would like for her to be doing that she is missing. I think that Martha really wants to do a good job, but she doesn't understand what she is doing wrong. [I was uncomfortable, because I didn't want to sound as if I were taking sides with Martha, and since I actually felt personally involved with Martha—I wanted her to graduate on time—I wanted this to be a positive experience for her. I realized that I was not really being objective. My only choice was to play the role of a negotiator and try to give Ann's side as fair and as clear a hearing as possible.]

Ann: Pat, it's *obvious*—I've told her a thousand times. [Surely she just thought that she had told her a thousand times, or else her messages were indirect and Martha did not understand them. I thought the second, alternative explanation was more probable.] She knows what she should be doing. She just doesn't want to do it. She's too interested in talking to the patients, and in seeing what's going on. She doesn't stay in the room where she is assigned. [Ann's voice sounded exasperated.] I just don't think a conference is going to do any good. [Ann's absolute sureness that "it's obvious" made me think that she had probably tried to give role messages to Martha but that they been so indirect, Martha had missed them.]

Pat: Ann, it may be obvious to you, and it may be obvious to me, but it is not obvious to a beginner. This is one of the things that I have become so aware of since I've been teaching. All the things that an experienced nurse takes for granted aren't apparent and don't even occur to a beginner. Martha was very upset the other evening, and I'm not sure that she even heard what you were trying to tell her. I would like a chance to sit down with you and Martha and see if we can put things in language that Martha can hear.

169

Ann still seemed unconvinced but agreed to a 30-minute conference on Monday night, provided that the place "was not jumping" and that she had time.

Monday was too busy. (I wondered if Ann were avoiding the conference, and whether or not it would ever take place.) Ann was curt and reluctant to schedule a conference on Tuesday, but I told her that I would come over any time that was convenient for her. I told her it would be more difficult for me to come during the dinner hour, but she said, "Well, that's the only time I can do it, right after my dinner." I agreed to a 6:30 PM conference. (Now I was convinced that she was avoiding the conference. I didn't really understand why.)

In our regular clinical conference on Tuesday, Susan, Martha, and I went over the purpose of the meeting with Ann. Our goal was to find out what Martha was doing or not doing that was so irritating to Ann. Also, we wanted to get some information about Ann's image of the ideal emergency room nurse. We hoped to come up with some questions that Ann would be able to answer and that would give Martha more of Ann's perspective of the nurse's role. Much of this clinical conference was spent in developing "answerable questions." I then gave my interpretation of the events so far. (I wanted to show that I had gained some objectivity during the time lapse, and I wanted to clarify that I thought Ann might have some important things to say. I was still in the role of the negotiator.)

Pat: Let me clarify my view of what might be happening. I am assuming that you have not heard or sensed some of the role messages that Ann has been sending to you, Martha. I think that there must be some omissions and infractions on your part that you are not aware of. Maybe you have crossed some "taboos." [We had just discussed an article on culture shock a couple of weeks earlier.] Perhaps there are subtle things other than "talking to patients too much" and "missing some vital signs." I don't think Ann has these infractions defined. Perhaps it's your demeanor. If we get enough information from her, then we might be able to make some inferences about what you are doing that is "bugging her."

Throughout the conference both Susan and I tried to be supportive to Martha. Susan pointed out many things that Martha had become proficient in. She also expressed anger that Martha was being singled out. Martha vacillated between anger and self-doubt. (Even though we were Martha's friends, there were times in which I wondered if Martha felt that she was on trial. If so, our reassurances might have only been added evidence that we were sitting in judgment of her.) Martha wanted Susan to sit in on the conference, and we all agreed that another person might help clarify what was going on.

THE CONFERENCE

Ann was late. The conference was held in a small women's lounge across from and outside the emergency room. Ann reiterated that she didn't have more than 30 minutes. (I still didn't know why this conference was so distasteful to her. Did she feel insecure, as if she were on trial?) I started the conference.

Pat: Ann, it occurs to me that the students and I may not know what the characteristics of a successful nurse in the emergency room at Brent are. Could you describe them to us or tell us about a new staff nurse who has been very successful in the emergency room? Someone who never had any emergency room experience but who was able to learn the job without too much difficulty?

Ann: No, I can't. We've never had a new nurse without any emergency room experience. [She was curt. I wondered if she felt defensive. My rehearsed question might have threatened her. Or it could have been that she thought the question was irrelevant. I thought it was possible that she hadn't known any inexperienced nurses, but I wondered if she could have been so positive without giving herself a minute to think about it. At any rate she discarded my question.]

Susan recovered the conference by asking, "Can you tell us four or five of the important things for a nurse to do on the evening shift?" (Martha was sitting quietly, smoking [she does not usually smoke]; her hands were trembling, and I inferred from this that she was very nervous. I wished I could make it easier for her. I was glad that Susan was here to take some of the pressure and focus off of Martha. Also, it was a good learning experience for Susan.) Susan's question was better received. Ann sat back and raised her hands in front of her before she began to speak.

Ann: Okay. [She counted off one finger with her right hand as if to number the first task as number one.] Staying in the room where you are assigned. Its very important for you to stay where you belong; people depend on you to be there. Two, [she counted off a second finger] to stock supplies at the beginning and end of the shift. Nothing makes you any madder than to look for something when you need it and not be able to find it. If there's an emergency, we have to have the supplies. Another very important thing: Don't butt in during a trauma in the trauma room. [The trauma room is a room set aside for major traumas; it is set up for all major emergencies at all times. Ann was being very selective. Her comments seemed very pointed. Martha or Susan or both had violated these unwritten rules at one time or another according to their reports to me and my observations. I wonder though, if Ann would make these same points if someone else asked the same questions as a newcomer. Then maybe she wouldn't answer them with the same emphasis.] When there is a major trauma going on, that one nurse assigned in there is all you need. With all the doctors in there, there are so many bodies that if a bunch of nurses go in there, things get very confused. If you have two nurses in there you end up drawing the same medication at the same time and that's so maddening. So ask if they need any help, and if they don't, leave them alone.

Martha: When I ask, 99% of the time the answer is "no."

Ann: That's because one is enough and it's just too confusing if you have more. [The animation in Ann's voice and gestures had picked up. If she had felt defensive before, I didn't think she did now.] And another thing, if you do go in to watch in the trauma room, don't watch what the doctor is doing. Don't be over looking into the chest cavity, watch what the *nurse* is doing. If you are going to be a nurse, then watch what the *nurse* is doing. She has already got all the equipment set up and everything ready. Most of the time she is busy filling out all the papers. Filling out the papers may seem like a petty thing to be doing, but when you take that patient up to surgery, if those papers aren't there, everything stops. So if you want to be a nurse, watch what the *nurse* is doing. [Ann stressed the important words by saying

171

them louder. I didn't blame Martha and Susan if they had been less than excited about watching someone fill out papers, important though they may be.]

Okay, another thing [Ann had moved to another point and another finger.] Taking vital signs. The patients in the ward have to have their vital signs taken two times in the evening, every 4 hours, whether they need it or not. Granted, we do have some boarders in there, but vital signs have to be taken. [I wanted Ann to give her rationale, but she didn't. I wanted to give her directions some sanction and support; so I said:]

Pat: Routine vital signs are especially important in ER, where you don't have much of a base line or a history to predict potential changes. [Ann acknowledged my comment by cocking her head to one side, and then she continued her listing. Her point really seemed to be: Vital signs have to be taken; a lot of times, they are unnecessary, but they have to be taken. It occurred to me that Ann doesn't share my compunction for stating my rationale for doing something.]

Ann: Then if you have any extra time [her hand gestures indicated that she was on the last item—she'd used her last finger, and her voice inflection gave the feeling "and last of all"], clean up the room, because everything always needs cleaning up around here. [A rationale for cleaning? I wondered why, maybe there had been some resistance to cleaning?]

At this point Ann looked at her watch and stated that she had to leave. We thanked her, and she nodded and said, "Okay," and left. After Ann left, the air in the room was heavy. Both Susan and Martha were sullen and looked depressed. I was pleased with Ann's exposition of her priorities, but I felt sorry for Susan and Martha and did not know how to convey to them the value of their new knowledge of Ann's priorities. They were in the throes of "reality shock." I broke the silence by giving them an example of the pressure and rejection I had once received because I did not know or act upon the unwritten "code," that patients should be in bed by 9:30 PM—as soon as a new graduate explicity told me this "code," I acted on it and became a well-accepted member of the group. Martha perked up a bit.

Martha: That is exactly what we are talking about. The things that are so important to the staff that we don't even think of. [I was relieved that Martha made the connection; I was sorry that I could not think of a more recent example, but the old one was the only one that came to mind.]

Pat: Yes, but figuring out what is important to this system doesn't mean that you have to give up your values. It just gives you a chance to look at the differences more objectively. [I was hoping that this conference could be used by both Martha and Susan as an example of the kinds of resistances that they would continue to meet, a reality inoculation. But I was worried that Martha's "inoculation" had come too late and in too strong a dose.]

Susan: [She looked thoughtful.] You know, Ann's priorities make sense in terms of moving patients through here, and it is very important to move patients through, so that you don't clog up the system. If the hall gets very full, then there are a large group of unknowns. [Perfect! Susan was beginning to see Ann's perspective!]

172   Pat: Right! Ann has reduced her concerns to the lowest common denominator.

She is worried about five main responsibilities. [We reviewed the duties she had enumerated.] She has excluded all extraneous things, such as talking to patients. She has delegated that task to the psych unit. [I made the last comment tongue-in-cheek style, since this attitude of not talking to patients is so foreign to my philosophy, the school's philosophy, and to Susan and Martha's values. Also, I wanted to show that I did not agree with Ann's perspective completely even though I could understand it.]

Martha: And when they are through with their priorities, they play pinochle. [Martha sounded disgusted; I think that she still had trouble even hearing Ann's values. She couldn't remember several of Ann's points; this could have been due to anxiety or she may have been so thoroughly in disagreement with Ann that she tuned her out.]

Susan: But Ann says that people work so hard when it's busy that they deserve some diversion when it's not busy. [I was pleased that Susan could state Ann's position, and consider it. I still didn't think that Martha could.]

Pat: Ann, too, has a right to be the way she is, right Martha? [I prodded Martha a bit, but I hoped my tone of voice conveyed a shared understanding with her. Martha had previously talked with me about the hassle she has had in school, because nurses tried to fit her into the same mold as everyone else.]

Martha: [She looked surprised.] Right, I haven't been giving Ann very much room to be who she is. [We all laughed a bit at the awkward "other shoe."]

Pat: A simplified, focused framework, is important for a crisis situation. It is impossible to be effective and maintain a very complex framework that takes in every stimulus during an emergency situation. The problem comes because it is difficult then, to switch from that simple framework to a more complex framework when there is time for it.

Susan: Yes, it's easier to just play pinochle and forget about the people when there is time.

By this time we all felt uncomfortable, because Susan and Martha were expected to be "on duty." The conference ended without final resolution. But it was talked about occasionally for the rest of the quarter. Martha showed marked improvement by just managing to stay in the system without causing any more major confrontations. She was careful to noticeably stock the cabinets at the beginning and end of the shift and to follow the other suggestions Ann had given. She did continue to talk to patients, and Ann eventually conceded that maybe she was wrong, that her advice "not to talk so much to patients" may be irrelevant at some times. However, at the end of Martha's clinical experience, Ann still voiced, in her words, that she was not impressed with Martha.

SIX MONTHS AFTER THE CONFERENCE

Martha and Susan have graduated, passed their state boards, and are now working. Martha is working in a small emergency room part time and going to school full time. She is taking arts and science courses and is unsure of her future. She is uncertain whether she will continue in nursing. Susan is working with a community health project.

I asked them to reflect on their experience and on the conference 6 months later.

Martha's impressions

Martha: We didn't ever fit into Ann's value system. She made a lot bigger impression on my life than I did on hers. However, as soon as I started fighting her—challenging her by making her define and validate what I had done wrong, our relationship improved. Actually that was a mobile unit for everyone except the RN.

Pat: Mobile?

Martha: Yes, everyone could advance and increase their domain except the RN's. RN's couldn't do anything that they weren't already doing, but the orderlies, the aides or the LVN's could learn to do new things and progress in their knowledge, even though they had tight job descriptions. In a pinch, or if they were interested, they could always learn to do something new and gain permission to do it. But everyone really got up tight if the nurse wanted to increase her sphere of activity, like do a blood count or check a blood sugar or talk at length with a patient. That's what got to me the most, I think. Just when I was the most excited about learning, about diagnostic concepts in the emergency room, Ann would really put a wet blanket on my learning. If I would ask about what was happening to a patient or why they were doing something or make a suggestion, she would always mention taking a blood pressure, or charting it, or passing a bedpan. Sure, that's important, but it was easy, and I could handle that without the constant reminders. She destroyed my image and took away all the exciting parts. She made me feel like a blood pressure machine or a bedpan passer.

Another thing I did that irritated Ann was that I never knew what level or state the papers were in. I didn't care about the papers, and this irritated Ann. I didn't think it was important to my learning goals to learn about the paper work.

That was another thing that irritated Ann. She didn't think I should have learning goals. I wanted to learn all about everything. The whole idea about treatment—not just 20 cc of glucose in a syringe handed to a doctor, but "Why glucose? Why not Sodium Lactate?" Ann would say, "Just do it, it's easy." But I was so interested in why. Every chance I would get, I would be sitting in a corner, reading. The difference between where she thought I should be and where I thought I should be was so great. She didn't think it was my place to plan my own learning experiences. The ultimate put-down was that I should not be talking to patients so much. I don't think that my *talking* to them bothered her nearly so much as my *liking* them. I enjoyed learning about their lives. Her philosophy was, "You are not the same person at work as you are when you are not working. You don't treat people the same." For example, if you sit down to have a cup of coffee after work with someone, then you act differently. You can be your "off work" self then. That approach doesn't make any sense to me, but a lot of people think like that, I guess.

Alice, another RN, was always irritated with me, too. I would try to understand her point of view, but finally she said to me, "Don't care so much about what people think. Don't take criticism so seriously. You always look as if you really take things to heart." Alice was often assigned to the trauma room. You could really tell which people were rewarded by the room assignments they were given. The top prize was the trauma room, then the male ward, then the pediatric and ingestion rooms, and last on the totem pole was the female ward. No one liked to take care of the women.

Pat: Did you work in the female unit very much? [I asked this thinking that it perhaps would have increased her popularity if she had chosen the least desirable unit often.]

Martha: No, because Susan really liked working in there. You know, Alice and Ann were always talking about how things had changed. They told their student stories with such relish, even though they were complaining. They would talk about how awful it was to wear the horrible outfits—crinolines and starch—but they said it as if it were a wonderful recollection! They would talk about delivering a baby at 2:30 AM or being on a huge ward all by themselves. They thought the 3-year diploma program was the only way to go. [Apparently, this had made a lasting impression. I had only asked about her reflections on the conference.]

Susan's evaluation

Susan: Ann didn't help us at all. Her message to us from the beginning was, "Just stay out of my hair." My response was to reflect her avoidance. I avoided her, too. But Martha tried to get in, to be accepted. I think that they just kept telling her by their actions in many strong ways, "Haven't you got the message yet! Stay out!"

Ann mainly denied that there were any staff difficulties, even though they had to have the large staff conference for the other shifts to complain how impossible it was to work with the evening shift. The other two shifts had been writing all their complaints on pieces of paper for weeks. I remember asking the head nurse what was on the pieces of paper, and she said that they were of "no concern to me"! I think we were banned, much like "company." We were considered "company," and they were having a "family" dispute that was not fit for company to see.

Ann avoided seeing or dealing with the human element at all—staff or patients. She ignored the whole thing. She liked to think that everyone was a team, but she really didn't deal with the situation.

By the end of the 6 months, a lot of people had changed. June and Irene were new RN's. June was a baccalaureate grad and decided to stay out of the "inner circle."

Pat: By inner circle, you mean Ann and Alice?

Susan: Yes. But June rotated shifts. She was really nice to us. But Irene decided to join the inner circle. She treated us like students, and she resented us knowing more than she did. "After all, we were just students." But we had been there longer, and we did know some things that she didn't.

I think that Ann compared us to the 3-year girls. The 3-year girls always had caps and name pins and white stockings. They fit the formal, old-guard nursing image—they were behaving "professionally." She always thought that they were better in their techniques. But June and others said that we were actually better. I think Ann resented that we could wear pants suits and have so much fun. She and Alice were always telling horror stories about their nursing school experience—delivering three babies at the same time, and so on. They reveled in these stories. I think that our easier time and all our fun cheapened their RN image, and they didn't like that.

The emergency room has made a lasting impression on both Martha and Susan, with its stories about the old, more difficult days, value conflicts and differences, and its strong message: "You'll never make an ER nurse; you talk to patients too much." I wonder if Martha will stay in nursing. I wish she would have had an earlier realistic warning, such as "talking with patients" is still not acceptable behavior in some hospitals. In fact, that's one of the challenges.

SUGGESTED QUESTIONS FOR DISCUSSION AND ANALYSIS

For undergraduate students

1. Describe the value system of Martha; of Ann; of Pat.
2. How was each trying to get her viewpoint across to the other person?
3. What do you think of the way Martha handled the initial accusation by Ann? Would you have done it differently? What do you think the consequences would have been?
4. What kinds of things might an instructor have said or done to help you if you had been in a situation like this?

For graduate students and teachers of nursing

1. How would you have handled this situation if you had been the instructor?
2. Within 6 months of graduation, Martha is seriously considering leaving nursing. Will this be a loss to the profession? What do you think could have been done to salvage Martha?
3. In terms of the dominant values and cultures of most nursing schools and nurse-employing organizations, Martha would be described as a deviant. What theoretical formulations would be helpful and would provide some cues on how to constructively handle deviant behavior?
4. Increasingly, nursing students are objecting to being placed in a mold, or being molded to fit a particular image. What does this mean? Education is a socializing process. How can one be socialized without being placed into some preconceived mold? Does socialization always mean "fitting a mold"?

section E

Nursing faculty and the impact of organizational setting

The nature of the nurse's work changes not only in respect to who the client is—patients in the case of the nurse practitioner, or students as in the case of the nurse faculty member—but also in respect to the primary and secondary settings in which the work is performed. For the nurse faculty; the school is the primary setting; the clinical setting or hospital is secondary. The following observations by Glass while she was a doctoral student provide the opportunity to analyze the various constraints placed upon the nurse faculty because of these differences in clients and primacy of setting.

177

12. A guest in the house

Helen Glass, RN, EdD

A particular concern of professional schools of nursing in universities is the preparation of practitioners, individuals who can move rapidly into work-oriented situations to render their essential services. Education to do this takes place in an institution designed to provide a broad base of knowledge of major areas of learning—natural sciences, social sciences, humanities, and fine arts.[1] In addition, the plan for professional education includes development of the art, science, and skills of nursing in health agencies, chief of which has been the hospital. Nursing educators are confronted with a situation in which it is necessary to move from one type of institution to another in carrying out the educational program with students. The organizations in which teaching takes place cause constraints on the nursing educator as she teaches. The teacher finds herself caught in cross-pressures. These arise between her role as teacher, founded in the educational institution to which she belongs, and her role as guest in the setting, founded on the relation of the educational institution to the agency setting. When, in the role of nurse educator she comes into an agency setting, she finds herself taking the role of guest as well as teacher. It has been suggested that teachers in the agency setting are ambassadors without portfolios.[2] Most see themselves as "guests." "And, of course, we are guests in the clinical setting." (Field notes: September, 1970.)

Teachers come with their own expectations as to how they will be received. They feel "comfortable or uncomfortable," they "belong or they don't," and feel "welcome or unwelcome" depending on the reception they receive in the setting. And the expectations the teacher has are either in line with, or different from, the expectations that the head nurse and staff may have for them. "A staff nurse in the intensive care unit said to the teacher, 'Well, you're never around.' To which the

With minor revisions from Glass, Helen: *Teaching Behavior in the Nursing Laboratory in Selected Baccalaurate Nursing Programs in Canada,* New York, Teachers College Press. In press.

teacher replied, 'We're here as much as we can be.' " (Field notes: October, 1970.)

Given the socially defined position of "guest" in an agency setting, the teacher, in her role of educator, becomes involved in the cross-pressures that are presented by the need for reconciling the differences between the status-positions of guest and educator. This is further compounded by the dual status-postion the teacher occupies as nurse, as well as educator. She attempts a delicate balance in relation to the constraints exerted by persons occupying other status-positions, such as head nurse and staff nurse, within the nursing administrative hierarchy, and the doctors and others in the medical hierarchy. Further constraints arise in relation to spatial and temporal properties, territorial rights, and obligations, such as routines, rules, and procedures, and the inevitable mistakes that are a property of the work-oriented world. The cross-pressures result in a double standard ideologically and pedagogically, as she strives to maintain the balance for her accompanying guest—the student.

STATUS THREATS

Early in the observations the researcher was aware of constraints relevant to status in the areas that teachers had selected for educational experiences for students. The following scene, which was overheard by the researcher and a student, illustrates this. The dialogue took place at the head nurse's desk between the head nurse and the teacher:

Head nurse: Dr. [X] does not appreciate being interrupted. We just don't do this with Dr. [X]. Would you do this? [It appeared that a student had asked directly of Dr. [X] for information about a patient's drugs—a patient for whom she was caring.]

Teacher: I had a conversation with him in the elevator, and he seemed friendly.

Head nurse: He is so preoccupied—if every student were to go to him with a problem, it would be impossible to handle it.

Teacher: I can understand, but I think she is feeling she can go directly to a doctor for information.

Head nurse: She may need to realize the organizational setup here—like if I went to Miss [Director of Nursing] without going to the supervisor.

Teacher: I like to see them go to the doctor. She saw Dr. [X]'s name, and she doesn't know the doctors apart. Then when Dr. [X] appeared, the name was on the chart, and she had a question and asked it.

Head nurse: Especially with Dr. [X], he is not just a consultant, he has many other problems. It has to be urgent before *I'll* go to him.

Teacher: The student got a full answer from him—she had a good discussion with him.

Head nurse: Do you think you should explain the difference between him and the other doctors? Another thing—the desk would like to know what's going on.

Teacher: We can discuss it.

Head nurse: I wouldn't be concerned with one student going, but if he was interrupted several times a day . . .

Teacher: I can understand his situation. (Field notes: October, 1970.)

Teachers in university schools of nursing are considered colleagues of doctors teaching in the university, by virtue of their faculty status. Historically, nurses have been assigned a status lower than that of the doctor, but recently, through upward mobility of the nursing profession and the movement of professional nursing   179 education into the university, nursing educators have achieved the status of other educators. The head nurse has traditionally been assigned a status lower than that of doctors in the hierarchy of the hospital setting.[3] The nurse "helps" the doctor, thereby borrowing, so to speak, from his prestige.[4] When instances as the above occur, the head nurse is threatened by her "guest's" functioning from a different perspective than her own. The teacher handled the matter with as great delicacy as possible. She "kept the peace" with the nursing staff by lowering the threshold of threat, as shown by conversation the researcher recorded later in the day between the head nurse and the teacher. One can see that the teacher had come to a compromise with the head nurse:

> *Teacher:* I'll be talking to the student. We'll talk again Thursday. I hate to discourage the student going to the doctor. He seemed very open to suggestions when going up in the elevator, so perhaps if I see him and talk to him. . .
> *Head nurse:* You talk to him.
> *Teacher:* If he says okay—fine.
> *Head nurse:* I hesitate to have everybody go to him.
> *Teacher:* If he did feel that way, we could decide then.

Later, when the researcher was discussing the episode with the teacher, the latter stated:

> The head nurse seemed to think it was all right for every other doctor. Dr. [X] is so busy, even she would hesitate. Well, I thought that was the crux—the old system of hierarchy. She had never been able to get through it herself but why should others be hampered? (Field notes: October, 1970.)

Compromise is a way of "keeping the peace" when one is a guest. Strauss speaks of negotiated order in hospitals:

> Both the division of labor and the daily work of treatment are accomplished through processes of negotiation. . . . In short, through repeated negotiations among personnel with different statuses within the hospital, agreements are reached about what is to be done daily and by whom.[5]

The head nurse is charged with maintaining order, and to do so, she has a set of rules, both written and unwritten. When a guest comes into her setting, the head nurse lets the rules be known. The guest is obliged to become aware of the accepted order and to discuss with the head nurse any deviations from it that occur and that may have implications for teaching.

While the head nurse is charged with maintaining "negotiated order," the teacher is equally charged with maintaining her own order and negotiates to do so. One teacher stated:

> Sometimes you have to curry favor in order to be able to do what you want. It is just a fact. The relationships are poor here, and the desired learning just cannot take place until those relationships are reestablished. (Field notes: November, 1970.)

Teachers work hard at maintaining relationships as guests. They speak of "public relations" and "maintaining the status quo." They judge the relationships by the freedom they are allowed in their teaching. The field notes describe this

situation on a psychiatric ward:

There is a comfortable atmosphere on this ward. The head nurse is warm and friendly. He discusses the patients with the teacher and tells her what he is doing in working with a patient when the students are not here. In this case he is using "humor." This gives the teacher some idea how the staff is working with the patient and enables her to work with her own student in such a way as to complement the care being given on the ward. The teacher remarked, "it is very comfortable here—the best ward I have." (Field notes: November, 1970.)

Cross-pressures tend to arise for the teacher when she deals with others in the service agencies while carrying out teaching activities. In the university she reacts within that social system with her own colleagues and with others in the other schools and faculties, among whom may be doctors, physiotherapists, and social workers. When she moves into a service agency, she is interacting with some of the same persons, particularly with the doctor, who may or may not have the same expectations of the teacher. He may view the nurse, teacher or not, from long-established expectations in terms of the doctor-nurse status relationship. It was evident from the observations that doctors and teachers communicate very little while in the agency setting. When communication does take place, it is well considered beforehand, and often a planned approach is used. This is especially so where relationships are at stake.

The teacher cited an incident that had occurred with Dr. [X] when, during rounds, a student had been sitting on the bed of a patient for whom she was caring, and Dr. [X] had said something about, "So, now we are teaching students to sit on beds while they care for patients." The student had been most uncomfortable and had come and told the teacher about it. She said her first reaction was one of anger, but then she simmered down and waited and made an appointment with Dr. [X] and when she saw him, said, "You know, Dr. [X], when my students do something like that, I wish you would tell me about it first." She said he was most embarrassed; he reddened and said he didn't mean anything. She said she was glad she had waited to bring his "ridiculing" to his attention, and that, had she done it at the time it occurred, she would have been too angry for it to be effective. (Field notes: October, 1970.)

Teachers don't always know the doctors and may have to make inquiries from the head nurse or staff as to who they are, especially if they wish to speak to them about a patient, or the student's care of that patient. The teachers' meetings with doctors are quite formal at times.

Where other staff are concerned, again there appears to be little communication with teachers, except for matters relating to students and their patients. It seems that attempting to be part of the ward, while a guest and teacher on the ward, poses some problems for the teacher and her student. While episodes were not numerous by the very fact of minimal communication, one or two will serve to point out the reactions of others on the ward to status positions the outsiders hold and the lack of authority commensurate with that status. A teacher on a surgical unit in a hospital described a situation in which she was involved. She stated:

Like, a fellow said he was having acute abdominal pain, and the nurse asked him to let them know. I was the first nurse that happened by. So I had to go and tell them (staff). I wasn't too concerned because I knew this fellow and had heard the report on him, and they think his pain is a little more in his head than in his abdomen. But I had to go and get the grad. Or

> when people come from x-ray to collect someone, and you don't know the patients, and people ask you. This is why I'd just like to have a great label on—'I'm an instructor.' Or a doctor comes and wants to give you an order, and is it really your function to receive orders? (Field notes: October, 1970.)

In summary, the teacher is caught between pressures from the university for which she works, which expects that she will excercise political astuteness in maintaining a place in the agency for laboratory practice, and pressures that arise from her status as guest in the agency, where she functions as a nonmember of the status order, and at the same time, with the head nurse's negotiated order. She also has to negotiate orders for herself and her students in order to accomplish the teaching. Verbal communication is limited with doctors, who belong to another status order, but the nature of the activities in which she engages brings her into close working relationships with the doctors and other workers. In such situations the nonverbal dimension of communication plays a prominent part. Space or territory for the teacher, as guest, poses additional constraints.

TERRITORIALITY

Closely linked to the concept of guest is the teacher's view of the space she occupies, her territorial rights and obligations. The teacher is seen as a guest from outside and must be accommodated when she comes into the setting, by reason of the agreement that has been negotiated between the university and the agency. When a teacher brings a group of students into the agency setting, she takes up space and requires allotment of some space for purposes of carrying out her teaching function.

The researcher found no instance of assigned space on working units, and it was evident that space was a precious commodity. It was customary to share with other groups requiring space. During observations the following was recorded:

> When I reached the intensive care ward, I looked for the teacher and was advised that if I wished to come in, I would have to put on a gown. I asked the nurse with whom I was speaking to let the teacher know I was there. The teacher came out to meet me and took me to the classroom on the ward, where there is a cupboard that they share with others on the unit. I was struck by the overcrowding and the fact that this was the only cupboard for everyone who was using the unit. I asked the teacher about space for instructors and students. She expressed great frustration with the lack of classroom space or even space to store teaching materials. They had no space and no office of any kind. (Field notes: October, 1970.)

There seems to be a premium on space in all agencies. Teachers hold interviews, classes, and conferences with students in everything from conference rooms to interviewing rooms, and so on. They "fit into the system." Territory that is their own is practically nonexistent. They are provided rooms a distance from the work area, usually in residences or in the basement of the agency where locker rooms are often located. Tables may be made available, but in none of the agencies studied was there sufficient room for each individual teacher or student to function independently in her own space. This is not to say that there were not attempts at accommodating the guests. Two agencies used by one university the researcher visited had made provisions for classrooms, a library, and offices. These were clearly marked as belonging to university faculty. But, generally, while in the agency, teachers have no territory that is their own. At best, they retreat to complete the work-team relationship and discuss the field experiences with the student, and at worst, they are crowded into inadequate space or move from space they occupy temporarily when required to do so by agency staff. There is everywhere evident a distinct lack of space.

The phenomenon intrigued the researcher, and conditions were noted under which the teacher would be able to use the rooms that were multiply allotted. They were used by teachers when "no one else was using them at that hour"; mostly, they were sitting empty or were the distinctly marked property of others. There were many rooms labeled for doctors, and these were kept free for their use:

> One morning the teacher arrived on the surgical unit with her students. It had been their custom to have their preconference in a particular room. Today it was to be occupied by the doctors and others for a conference. The teacher explained that "doctors have priority when they are here." (Field notes: October, 1970.)

It is evident that status-position is a factor in the use of space. The teacher, as guest, has minimal status, and when related to that of the doctor, it is lessened still further. This is not the only aspect of territoriality that offers constraints. There are other forces, mainly related to control of territory, that bring about added pressures for the teacher.

Teachers talk about the territories they occupy and in which they select patients for whom students care. The selection of such territory is controlled by administrative faculty at the university school. Teachers attend faculty meetings at which they voice preferences for particular agencies for experiences for their students. It is apparent that they are not always pleased with the territory assigned for field practice. This is so for several reasons. First, what they would like to have is not available to them. The arrangements and decisions about experiences that are made at the university nursing school administrative level may effect discontent with territories assigned. Second, certain territories are in use by other nursing schools and are, thus, not available to the university faculty. Third, control of where they will have their experiences is in the hands of the agencies. Certain territories are off limits to them:

> The students do not have an opportunity to go to conferences themselves at Home Care, but the teacher arranges that the coordinator of the Home Care program talks to them about the services offered. (Field notes: November, 1970.)

Sometimes they are off limits because of crowding in the areas. Either students from other schools are there, or the beds or cribs are crowded together, and staff members are so numerous that there simply is no room. Other times, agencies have their undisclosed reasons for barring access to wards or services. Teachers will try to accommodate to these kinds of difficulties, sometimes altering practice times to be able to use space to advantage.

It is not only the nursing staff that determines the territories teachers will use. **183**

Doctors, although not a part of the administrative hierarchy of which the nursing service is a part, still exercise considerable influence. They often control where students can go. The teacher may have to obtain permission for the student to attend certain clinics, conferences, and team meetings, especially in psychiatric nursing situations, and it depends on whether the doctor will give his permission for the student to attend. Teachers are careful to let doctors know when a student is working with a patient in public health or community nursing because of the control doctors exercise there. The control, then, of selection, nature, and duration of the experiences for learning is not always in the hands of the teacher. Her territorial rights, where care of patients is concerned, are limited by circumstances over which she has little control.

The teachers in the particular areas of the program have definite ideas as to territories they would like to use and when they would like to use them. Thus, within certain areas remnants of "rotations" exist, as teachers "rotate" students through, for example, prenatal clinics, labor rooms, delivery rooms, postpartum wards, and the nursery. In psychiatric nursing they "rotate" through a mental health clinic, acute, intermediate, and convalescent units. In the medical-surgical areas there are increasingly seen varied kinds of intensive care units that teachers select for practice. There is an effort to find the best territories in which to obtain rights, and teachers size these up quickly. In the community there may or may not be a need to "rotate" a student through school, the visiting nurse service, and nursing departments in public health agencies. Territories differ according to whether the family desired for student learning is a family expecting a new baby, a family with a patient with a long-term illness, or a family with a patient requiring immediate physical nursing care. In the school, teachers are expanding territories into the community. Experience areas for learning include neighborhood mother-hood clubs, La Leche Leagues, and community services of all kinds. In the first year of one of the programs a total of 56 agencies was visited by 45 students in 283 visits. Teachers seldom accompany students into community territories except in the case of public health agencies and the visiting nurse services, which in Canada is usually the Victorian Order of Nurses for Canada. Doctors' offices are increasingly included in the newer territorial acquisitions.

A facet of territoriality is the large amount of territory the teachers are often called upon to traverse in keeping track of groups of three to ten students, the usual range of group size. Teachers might assign students in wards of semiprivate, four-bed, and private rooms. Corridors are long, and students are separated from one another. The teacher, as a result, takes on flip-flop activities or thrust activities. Flip-flop activity is engaging in actions such as stopping old activities and engaging in new ones, or it might be questions about old ones; thrust activity is bursting in with the initiation of a new activity without engaging in any action to ascertain the target group's readiness to receive the induction.[5] In psychiatric institutions students might be assigned to several different wards several hundred yards and several floors apart. When the teacher assigns students to such areas, the scope of her territory is greatly extended. This occurs because the control of the number of students to a unit prevails at the discretion of the agency. Or it might be that, to provide varying experiences, teachers seek the use of different territories housing different types of patients, a factor that in hospitals is medically determined.

Territorial rights for the teacher in agency settings, then, are varied and controlled in many instances by factors other than the teacher as she selects experiences for students within that territory allotted to her. The status she holds as guest reinforces her position of ineffectiveness in bringing about desired changes for teaching purposes in settings or the use of new settings. Negotiations for territory, for rights and obligations, are essentially negotiations for order. The scope of the territory with which she is involved and the need to group students to accommodate to the agency settings require that she extend her time in the agencies, so that time becomes a most significant factor in her activities.

TEMPORALITY

The concept of time as a significant influence in the teacher's life as a guest in the agency settings became clearly evident during observations and in discussions with the teachers. Cross-pressures arise by reason of conflicting demands of the teacher's associations with two and more institutions. When in the university, the teacher is subject to the scheduling of the program of study and the demands of the administrative activities with which she is involved. She must adjust time to accommodate these, as well as the student's activities and needs, and also to accommodate to agency time. As she accompanies students or arranges time for student practice in various agencies, scheduling becomes a particular concern. Time is a valued commodity, certain times being more valuable than others, and by reason of her guest status, the teacher feels certain obligations. Time for the teacher is a task master.

Being a guest requires keeping the host informed as to the time the guest will be there, plans for the stay, and the length of the stay. The university teachers go to great lengths to inform the host of their plans. Planned orientations are conducted by the teachers. These are usually meetings with head nurses before the actual practice sessions for students begin at the start of the term. At this time the teacher indicates desired times for practice to fit into the program of study and the schedule the students and she will have to keep at the university. And students must fit classes into time tables of arts and sciences and other faculties where they take courses. Some faculty professors teach the formal classes in nursing at the university as well as provide clinical instruction, and they have "tight" schedules. The meetings between head nurses and teachers are concerned with the objectives of the program, types of practice desired, and so on, but scheduling is the most important factor. Teachers are conscious of ordering their own and students' needs in planning the time for practice as well as "fitting into the system."

Not only does scheduling have to be planned in terms of days, hours per day, and days per week, but it also has to be planned in terms of weeks per year. In selecting hours for practice, the teacher has to negotiate not only with the head nurse but also with teachers in other programs, especially if, for example, a hospital in which practice is desired has its own school of nursing with students requiring practice. Sometimes these negotiations take place under the jurisdiction of directors of nursing in the agency, directors of nursing education, clinical coordinators of different services, such as "obstetric nursing," or inservice education directors. Sometimes direct contacts are made by administrative faculty in the university school, usually the coordinator of the basic program. In all three schools studied, this person played a prominent part in selection, arrangements for, and general public relations with the agencies. Scheduling, too, took on a characteristic of a status rite under these circumstances. Once preliminary negotiations were over, the teachers were left to plan time with the agency and to keep the coordinator informed.

The value of time also enters into scheduling. Wards in hospitals, for example, are busiest at the beginning hours of the day, when doctors arrive on the scene for surgery, medical diagnosis, and treatment. This is when "the action is," and action slackens off on general medical and surgical wards as the day wears on, and doctors and other therapists are not in attendance. In other areas, such as intensive care units and "premie" nurseries, which are considered high-risk situations, residents and internes are either in constant attendance or are readily available, and there is less slackening of the action. A readily discernible norm in scheduling was for the teacher to select "action-oriented" time.

Teachers arrange for nursing practice to begin just prior to the time when the action commences—7 to 8 o'clock. Some do so for reasons of hospital schedules. "Coming on" has something of the connotation of "duty," and, indeed, teachers say they come at this time so they can "fit into the ward routine." Others say it is so students can experience the hospital schedules of giving "basic care." This is the term for morning ablutions and other activities patients indulge in each morning in the hospital that are particularly related to hygiene and nutrition. During this time patients are "done up," a term that has survived through the ages of nursing and that originated when patients had to be shining and in rows for doctors' rounds.

Teachers are conscious of commitment to the agency in the scheduling of time. Sometimes negotiation is possible; other times it is not.

> The two teachers I talked to today told me they feel obligated to the unit when they say the students will be there. One of the teachers, I had talked to earlier, and she had told me that in [X] Hospital, it was stipulated by the hospital that if they say they are coming, they are committed to "carry out the assignment." (Field notes: November, 1970.)

There are evidences of nonnegotiable demands such as in the above agency, but there are also negotiable demands in terms of time spent in the unit and how it is used. Teachers have their own ordering to do in terms of time, as do head nurses. They are also likely to negotiate in terms of the value of the time that they spend in the agency, even though they feel a commitment. One teacher said:

186   In no way does anybody at [X] Hospital expect you to be a staff member. They expect you

to be somebody entirely different from the staff. But this is quite different from [Y] Hospital. There I tell the head nurse exactly where I am going, what I am doing. At [the first] Hospital it isn't expected. When I tell them where I am going, they almost say, "Why are you telling me?" (Field notes: November, 1970.)

One of the most devastating experiences for teachers is in terms of commitment scheduling when students are ill and do not turn up for practice or are late arriving on the unit. When students are late for classes at the university, this is their own concern, but when they are late or absent at the agency, the teacher has to "smooth the feathers." This excerpt from field notes is illustrative:

I met the two teachers at the locker room at 7:00 AM. One teacher stayed with me while I changed since we were going to the postpartum unit. She did not have any students as yet, and only two had arrived for the other teacher; she was expecting four. I left to go to the latter teacher's unit, since these were my plans for the morning. It was 7:15 when I arrived there. The teacher was talking to the two students at the desk, and they were all in conversation with the head nurse. The phone rang; it was for the teacher. Two students had slept in, and since it would take them over an hour to arrive, the teacher decided it was not worthwhile for them to come. She spoke to the head nurse about this. She, of course, had been prepared for four students and had selected four patients for them. The head nurse said, "What kind of nurses will they make when they graduate?" The teacher looked upset but said nothing except that she was sorry. The other teacher came along at this point—she is senior to the first teacher and is "in charge" of the practice. She was skeptical that it would have taken over an hour for the absent students to reach the hospital, but now that the decision had been made, she left it as it was. They were both visibly upset. They remarked that they had worked so hard to build up this relationship to what it was now—which was still considered to be "shaky." "Now this kind of thing happens," was a remark made. Both teachers decided that a discussion with students was forthcoming, since they felt obligated to the unit, and when they told the head nurse students would be there, they were committed to carry out the assignment. (Field notes: November, 1970.)

Temporality, then, is concerned with scheduling and ordering and with negotiating as an aspect of scheduling. These must be done in terms of agency, teacher, and student schedules. Action-oriented time tends to dominate scheduling, and commitment to the agency is a facet that has a distinct influence. Negotiable and nonnegotiable demands are brought to play, and illness and absence have devastating repercussions for the teacher.

MISTAKES

When asked about mistakes in the agency environments, teachers agreed students should be allowed to make mistakes, that they are not "infallible," but they tend to try to have students avoid mistakes because of consequences not only to the student but also to the patient, teacher, and school. As a guest in the agency, the teacher is concerned with three types of mistakes: performance, social, and educational, all of which she or the student can make. Because the teacher's ideology of the professional image is oriented to success in each component of the image, the teacher is placed in a dilemma as to how to handle mistakes. Her own patient orientation and commitment to nursing care of a high quality influences her in the directions she goes in handling mistakes. In addition, she is a guest and has a stake in keeping the door open to herself and the university school.   187

A social mistake is likely to hurt the professional image and create difficulties in the attitude or "climate" toward the guests. In the incident where students did not arrive for practice in an institution that expected they were "committed" to the service they would provide during their practice period, the response was, "What kind of graduates will they make?" There is a danger that such errors reflect on who the student is, for she is being shaped in the professional ideal.

Social mistakes have consequences for the teacher in that they may affect the attitude of the staff towards the guests. Where a student in a public health nursing course had inadvertently left her telephone number with a patient, the teacher said to her:

> This is something that, just because you are a student, would occur. I think it is better to leave the number of the district health nurse, rather than your's at home. I'm quite sure you won't be bothered by her, but this is something that is better for politics, too. You could either leave your name here for her to get in touch with you or she could get in touch with the public health nurse. (Field notes: October, 1970.)

Social mistakes, such as the one this student had made, could affect both the student's learning and the climate in the agency.

A performance mistake usually centers around the "right or wrong" way of doing things. It is tied up with the policy, rules, regulations, and ritual of the agencies in which practice is sought. Consequences are seen as having great importance: "If the student commits an error in the nursing skills lab, this isn't the same as if she does something right or wrong on the ward." (Field notes: October, 1970.) Not only are there consequences for the teacher related to the care that students give, but also the consequences of errors are or could be grave.

> The teacher was very concerned about students carrying out ward routines—she was showing them where things should be put as the students finished certain aspects of care. She told me she was concerned about consequences of error and the need for students to know the ward routine, because there were definitely consequences of error when one was made. She also stated that they "were constantly pouring oil on troubled waters" in regard to medications not given by students before they "go off," or given but not recorded. She checks very carefully so that this does not happen. She does not tell the student she does this, but she always does it. (Field notes: October, 1970.)

Here the teacher was concerned with consequences for the relationships with staff and was also concerned with the student avoiding difficulty, as once the students leave the ward, it is difficult for the staff to contact them in the event such errors are made. The teacher "runs interference" for the students to avoid occurrence of such errors and "buffers" them from the ire of the staff should a mistake occur.

The third type of mistake is that centering around the student's learning. The above incident indicates concern for the student's learning, and educational mistakes are sometimes allowable, sometimes not. It depends on the consequences the mistakes have for the student as the teacher sees her progressing along her "educational way." Since this is part of the professional image, educational mistakes have consequences for that image, and also, if serious enough, would jeopardize the status of the teacher as guest.

REFERENCES

1. Russell, C. H.: *Liberal Education and Nursing,* New York, Teachers College Press, 1959, p. 80.
2. Olesen, V. L., and Whittaker E. W.: *The Silent Dialogue,* San Francisco, Jossey-Bass, Inc., 1968, p. 141.
3. Coser: *Life in the Ward,* pp. 16-17.
4. Strauss, A. L., Schatzman, L., Bucher, R., Ehrlich, D., and Sabshin, M.: *Psychiatric Ideologies and Institutions,* New York, The Free Press, 1964, p. 343.
5. Kounin, J. S.: "An Analysis of Teachers' Managerial Techniques," *Psychology in the Schools* 4:221-227, 1967.

SUGGESTED QUESTIONS FOR DISCUSSION AND ANALYSIS

For undergraduate students

1. As a student what do you think about the concerns and problems as discussed here that teachers may encounter in an effort to provide a learning experience?
2. From your perspective as a student do you see those problems teachers may encounter as avoidable or as inevitable ("built into the system")? Explain your choice.
3. How do you think students' mistakes should be handled? Do you think making a mistake "damages" the image of a nurse?
4. What are the criteria for the uses of space in hospital settings; that is, who uses what space and why?
5. Identify examples of the stereotyped thinking of the physician and nurses in the various clinical settings with respect to the teacher and her students. Discuss how this affected the performance of the teacher and the students.
6. Identify the various orientations to patient care described here. Do you see a relationship between orientation to one's work and the work setting?
7. Explain as many factors as you can that shape one's orientation to the work he or she does.

For graduate students and teachers of nursing

1. In what ways might cross-pressures experienced by teachers in clinical settings be mitigated?
2. Should teachers always be in the clinical setting? Are there any alternatives to the teacher's presence in the clinical setting?
3. What might be some ways to both bridge and lessen what is commonly referred to as "the gap" between nursing service and nursing education?

part II

Outside the hospital

This discussion considers four features that influence the work of nurses in environments outside the hospital: medical versus nonmedical values, the nature of the illness and of the problems, organization of services, and the nature of the population served. Admittedly, nurses' work occurs in many nonhospital settings, such as schools, industrial plants, health centers, and so on; however, the papers presented in this section deal mainly with the nurse at work in the clinic, in the patient's home, and in informal neighborhood locales.

MEDICAL VERSUS
NONMEDICAL VALUES

As we saw earlier, the hospital is organized in accordance with medical values, which, in effect, influence the total hospital atmosphere. Because the hospital organization reinforces medical values and gives them top priority, their transmission to and general acceptance by patients are facilitated. Consequently, both physicians and nurses are able to exercise a measure of patient management and control unknown to their counterparts in work environments outside the hospital. For example, in work settings such as schools, industrial plant's, or a patient's home, medical values are not primary. The patient (or client, as he frequently is labelled in these settings) is not only less clearly a patient, but he, too, may not consider health to be his primary value. The opportunity, therefore, is greater in these environments for the nurse's influence and management of the patient to be more tenuous.

Clinics, however, while oriented to medical values, are unable because of limited contact with patients to inculcate medical values as primary within the patient's value system. And, too, nurses in clinic settings encounter problems in management and control similar to those in totally nonmedical locales.

NATURE OF THE ILLNESS AND OF THE PROBLEMS

Generally, persons who require the care of the nurse in their home or clinic are as a rule not as acutely unwell as one would find in a hospital. Issues of immediate cure and healing that are largely dependent on medical intervention do not take precedence here. This shift in emphasis on the nature of the illness results in differences in the nature of the problems encountered in these settings. For instance, the problems generally encountered, such as fragmentation and discontinuity in care and services, social isolation of patients with long-term illnesses, inadequacies in services and facilities for disabled persons, and so on, are inclined to be resistant to dramatic or quick alteration. A substantial change in the nature of these problems is greatly dependent on nonmedical events, such as legislation governing the appropriation of monies, changes in public attitudes, innovation in education for health professionals, or even reorganization of some aspects of the health delivery system. Consequently, the degree of success of the nurse's work with respect to such goals as health maintenance, rehabilitation, disease prevention, and improvement in the quality of living for persons in this group are influenced by these nonmedical factors as well as by her degree of expertise in nursing skills and knowledge.

ORGANIZATION OF SERVICES

Unlike the hospital, the facilities for care and services to patients in environments outside the hospital are not located, so to speak, under one roof. Rather, facilities are dispersed over a wide geographic area. This situation in and of itself would not be a problem if the system of helping agencies were a closely knit network where relevant information about patients could be shared among agencies and health professionals working with the same patient or patients. But, because the helping agencies are in effect a collection of separate entities, problems for the nurse in coordinating their services and at the same time maintaining continuity in care are almost insurmountable under the present arrangement. It should come as no surprise that there are grave discontinuities in care and wasteful duplication of services or, in some instances, no service.

NATURE OF THE PATIENT POPULATION

The people who generally make up a sizable number of the patients receiving services and care in these contexts are those persons who traditionally have not been at the center of interest of health professionals (or of social attention) and who tend to be on the periphery of medical care. This population includes the chronically ill, the poor, the aged, some ethnic groups, and all others marginal to society, such as hippies, drug users, alcoholics, and so on. Working with such groups brings one face to face with life styles and living conditions so alien and unfamiliar as to produce "culture shock" for some nurses on their first encounters. Not infrequently, cultural values, beliefs, and concepts of illness valued by these groups are in direct conflict with those held by the nurse. The nurse's influence, already made tenuous by the absence of organizational supports, is further challenged by these cultural and social factors.

Without doubt, some of the features discussed here pertain to the hospital environment as well. However, because nurses can exercise only limited control over the patient in his community environment, the problematic facets of her work that result from these features are bound to stand out more sharply and prove more intractable than in the more ordered environment of the hospital.

The chapters to follow vividly illustrate these and other aspects of the work of nurses in environments outside the hospital.

Nurses in clinics and community settings

There is much discussion in current nursing literature about expanded or extended roles, or both, for nurses. Since our focus throughout the book has not been to suggest how nursing should be done but to describe how nursing *is* being done, we have purposely not addressed nurse role expansion as such. However, two entries that follow, by Peterson and Popell, are about situations where nurses are without doubt functioning in expanded roles. For example, in the Peterson chapter nurses not only establish a clinic in response to an expressed concern of a client population, but they also direct the running of the clinic. Popell describes still further a situation where nurses are in the role of entrepreneur; that is, the nurses maintain control over those factors that affect their area of practice, such as with whom they practice, how they practice, and payment for their practice. Popell herself is a good example of a nurse in an entrepreneurial role in her capacity as president of a nurse consulting firm that she established.

13. A nursing Camelot: a legend of two nurses and the clinic they developed

Evelyn T. Peterson, RN, MA

Autonomy, both its relative lack as well as its total absence with respect to the work of nurses, has been mentioned at several points within the text. The following piece, a shining example of autonomy, was written especially for this book, not so much to disprove those earlier comments but more to illustrate what nurses can do given a particular set of circumstances. For example, in this situation (1) both nurses and clients shared similar values and perspectives, (2) the nature of the problem was highly responsive to attention, (3) all services relevant to the problem were easily accesible, (4) communication among the professionals, volunteers, and clients, was open and responsive to corrective measures, and (5) last, but perhaps in its own way most significant, the client population consisted mainly of socially conscious, articulate young persons who viewed the delivery of good health care as a right, not a privilege.

In the late 1960's two nurses helped create a contraception clinic at the University of California, Berkeley. At that particular time there were certain social events on the campus that radically modified the nature and direction of student life. The following discussion is about the relationships and interactions between the social context (University administration, physicians, surrounding communities,

I am grateful to Rose Ann Parkard, RN, MS, the first nurse employed in and my co-worker in the Contraception Counseling and Education Clinic and to Henry B. Bruyn, MD, Director, Student Health Services, Cowell Memorial Hospital, University of California, Berkeley, for their helpful comments on this paper.

and students) and how the nurses' roles evolved. Its main purpose is to draw attention to the hitherto largely neglected aspect of nurse's work; that is: As much as professional ideology, the social context in which the professional work develops mediates what the nurse's work will be.

During the last years of the 1960's university students developed a heightened sense of the social problems surrounding them. In this they were different from students of previous years. They voiced their opinions about campus and worldwide issues. They openly questioned the American way of life. They were politically active on the university campus and in the community. They demanded autonomy over their personal lives, especially in social relations between the sexes. The last demand made profound changes in their living arrangements. No longer were they content to live in approved university housing. They shared apartments and lived in group arrangements such as communes. They recognized that the new living styles with new sexual freedom brought a concomitant need for contraceptive services.

During the 1960's the increasing world population and the dangers of overpopulation were becoming a public concern. The consequences of sheer population growth on the earth resources were quickly grasped by the university students. With an acceptance of restraints on having as many children per couple as in past generations was an ardent commitment by students to see that every child would be a wanted child. Pragmatically, the students realized that children could interfere with their career and life plans.

A referendum of the student body found an overwhelming support for birth control facilities on campus. The students almost continuously petitioned the university administration for the service. About 18% to 20% of the university's student body were married, but the contraception service was also needed for the large number of unmarried students who were requesting such information and care. There were about 10,000 women of child-bearing age on the campus. Many of those who were in need of birth control information had visited the local Planned Parenthood agencies. In 1968, 1,145 family-planned visits (53%) to the Berkeley Planned Parenthood Clinic and 4,600 visits (49%) to another, similar agency in an adjacent community were made by students. In addition, an unknown number of students visited other clinics and private physicians for services. These agencies, overwhelmed by students' requests, were forced to cut back on services to people for whom they had been originally founded.

At the request of the Director of Student Health Services one Planned Parenthood agency set up an ancillary clinic as a stopgap measure in the YWCA directly across from the campus. Its services were almost immediately oversubscribed. Pressure from the students for the clinic continued. They felt it was old-fashioned and hypocritical not to provide this service on campus. The students also saw the clinic as an opportunity for the university to respond to their requests as the university administration rhetoric so often declared that the university was capable of doing. However, the university health service was unable to do so because of bureaucratic and financial limitations.

197

The Student Health Services at the University of California, Berkeley, is unique in the comprehensiveness of its outpatient and inpatient services. It is actually a small hospital with all the supporting services of such an institution, including surgery, orthopedics, x-ray, and complete laboratory facilities. When the students were pressuring the administration to add a birth control service to the already comprehensive services available, there seemed to be no reason for not doing so. However, since the health service was running a deficit budget, a new program would have meant an increase in student fees (which support the health service) or the closing of another program. Such an increase in fees would have meant a lengthy fight through the bureaucracy of the system and certain delay in opening any type of contraception service. Closing another program was not seen as an improvement in service and was not considered. The only option open and the one finally agreed to by a majority of the students and the health service administration was to open a contraception clinic supported by funds obtained by charging the clients who used the service. This was also a politically astute decision, since there could be no public disapproval of using university funds to support "birth control programs for unmarried students."

By spring of 1969, after years of discussion and pressure, it seemed that the clinic would open. Fortuitously, a professional nurse, enrolled as a graduate student in the university's School of Public Health and known to the Student Health Services Director, was interested in beginning work on such a clinic as part of her 2-month field work placement. She was able to pull together the different factions who had an invested interest in seeing the clinic develop: The Student Health Services Director, Planned Parenthood agencies, and the students. Under her leadership the clinic opened.

So the clinic began its existence and continued under the auspices of nurses. That summer the Contraception Counseling and Education Clinic was inaugurated using the student health facilities and with a professional nurse employed to supervise its functioning. A second nurse was employed to coordinate the delivery of the core service, that is, the birth control education and examination clinic sessions. Both nurses held postbaccalaureate degrees, had nursing experience, had worked as volunteers for planned parenthood agencies, and were strongly motivated to attempt new methods of delivering health care. Both had expostulated on new concepts of care that would give more control to the patient in planning for health needs. The clinic seemed to be an opportunity for the nurses to take leadership in setting up a service with lessened emphasis on the medical aspects of the clinic and more on the client's perspective of what was needed. In this situation this goal seemed to be one that could be reached because the client group had clearly articulated their demands. They saw themselves as clients of such a clinic but also as having a voice in the details of planning and operating the service.

Professionally and administratively, the nurses functioned under the Student Health Services Director (a physician). They were given sanction to develop the clinic to fit the needs of the students. Two clinic components allowed for this freedom: (1) a contraception service was not one that the university health services could deliver, and (2) the money to support the clinic came from outside the usual university funding. The fee the students paid for the contraceptive services put its programs outside the university financing, and consequently, there was no economic threat to ongoing programs.

Taking these conditions into consideration, one can understand how it was that the contraceptive clinic was outside the usual administrative constraints of the university's regular health facilities. Other clinics were functioning with medical and nursing staff who were busy with their own work and not interested in adding to their work loads a new, untried service. Community health services had long looked at students as recipients of health care from the university. Consequently, they were not interested in developing specialized services for students, since they believed this was the responsibility of the university.

What did this mean for the nurses' work? For the nurse supervisor it meant no official orientation to the hospital, clinics, or the university itself; she began her work in limbo. Most of the information needed for the clinic's development was obtained from the nurse's own explorations into the bureaucracy of the university and its health facilities, from the students who worked in the clinic, and from the clients themselves. This situation had some disadvantages in that at times it was more time consuming to find one's own way through the labyrinth of the university functioning, but the advantage was that one could develop and plan with the potential clients for services they desired without interference. A pregnancy counseling program requested by the students, for example was initiated by the nurse and was functioning before she realized the number of constraints that might be placed on such a program. This program had the enthusiastic support of the students and was organized to help them with problems concerning pregnancies. No medical services were given through this program. It was a counseling and referral service under the supervision of the nurse, and as such it was completely oriented to the social-psychological needs of the students.

For the nurse, whose primary work was direct patient service, being free of the constraints of the ongoing health service clinics meant that the contraception clinic's plans could be changed while in operation. Because of the time and place of the clinic, it was not meshed with the other health service clinics. Thus, if the patient came with special or unusual problems, he or she was seen by the nurse, and she routed the patient to where he or she would receive the needed care. Changing the clinic pattern so that the patient could get his or her problem cared for was sometimes necessary. The student volunteers supported such changes. The nurse was the central person in the clinic, and it was to her that the volunteers directed their questions on birth control and on patient care. All referrals to other agencies were made through the nurse. The path of the patient through the clinic was episodic in that the patient moved from one room and one volunteer to another room and another volunteer as he or she progressed through the clinic. The only individual observing the patient throughout all phases of the examination was the

199

nurse. All information regarding the patient's problems and needs were filtered through to the nurse, and she initiated action to see that those needs were met. There was complete freedom to discuss with the patient what his or her problems were, or what the patient saw the clinic helping him or her with, and to follow through to see that the clinic did respond to meet the patient's needs.

The physicians employed by the clinic were interviewed by the supervising nurse. Decisions on employment were by mutual agreement and approval of the nurse and the Student Health Service Director. Each physician was told of the clinic's emphasis on the team approach, with the team consisting of the volunteer students, the nurses, and the doctors. The physicians were expected to participate in the postclinic conferences, at which time problems with the clinic and new ideas would be discussed. This meeting was lead by the clinic nurse. In this way, physicians were screened so that only those who were interested would seek employment or be employed. If the physicians did not function as part of the team after pledging their cooperation with such an approach, they did not continue in the clinic employment. The student clients and volunteers were critical and not hesitant about making their opinions of professionals known.

The physicians who worked for the clinic were those who were outside the mainstream model of private medical practice. Women physicians who worked part time because of family responsibilities, student physicians who were enrolled in the School of Public Health, physicians who were residents at the local medical school, physicians who worked for the Student Health Services, physicians who worked for Planned Parenthood agencies, and maverick young hip physicians who worked part time at many different positions were the varied types who came to the clinic. For each clinic session two physicians were employed for 4 hours. The fragmented contact the physicians had with the clinic and the fact that they did not look upon this work as primary to their medical careers but as stopgap positions lessened the possibility for medical control of the clinic. At the same time it allowed the nurses, who were the constant persons in the clinic and who had a professional interest in expanding their roles, to grasp leadership in the operation of the clinic and to set its functioning in accordance with client-oriented values.

Although the clinic was patterned after the Planned Parenthood clinics, the clients were far from the type of patient for whom Planned Parenthood was originally designed. The clients were primarily healthy young women and men. They were intelligent, articulate, and interested in their care, and they were motivated to take an active part in it. They were concerned with all facets of the medical examination and the contraceptive methods available to them through the clinic. They talked about their desires for help in improving the quality of their sexual life. They asked questions and pushed for direct and honest answers and were not satisfied with glib professional jargon.

Being accountable directly to one's clients was a new experience for both nurses. In most work situations the nurse is accountable to other professionals: doctors, other nurses, or the hospital administrator. Besides the contact with students in client and volunteer relations, there was a formal channel via the Student Advisory Committee. How did this affect the nurses' work? The sophistication of the clients about their needs and making them known to the nurses allowed the nurses to use time, usually needed to ascertain the patient's wants, to respond to those wants. It meant weekly program evaluations by the nurses and volunteers, with decisions on changes to be made and changes to be implemented quickly. Nurses also received direct feedback on the students' pleasure with the clinic and its treatment of student clients.

A problem for any new service moving into an institutional setting where all facilities are in use is where it will locate. The contraception clinic was offered space by the Student Health Services if the facilities were used at hours when the old, established clinics were not in operation. This meant evening clinic sessions, but it was still a most desirable situation in that all the facilities of the Student Health Services would be looked to for help. Such ancillary services as the laboratory, record room, and emergency room would be available for use. A fee would be paid for the use of the space.

The gynecology clinic rooms were offered for the physician examinations. The Student Health Services' psychiatric department offered its facilities for classes and interview rooms, again a desirable situation in that the space provided exactly what was needed, a large room and several offices. A commitment was made by the contraception clinic to furnish its own supplies and equipment and to return all rooms to their former pristine condition. This meant that in some way the equipment and supplies had to be moved in, used, and then removed. Putting the clinic on wheels was the answer. Carts were employed, one for all the paper, pencils and educational material used by the clinic, one for all the equipment needed for physicians' examinations, and one for the birth control methods that were to be sold at the clinic; carts were used for everything except the money, which was carried by hand. So this "clinic on wheels" rolled out at sunset and was gone by morning.

There were, of course, some small problems, such as not returning pencils to desks and not completely throwing away all the debris of the clinic. One group of men who also inhabit institutions at night, the maintenance men, became our mentors in returning everything to its proper order. Slowly we learned what went where. Later, when the clinic was given a permanent place of its own, it lost some of the conspiratorial flavor that pulled professionals and volunteers together in its early weeks of functioning.

SUGGESTED QUESTIONS FOR DISCUSSION AND ANALYSIS

For undergraduate students
1. Look back on history and choose a nursing leader who was a nursing-cultural heroine, and develop what the social context of her life might have been. What were the influences in her life that made it possible for her to accomplish what she did? Which is most important, the cultural milieu or the individual's motivation to work toward establishing a new program? Support your choice. **201**

2. As a student, what has been your experience with volunteers? In what manner did the presence of volunteers affect the nurses' work?

3. Historically, what has usually happened to new health programs that began outside the mainstream of health services? What other purposes besides giving direct contraceptive services does a clinic like this serve when it begins functioning in the midst of a long-established, more conservative service?

4. If you were to begin a birth control clinic such as this in a small rural town, what would you need to take into account? Who would you see as allies in the development of such a clinic? How could you finance it? Where and how would you use physicians? What other staff would you employ? What services would you offer? Who might your patients be? Who would be the volunteers? Do you think they might be from the same public as in this clinic? If not, why? How do you think the nurses' work might differ?

For graduate students and teachers of nursing

1. Do you feel you were prepared for or are preparing nursing students for leadership functions such as those described in this article? The nurses in this article were prepared at the master's level. Would graduate preparation be more important for a nurse working in a university health service than, say, in a grade school health agency? Why?

2. Critique the chapter and identify another perspective from which the article could have been presented. To what audience would you direct the paper? What difference would it make? Briefly outline how you would have written about an experience such as this.

3. After reading this chapter one becomes aware of the time involved in translating identified health needs into action—the contraception clinic had a long gestation period. Should nursing take a more active role in helping to translate health needs into services? What are the difficulties a nurse might face in doing so? Would it affect her work? Would it change her relationships with her clients? In what manner?

4. With the introduction of nurse practitioners into the clinic what changes in the present nurses' work do you predict will occur? What can be done to expedite such changes? How should the nurse-practitioner be prepared? Where, in an academic setting or on the job? Do you foresee any legal problems with the use of the nurse practitioner?

14. The nurse as leader: the Lamaze experience

Catherine Popell, RN, MS

"Lamaze" is a term used to describe a form of anticipatory teaching done in a step-by-step, systematic fashion with couples in preparation for the imminent birth of their babies. Because the Lamaze method is based on the assumption that giving birth to a baby should be a joint, cooperative effort of mother and father, both prospective parents attend and participate in all the sessions together.

The reader should make special note of the ways in which the nurse-leader attempts to establish a particular social-psychological climate within the group. There are other subtle happenings occurring within the group meetings that could be viewed differently by the various members. The reader should note which of these are "seen" and handled by the leader and which are not, perhaps for reasons of taking them for granted.

The Lamaze nurse-instructor is self-employed. Her objective is to help couples have a satisfying birth experience. Each instructor must be accredited by the American Society of Psychoprophylaxis in Obstetrics (ASPO). She receives her late-term pregnant couples through referrals from obstetricians, hospitals, other instructors, or past clients. Each woman must have written permission from her physician to attend class.

As an independent practitioner, the Lamaze instructor is paid directly by her private clients and by local high school districts for classes she conducts through adult education programs. While private rates vary somewhat, the typical charge in the San Francisco Bay area is $30.00 per couple for six weekly 2-hour sessions. Each private class normally contains seven couples. Some instructors charge extra for labor coaching or for instructing one couple.

Many Lamaze instructors have agreed to conduct programs through adult education programs because this medium allows them to serve a segment of the market that could not afford private rates. Clients pay a minimal amount, averaging $3.00, to the high school district, which, in turn, reimburses the instructor. The class size ranges from 12 to 15 couples.

Whether in private or adult education sessions, the Lamaze instructor controls the content of her course. She places greatest emphasis, of course, on the Lamaze techniques of childbirth, but she may add subject matter according to the needs of her clients. Breast-feeding and early infant care have been common additions. Most instructors invest in their own audiovisual materials and often invest jointly in films for presentation to large audiences.

Locally, several Lamaze instructors have arranged to use a church hall one morning per week for a drop-in coffee klatch center for new and expectant Lamaze mothers. One instructor is always present as a resource person. These instructors realize that their clients have needs outside the scope of the normal course content and have tried to meet these needs.

The nurse-doctor relationship is on a colleague basis. She consults with, and is consultant to doctors in the area who are also members of the ASPO. In addition, she "lobbies" with hospital personnel for appropriate services for her clients. If she hears from clients that a particular hospital or shift of nurses is antagonistic toward Lamaze-prepared couples, she intervenes and discusses problems with the obstetrical nurses or other appropriate personnel, or both. In her advocate role, she must also be aware that, at times, clients may be unrealistic in their expectations and demands on hospital personnel.

The following observations of three Lamaze classes were conducted with the cooperation of Janet, an accredited nurse-teacher.

My first observation was of the initial meeting of Janet's adult education class, which was held in a local church. Janet's objectives were to begin to establish trust between herself and the class and to put the couples at ease with one another. She assessed their level of knowledge and discussed with them any questions, problems, or "old wives' tales" that they raised. Janet then gave a brief description of labor and delivery. Prenatal exercises, as well as techniques used in the Lamaze method of childbirth, were also introduced.

I returned the following week to observe Janet teaching the Lamaze techniques of relaxation and breathing to the same group.

The final observation was of the last session of another class, a private one given at her home. For the last session, Janet invited two couples from a previous class and their babies. Each couple discussed with the class their labor and delivery. Janet's goals were to reinforce her own teaching that the Lamaze method can be helpful in a variety of labor and delivery situations and to emphasize that no two labor and delivery experiences are the same. The parent couples also discussed their lives with a new baby.

Wednesday, 7:30 PM

As I drive into the churchyard, I can see through one of the classroom windows that the class is about to begin. By the time I enter, all couples are seated.

The room could easily be divided into two classrooms. In one half is a large circle of chairs with small tables in front of them. A portable blackboard and an oblong table behind it create an artificial separation from the rest of the room, which is bare except for a few scattered folding chairs, on which rest pillows and blankets brought by the couples. A large table covered with tiny blocks of clay indicates that the Sunday school class is working on a project. The blackboards on the walls are covered with early Biblical names.

Janet's large coffee urn and myriad of books are on the table behind the blackboard. She has a loan system for the books that enables her couples to read as many as they want during the 7 weeks of classes. (I have taught a class with Janet and know that these materials belong to her. The books are on subjects ranging from conception through early child care. Reports on labor written by past class members are also available.)

There are ten couples in the group, a Lamaze teacher candidate, and a "helper" for Janet. (The helper is a former client of Janet's who delivered 9 months ago and expressed a desire to assist her in her classes.) Everyone wears a name tag. With the exception of one man who seems to be in his late 40's, all appear to range in age from the early 20's to late 30's. One man is asleep, with his arms folded across his chest. He nods slowly. Without opening his eyes, he picks up his head, but soon it is back on his chest again. He looks exhausted. His face has deep lines, the kind caused by repeated exposure to sun and cold weather. His wife does not try to wake him. She seems quite content just to have him present. She probably knows that once class starts he will wake up, which he does.

Janet takes a seat in the circle and begins: "I'm glad you could all make it tonight. I like to begin by having everyone introduce themselves. Let us know when the baby is due, if it's your first, and anything else you would like to add. I'll begin with myself. I'm Janet [X]. I prefer to be called just Janet. We have two children, the second of whom was delivered using the Lamaze technique. I've taught childbirth for many years; first, the Grantly Dick Read Method and then the Lamaze. . . . " (I'm surprised that she doesn't mention that she is a registered nurse and a midwife. I think it would make the class feel more confident.) She looks to the group, and as she leans forward to see the name tag of the man seated next to her, she says "Let's continue with—is it Joe?" "Yes, my name is Joe, and I pass to my wife," he answers. (Some laughter among classmates.) I have observed in some of my own classes that many men are reticent in the beginning and let their wives do most of the talking. "My name is Josephine, and I'm scared," Joe's wife says. (Laughter from the class.) "You're in good company. There are very likely others here who feel the same way," Janet tells her. (Some creaking of chairs.) "That's one of the reasons I want to take the class. This is our first baby, and I'm due in the middle of March," Josephine says and turns to the woman next to her. Lydia introduces herself; this is her first baby, due March 18. "I'm a fourth grade teacher and all my children have been sharing this experience. I've been using this as a good sex education tool. They love to feel the baby kick," she says. Janet interjects, "I hope you go back and show them the baby after it's born." "Oh, I'm going to.   **205**

They would never forgive me if I didn't." Lydia then turns and looks at her husband. "I'm Bob," he says, "I really don't have any more to add." (Another backstage hubby.) The next woman looks quite tired. (I wonder to myself whether she's unable to sleep in late pregnancy or just has lots of work.) I'm surprised by the enthusiasm in her voice as she speaks. "This is my first baby and my husband's third. His other children are teen-agers and are living with us now. I'm not too sure what to expect and consider Mel the expert. He helped deliver his youngest child." Mel, in his late 40's and the oldest man present, offers, "It was a freakish thing that happened. The nurses weren't around and the doctor needed some help fast, so he asked me. And in those days it was rare to even be in the labor room! It was the greatest experience! I wasn't frightened at all. It was terrific! He's 16 now." (I think to myself, no nurses in the delivery room—how frightening that must sound to the other couples! I can't imagine what happened.) Janet must have the same feelings; she says, "That's a very uncommon situation." Mel adds, "It was in another state, and the doctor explained that it had never happened to him before. I don't remember exactly what it was all about." As I look around the circle, none of the couples appear worried. Maybe I'm overly concerned. In writing down a few notes, I miss the names of the next couple. The husband looks like a clean-cut college student, except he is about 10 years too old. I manage to catch something of their story about an earlier delivery that they found unpleasant. The wife says, "I was the last to find out what I had. I kept moving my head back and forth and saying I didn't want to be put out, and the doctor kept chasing my face with the mask. When he put it over my face I was knocked out. I really think I could have managed the delivery fine." Her husband adds, "Besides, it doesn't cost as much if there's no anesthesiologist. They charge about $175.00." (I hear one audible gasp, and several people shift in their chairs.) "The cost of an anesthesiologist depends upon the circumstances and the medication used," Janet interjects. "It's difficult to give a blanket rate for all anesthesiologists." The husband continues, "I haven't decided yet if I'll go into the delivery room." I see a head nod in agreement across the circle. "I hate the sight of blood." At this point Mel leans forward, contributing, "No one could be more frightened than I am at the sight of blood. I cut my finger and faint! But seeing my baby born wasn't the same. It didn't bother me. I cut my finger now and faint!" (Laughter.) "It may be the same for you."

Another husband, Don, interrupts. He looks more perplexed than angry, but his voice has a sharp edge to it. He turns to the woman who protested the use of medication. "The doctor wanted to give you something. Doesn't he know what is best for you?" "What is best for him!" she almost shouts back. Janet begins speaking. Immediately all heads and eyes turn toward her. "A doctor relies on his experience when he suggests the use of medication. It is important that together you see your doctor and discuss choices with him. Every delivery is individual. Only you will know exactly how you feel. That's why it's important to have talked with your doctor beforehand." Any tension that this exchange caused is eased considerably. Don suddenly looks young to me. I realize this is the youngest couple in the class. His next question is directed to Janet. There is no sharpness in his voice; in fact, it sounds more like a schoolboy talking to his teacher. "How can I talk to the doctor about medication? I don't know what Betty will need." "We will discuss all the commonly used medications in one of our class sessions," Janet explains. "It will give you enough information to talk with the doctor." Betty begins speaking, "If we take this class, I can't have any medications, can I?" She is looking directly at Janet, who responds, "You can have medication if you need it. This course teaches techniques that help most women cut down on the amount of medication they need. Some women don't require any."

I am amazed at the questions and exchange of information that already have taken place and decide to jot down a few notes while the introductions continue. In the middle of my note taking I overhear, "I saw a film on childbirth and was horrified!" (I've heard that statement before!) I start observing again. A woman is speaking. "My doctor doesn't really seem interested. He just said, 'Whatever you want to do is okay.' " Janet asks if anyone else has spoken with his doctor or resident. Josephine answers, "I see a different resident every time I go. The last time I asked a question about pain in my legs. He said, 'What do you expect?' " "That's a lot of damned help," Janet comments. (Laughter.) (I am feeling angry toward the resident and have a great desire to explain what can cause the leg pain, but I know that Janet will cover the material in one of the later classes.) As Janet begins a discussion of the necessity of a good relationship with a doctor, I gather my materials and quietly leave.

Wednesday, 8:30 PM

I arrive during the last half of class in order to observe Janet teaching exercises. She acknowledges my presence with a nod, but doesn't interrupt what she is saying. The classroom doesn't look so bare this evening. Couples, shoes off, are on blankets spread around one half of the room. Each woman is lying on her side, with a pillow under her head and another pillow supporting a leg. Husbands are either sitting next to their wives or are lying down also. Janet is reviewing relaxation with them. (In this exercise the woman concentrates on complete relaxation. The husband assists her through work and touch.)

Janet instructs, "As I talk, I want you to concentrate on relaxing each part of your body," Her voice is soft and soothing. "Relax your head. . . jaw. . . shoulders. . . arms are limp. . . feel the weight of your body sinking into the blanket. . . ." There is a wide variety of responses by the husbands. One is sitting on his heels in front of his wife; one hand is on her shoulder, the other on her knee. He doesn't move throughout Janet's dialogue. Another husband is lying down facing his wife, with his head resting on the pillow. He softly caresses her shoulder, waist, and hips and then begins again at her shoulder. Janet stops speaking and lets the couples continue on their own. She begins to move among them. One woman is on her back. Squatting, Janet speaks to her softly. The woman rolls to her side, and Janet shows her husband how to arrange the pillows. She gently massages the shoulders of another woman. When Janet leaves, the husband imitates the gentle caress. I hear tenderness in the voices of the husbands. Spontaneous giggling between couples occurs twice in this 5-minute period. Janet continues to observe the couples. She squats and speaks to one couple, but she is too far away for me to hear. She works her way back to the outside of the group. Janet continues, "Now we'll practice the slow-breathing technique learned last week. Husbands, you will time two 60-second contractions with a 30-second interval. Remember to begin and end with a cleansing breath." The couples stop to listen to Janet. The room becomes very quiet, punctuated only by scattered, soft "Contraction begins" from various parts of the room as each man begins timing his wife's "contraction." Everyone is serious. The women are staring at chosen focal points. Some men begin again with gentle caressing. The minute and the "contraction" ends. Some men shift positions.

When the second practice contraction is over, Janet asks if there are any questions. Some women sit up. One asks, "This is kind of off the subject, but when we are in labor, do we lie on a bed, a table, or what?" Janet explains, "In the labor room you'll lie on a bed. It can be adjusted to different positions." There is a brief exchange of questions and answers, "Is the delivery room table soft?" someone asks. Janet explains, "It has about 3 inches of padding, and it's softer than most doctor's tables used for pelvic exams." A woman pipes up, "Good, I thought it might be like the floor!" (Laughter.) Janet understands the woman's real question. "I have you practice on the floor because it is the most practical place here." The woman nods her head and sighs, "Oh."

"You can roll up. . . things. . . and go over to the tables; we won't need the floor anymore." Janet begins to laugh and shares with the group what she almost said. "I almost said you can roll up the floor and put it away." This time I hear some guffaws. Blankets and pillows are quickly gathered up and placed on chairs. Within a matter of minutes everyone is sitting down.

Janet asks, "What things have been bothering you now that you're at the end of pregnancy?" (What a loaded question, I think!) Silence and tenseness are in the air. Janet modifies the question. "Is it harder to sleep? To move about?" A visible relaxation of the group is taking place. "More indigestion? Hate-to-cook?" One man laughs and pokes his wife, "She hated that before she got pregnant." (Laughter.) Another husband adds, "My trouble is I can't get Roberta up in the morning. Some days she is late for work!" I gather from his tone of voice that this is a sensitive area between this couple. Defensively, the wife counters, "I can't get to sleep until 4 or 5 in the morning! I'm exhausted when the alarm goes off!" Her husband says, "But you shouldn't stay in bed." Janet says, "When the baby is born there won't be any more staying in bed for quite a while. It may be a help now to sleep late once in a while. The problem really is how to fall asleep earlier. What do the rest of you do?" From across the circle Vincent speaks up, "One night Jill couldn't sleep, so I heated up some body oil and gave her a nice massage. It really helped." (A clever idea!) The man next to him added, "The last time Sally went to the doctor, he told her to take a sleeping pill. I've always been against sleeping pills. He told me it would help develop the baby's liver." (Laughter.) (My first thought is that he must have misunderstood the doctor, but I'm not sure.) Janet explains, "I don't think your doctor was pushing pills. When one of his patients can't sleep, he has to make a choice. Is it better for her to begin labor when she is exhausted, or is it better for her to take the pills and be rested when labor starts? He chose the latter. It is difficult to handle labor if you're exhausted. I don't know about the liver jazz. I don't think I could go along with that." (Some laughter.) Janet then asks, "What is different these last couple of weeks of pregnancy?" Immediately a woman answers, "The baby drops." Janet stands up and moves to the portable blackboard. She writes "drops" on the left side of the board. On the right side she prints "Things to Do" and lists under it: "tour, preregister, pack bag, and pediatrician." She turns back to the class. "What else?," she asks. The class adds, "a sudden burst of energy," and "sometimes the uterus starts contracting." Janet lists: "nesting and BH frequently stronger," while explaining that BH means Braxton-Hicks, which is the name of the contractions felt at this stage. I take this opportunity to slip out.

Sunday, 7:30 PM

I walk to the door of Janet's home, knock, and enter. The view is dominated by a glowing fireplace. Since a crackling fire can easily mesmerize me, I consciously alert myself to the activity in the room. Two couples have already arrived. One pair is seated by a bookcase against the far wall. The other is standing in the middle of the room with Janet. By the intense but excited expressions on their faces, I know something is up. I overhear Janet saying, ". . . so he may drop by this evening if possible. He is quite excited. Things have been happening awfully fast for him this evening." I assume, and it is later confirmed, that one of the couples has delivered this evening. One of the men turns and stares at the fire. (Expectant fathers are often concerned about the birth of their baby, their wife's safety, and their ability as a labor coach. Perhaps one or more of these things is on his mind.)

"Catherine, I'm glad you could make it." Janet greets me with a wide smile. Both couples smile and say, "Hi." Even though I am not formally introduced to them or to the rest of the class, I experience what I consider to be an immediate acceptance and friendliness.

Janet takes this opportunity to give me some Lamaze material I had requested earlier. There is often an exchange of information and materials whenever two Lamaze teachers meet, even if it's just for coffee. I then sit in a chair tucked in a corner of the living room and begin to take notes.

Three couples arrive in succession. One has a tiny baby and an older woman with them. This is a returning Lamaze couple. Janet invites couples from previous classes to talk with expectant couples about their labor, delivery, and early surprises of parenthood. This is planned for the last class of the session. I assume the older woman is the baby's grandmother.

The living room phone had rung shortly before, and Janet, still talking, waves and smiles to each couple as they arrive.

The baby, bundled in pink, is held closely to the mother's body. The   **209** grandmother leads the way to three straight-back chairs and sits in the one nearest to the fireplace. The father sets the diaper bag on the floor and stands protectively by his wife as she sits down with the baby. He then sits down. They still have on their coats. It is quite obvious that they are not yet accustomed to maneuvering with their new offspring.

This is in sharp contrast to the second parent couple, arriving shortly afterwards with their 5- to 6-month-old daughter. They casually pass their baby back and forth as they alternately remove their coats. The mother unbundles the baby and then, in one flow of motion, takes a large rubberized pad, places it on the floor, smooths an infant quilt over it, and places the baby on it face down. She then sits back comfortably and chats with her husband.

Within 5 minutes everyone has arrived: five expectant couples, two couples with one baby each, one grandmother, and a woman studying to be a Lamaze teacher. Janet has managed to greet each person, answer questions, exchange information, and joke. She passes among them with great ease, stepping over purses and feet. Two couples have preferred to sit on the floor. The couples appear to be in their late 20's to late 30's.

Janet is beginning the class, "I'd like to introduce you to Sue and Joe and their daughter, Cindy, who is now 1 month old. This is Joe's mother, Mrs [X], who is visiting with them. Sue and Joe were in my previous class. Next to them are Alice and Ray and their daughter, Diane, who is 5 months old." The phone rings. Janet lifts the receiver and continues, "Will you share with us your labor and delivery experiences plus any suggestions you have for the class about those first few weeks after the baby is home? I'll let you decide who should start." Janet begins speaking to her telephone caller, and takes the phone into the kitchen.

The two couples agree that Sue and Joe should start, since their memories of labor and delivery are probably fresher. While Sue begins her description, I concentrate on observing the expectant couples. They have become almost motionless. One couple's hand caressing quickly changes to hand holding. One man leans forward, I don't notice any group reaction as Sue's baby wakes up and begins to cry. Sue bounces Cindy on her lap, then passes her to her grandmother, who continues to bounce her, but at a different rhythm. Cindy continues to cry. Grandmother gives up, crosses in front of Sue, and gives Cindy to her father. About half the expectant couples are now watching Cindy, who, as soon as she lands in Daddy's arms, takes one deep breathe and lets out a wail. Everyone laughs, but Dad. Cindy is quickly passed back to Mom. With ease and modesty, Sue begins to nurse the baby. Things quickly settle down, and Sue continues relating her labor, with Joe contributing. I find myself smiling over the noisy smacking sounds Cindy is making. Janet is back in the room and also smiling. I know she is hearing them, too. None of the other couples seem to notice. Their "all business" attitude reveals the typically high anxiety level of late-term couples.

My eye catches a sudden stiffening movement made by Alice, the other mother. A swift lifting of Diane off her lap follows. She must have picked her up off the floor while Cindy was crying. I gather she is feeling a little wet and warm. She holds the baby with her right arm about 6 inches off her lap, checks Diane's underside with her left, gives a quick touch to her own lap, as if to survey the damage, then quickly bends over and pulls a rubberized pad from the diaper bag and places it on her lap. She sets Diane back down, turns, and grins at her husband. Alice then leans to the expectant woman next to her and tells her what happened. The woman laughs audibly and tells her husband. Only one other couple appears to be aware of this "little drama."

My attention shifts as Janet begins speaking. "When labor is short, it is usually intense. It is not uncommon for the woman to become confused. Husbands, this is when you will really have to help. Your wife may forget what to do and will depend on you." From the parts of Sue's labor that I overhear I know she had a short labor and relied on Joe throughout.

Alice's labor was almost the exact opposite, very slow and controllable. "We were at home for the first 5 hours. I was lying on the couch watching TV. Finally we called Janet and asked what to do. She said,'Drink a little orange juice and walk around.' That picked things up. We were in the hospital in an hour." During this episode Alice looks at Janet, and so does the majority of the class.

Diane has been placed on the floor again. She is doing all of her 5-month-old exercises—scooting backwards, flying, smiling, and "stiff-arming" the floor. Again, none of the expectant couples seem to notice. Their prime need is to prepare for labor and delivery. They don't seem to have time to pay attention to anything else.

When Alice finishes, Janet calls attention to Diane's performance and adds, "Don't be afraid to put your baby on the floor. Get an old blanket and put the baby on it." Attention shifts to the baby's antics. There are spontaneous bursts of laughter when Diane starts "flying." She arches her back and necks, holds up her arms and legs, smiles, and begins to look around. She holds this position for about a minute. Janet asks, "Do you think you could do that?" I hear one husband murmur his amazement, and everyone begins talking. Janet announces break time and people begin standing, stretching, and talking back and forth. Janet immediately has four people waiting to speak with her. I signal my good-bye and thanks, and cross the room to the door.

SUGGESTED QUESTIONS FOR DISCUSSION AND ANALYSIS

For undergraduate students
1. Describe the nurse's leadership style. Do you think it is appropriate? How does she encourage the father's participation?
2. Cite some instances of discomfort expressed by members of the group. Discuss how these are handled.
3. Give examples of group-building functions and group task functions.
4. How do the responsibilities of the nurse to her clients differ for the nurse in independent practice from those of the more traditional hospital nurse?

For graduate students and teachers of nursing
1. Discuss how the group's level and direction of anxiety affect the learning process. How would this affect your teaching methods?

2. Compare the nurse-leader's responsibilities to her clients with her responsibilities to her clients' physicians. How well does she discharge these responsibilities?

3. Cite one technique that the nurse-leader utilizes to overcome the reluctance of some couples to touch each other in a group. What other techniques would you suggest?

4. What attention has the nurse-leader given to creating a particular social-psychological climate for her group?

5. Discuss the role of the nurse as entrepreneur with respect to its impact on the practice of nursing as it is traditionally done, in the employ of others.

6. Women who enter the Lamaze group are referred by a physician. If interested clients were allowed to enter without a referral, what might be the consequences to this nursing role?

Work in the field

Improvisation, "feeling one's way through," and being on the alert for the unexpected characterize the nurse's work in the field. These nurses, whose work brings them into community settings and patients' homes, are not immediately surrounded by organizational supports and constraints found in hospitals, features we saw earlier, which influence practice. What then shapes their work and guides their decisions in the often complex situations confronting them? The selections to follow contain much empirical data from which the reader may draw his own conclusions.

15. Surveillance in long-term illness

Charlotte F. Bambino, RN, PhD

In the analysis of these data by Bambino, the work of the public health nurse with noninstitutionalized chronically ill patients is presented from the perspective of the patient. These observations demonstrate particularly well the imbalance between the patient's definition and perception of need and the nurse's perception of the patient's situation. That is, all too frequently there are wide discrepancies between the patient's definition of his need and the nurse's definition of the patient's need. Incongruity between their respective definitions stems from many sources. One of the sources suggested here is that as the patient's physical condition improves, allowing him to bring his daily routines within his control, his focus and emphasis on what is needful continue to shift. Unfortunately, the nurse's perception, and hence her definition of the patient's situation, have not kept pace with these definitional shifts. Thus, we see some disheartening consequences for both patients and public health nursing in general. The reader should look further and draw on the introductory material to this section for other factors influencing the nurse's performance.

In this chapter I will describe clients' perceptions of professional service for surveillance in the home of long-term illness. The data are from an exploratory study concerned with how, when, and under what conditions clients with long-term illnesses perceive that the Public Health Nurse Home Visit Service (PHNHVS) assists them in family health care.

Professionals concerned with the delivery of health care services generally agree

Adapted from Bambino, Charlotte F., PhD: *Dimensions of Acceptance: Client Perceptions of Public Health Nurse Home Visit Service,* thesis, University of California, Berkeley, 1969.

that the continuing medical management of long-term illness is an important aspect of comprehensive health care. Orientations keyed to the control of the health condition with focuses on pathology and the concept of the patient as a sick, dependent person unable to cope with his needs have hindered professionals in looking at clients as human beings capable of assuming responsibility for managing their conditions of health. One of the consequences of these orientations is the tendency of professionals to "hang onto clients" through continued surveillance. (Although measures for control of some long-term illnesses are known, by and large, procedures for cure or prevention of them are not yet known to medical science. This latter aspect of long-term illness serves to routinize surveillance.)

From the clients' point of view, when the crisis is over and other tasks of daily living assume greater priority than the condition of illness per se, professional surveillance, particularly when prolonged and routine, tends to have little meaning for the clients. At times it may even increase the clients' resistance to future health care. Attention to clients as human beings with positive potentials for self-care and the understanding of client priorities can help professionals plan more objectively for effective delivery of health services as well as for utilization of health personnel.

ACCEPTED BUT AMBIVALENT

Clients who had considerable difficulty in identifying aspects of the present PHNHVS being rendered that was of assistance to them, or who referred to helpful aspects of their former experiences with prior nurses who had rendered service to the same client for the same specific problem of long-term illness, constituted the clients in the accepted but ambivalent category. In contrast to clients who overtly expressed no need for PHNHVS, these clients did identify aspects of this service that were helpful to them, as well as aspects of the service that were not needed.

Most of these clients had continued to receive service over a period of several years, although there were some who had received service only for several months. All these clients were in situations in which the medical regimen had been established. They were knowledgeable about their diagnosis and aware of the established treatment procedures, and their source of medical care and the relationships with their physicians were established. In contrast to clients who found the PHNHVS more helpful, these clients' conditions of illness that led them to seek and establish health care were not acute or stressful. Therefore, these clients may be viewed as having reached a plateau in which varying degrees of adjustment and management of the illness had been made. Various service workers, such as housekeepers, visiting nurses, physical therapists, and social workers, needed for the maintenance of this plateau and prevention of further illness had been obtained. All these clients had been hospitalized during an acute phase of their illness.

In contrast to those who found the PHNHVS more helpful, these clients did not perceive the nurse as a participant in the medical treatment plan. Her source of authority was still perceived in relation to the source of medical care used by the client after hospitalization. Clients' expectations of what the nurse was supposed to 215 do were vague and not related to prescribed treatment activities. "She has to come; it's her job; the hospital sent her; you know she is the nurse; she is a nurse, by golly, and she knows all about the records of sick people like me." Most client expectations of the PHNHVS were in the nature of an extension of medical control or one of surveillance, whether the authority perceived by clients was prescribed or imputed. "She comes along every so often to see how I'm doing." "She does that public kind of social work, and she has to make a report." Even clients who had experienced PHNHVS for 2 or more years did not know who the nurse was. Who she worked for was unclear. One woman whom the nurse had visited almost twice a month for 3 years said, "Oh you know, she was assigned to me, and she's just a friend." (This latter situation was not one of delegated authority, such as found in the treatment of a patient with tuberculosis.)

In general, in this category clients' perceptions of assistance focused almost entirely on those activities of the nurse in terms of nontechnical skills. Most of the clients tended to place emphasis on using the nurse's position as an intermediary within the system of medical care to resume or maintain control of their situations and to facilitate carrying out the prescribed regimen for care. The nature of the intermediary activity focused on the mechanics for coordination between health and other community agencies.

Those clients whose regimen had been established fairly recently where those who were not likely to have previously experienced PHNHVS. Their conditions of illness were new, and they tended to perceive assistance in terms of obtaining equipment, medications, medical reports, and appointments.

Those clients who had received long-continued service perceived the nurse mainly in terms of a "medical monitor agent," in situations of legal control as a "checker upper," and as a "clinic appointment reminder." A further aspect of the intermediary position of the nurse resulting from client experience with the PHNHVS, and sometimes not identified by clients, was a non–home visit activity in which clients used the telephone to obtain information "not important enough to call a doctor," or about a facility or appointment.

Although clients in this category did not perceive PHNHVS as needed at this time, they did perceive activities rendered by the nurse at an earlier point in time in a manner similar to those clients in the helpful category. Thus, client ambivalence stemmed from continued medical surveillance or control for their conditions of long-term illness. The following discussion describes some of the conditions surrounding the situations of surveillance in which the PHNHVS was rendered to clients. These situations were (1) when the regimen was established and surveillance was being established, (2) when surveillance was established, and (3) over a period of time when the nurse continued the PHNHVS as an agent of surveillance.

Regimen recently established; initial surveillance clarifying remnants of medical conflict

Clients who had returned home from the hospital and had received PHNHVS for a shorter time than those whose regimen had been completely established were still in the process of learning ways of carrying out their regimen at home. Although the source of medical care for follow-up was established, and prescriptions were clear, management of particular aspects of the regimen to be carried out or needs attendant to the illness influencing management of the illness at home had not been completely resolved. Unlike clients in the helpful category, these clients did not perceive the public health nurse as a participant in the medical treatment plan. The prescription had been learned by clients or care agents, or assistance of another type of worker had been obtained. These clients tended to perceive the PHNHVS mainly as an intermediary clarifying remnants of medical conflict. Rather than conflict in medical prescriptions, the assistance perceived was in terms of filling the gaps in the mechanism for coordination between hospital and outpatient community facilities used by clients for continued health care while at home.

Although assistance was identified by these clients, the import of the assistance was viewed as temporary in nature and not essential for continuance of service. As the client's control for management of his illness increased, the degree of import of the service was reduced. Acceptance of the PHNHVS (which clients had not requested) was influenced by the clients' perceptions of the authority of the nurse in relationship to the medical source of care used and the behavior of the nurse in rendering the service.

In relation to nonmedical needs, such as for housekeeping services and jobs and financial distress, clients' descriptions of assistance from the PHNHVS were limited to nurses' suggestions of appropriate community resources. A typical response in relation to these needs was, "There is nothing she can do about it." On the other hand, a new type of intermediary service, although frequently not recognized by clients as being of assistance, was a non–home visit service rendered by the public health nurse via the telephone. Three major types of assistance were in the form of information: (1) information about appointments or where to go, (2) information or advice not important enough to bother the doctor, and (3) remnants of medical conflict that clients were not able to interpret or manage.

A man discharged from the county hospital had been given medications and instructions for their use. However, arrangements for payments, medical authorization, and the route for replenishment of the medication were not clear. In this situation the man viewed the nurse as easing the struggle to obtain medications.

In another situation a client with tuberculosis did not struggle but stopped taking medications when the supply ran out. Rather then resisting taking medications, this man, having resumed his accustomed work role, with the acuity of his illness passed, found that the unclear route for obtaining refills for his medicines and the cost involved made the effort to obtain medications too much of a struggle. He viewed the nurse as guiding him to the appropriate resource and obtaining medical authorization for the medicines. He said, "She was nice, but now that I have my medicines there is no reason for her to come and see me, although I know it's her job, and it's just something she has to do." Another man awaiting his last sputum report, which would determine the behavior allowed by the regimen, said the nurse let him know about the laboratory reports sooner than he would have learned the results by the usual route. He said, "It was nice of her, the nurse, to let me know about the report, but there isn't any need for her to visit me. I don't know how she could help me do any more than I'm already doing. What I really need to do is figure out how I'm going to work out my payments for the house. . . . "

When there was no medical conflict and the situation was not legal in nature, clients often imputed medical authority to the nurse similar to that of a legal situation, even though, in fact, this was not so. A man who was under the care of a private physician and who had had a "stroke" that had left him with some immobility described the nurse's source of authority in vague terms not related to his particular physician. He said, "You know, she knows about all the records and things of all the people. She told me not to wait so long next time—before I go to see my doctor. She's a good gal. . . . I joke with her, but I've got all my appointments, and the doc told me I could call him any time in-between if I feel something isn't right."

Surveillance established

As previously noted, clients perceived the purpose of the nurse's visit in relation to the medical source of care used. When the procedures for nurse surveillance were clear, as in tuberculosis, clients described the nurse's activities in terms of the preventive aspects of the illness, such as telling them about their clinic appointments for their x-rays or continuing prescribed medications. Although clients were not able to describe assistance other than the prescribed procedure of "checking up" on their behavior, they did describe assistance from the *prior* nurse as being something concrete that she did, such as teaching about injections. When no mechanical procedures were involved, they described the activities of a prior nurse in terms of procurement of medications or a coordinative activity rather than "teaching about" medications or a disease condition. No client mentioned any assistance other than the prescribed one of nurse surveillance. Most clients described the present nurse as a "nice person" even though "there is really no need for her to visit."

Positive and negative aspects of both the behavior and activities of prior nurses were described in various combinations. The present nurse may have assumed authority for more frequent visits than the prescribed procedure. One man described a situation of this kind: "All the nurses are good nurses, and they know their jobs; they know how to give shots and all that. You can tell when the nurse knows her business. Mrs. S., who keeps coming now, just talks and that nonsense—no sense in her coming. She tells me I should put a hat on when I go outside." (In the record of three nurse visits the major focus of the nursing notes centered on, "Mr. [X] was outdoors with [or without] a hat on," or, "Today Mr. [X] was outside and had on an overcoat.")

In addition, the nurse may have also extended her role. A woman stated, "The nurse that comes now doesn't do anything, but she's nice, and I enjoy her; we just talk about everything in general. The nurse that used to come was good with checking with the kids about their medicines while I was in the hospital. But when I came home from the hospital, she started telling me how to treat my kids. I kicked her out and told her not to come back, because it was none of her business."

As previously noted, clients spoke of a nurse's behavior in relation to the manner in which she explained the legal requirements. "She was very nice, and told me what to expect about the number of sputums and all I was supposed to do. She talked with me, but I used my common sense about being near children and all that, like I was supposed to—you know, wait 'til I got my third sputum report, like my doctor told me."

There were situations in which prescriptions were less clear, and clients imputed authority to the nurse. Some clients obtained medical care via admission to a health department program in which the public health nurse completed eligibility applications. These clients continued medical care at a specific hospital. Care was financed from funds administered by the lealth department program. The patient's progress was routinely by the health department program. The patient's progress was routinely procedure that required intermittent hospitalization, such as a child with a heart condition (intraseptal defect). The frequency, timing, direction, and purpose of the PHNHVS were mainly determined by the public health nurse. Prescribed directives were less clear than those previously discussed. These clients (parents) imputed authority to the public health nurse in relation to the hospital source of care as a county program, and they felt obliged to receive the public health nurse in their homes. As stated by several women, "She [the nurse] was very nice; she came from the county, and she did everything she knew how to do to help with the appointments and all that, but there was nothing else she could do." "Well, you know it is a county program, and as taxpayers we are entitled to such care, and the public health nurse goes with the program. She was very nice, and I'm always glad to see her and chat with her, but I don't know why she visits—there is really no need for her to come. She did help us fill out those forms, but my husband and I could have done that. Besides, when something happens, I just bring Tim right to the hospital."

The lapse of time between clients' attendance at medical care facilities and the nurse's receipt of the routine client medical progress report influenced the time when the PHNHVS was rendered. During this interim, clients had already obtained assistance needed elsewhere. The PHNHVS was of little importance, and even of less significance, when the nurse assumed authority by her own general nurse prescription. One woman, whose 16-year-old daughter had a severe heart condition, described a situation of this nature: "The nurse that used to come always seemed to visit us after the doctor had already told us what to do, and she was just interested in how we were getting along. She kept telling Sandra, my daughter, what to eat or not to eat and not to drink so many cokes. Sandra didn't like her. The present nurse used to visit us, but now she just sends us cards to remind us about doctor appointments, and I guess that helps."

In other situations clients imputed authority to the nurse when the nurse did not have medical prescription. When neighbors or other community workers referred clients for PHNHVS, client response to this service was perceived in very vague terms and mainly in terms of the nurse as a person. "My housekeeper called her to see how I was doing. She's nice, but I'm doing fine. It's all right if she comes to see me."

Often clients imputed authority to the nurse in relation to the clients' initial contacts with the public health nurse for purposes other than the present conditions of long-term illness. A woman who had previously received PHNHVS for health supervision of her child and who was recently recovering from a heart condition still viewed the nurse in relation to her original use of the service for child care. The client did not see the nurse's assistance as related to her existing condition: "She's the baby nurse."

The nurse as an agent of surveillance

When the regimen consisted mainly of taking medications, clients saw little need for PHNHVS. They were aware of the importance of taking their medications, and it was an easy procedure to follow. When emergencies arose requiring hospitalization, or some changes occurred in the clients' conditions they sought care directly. Over a period of time clients learned which type of worker was of most help to them for their particular conditions and situations of illness.

If the regimen entailed long-term intermittent hospitalization with changes in treatment plans, the long-established client relationship with the doctor or locale of medical care usually taught the client the necessary procedure.

Frequently the timing of the PHNHVS was not in conjunction with the time in which changes in the regimen occurred. In the meantime, clients had managed the situation by themselves or with other sources of help, such as friends and relatives. Thus, clients viewed the PHNHVS as being of limited assistance, and the nurse visits consisted mainly of a rehash of what the client had already done. (Nurse records were replete with descriptive information about the client's medical condition and progress but dealt little with public health nurse assistance.)

In due time nonmedical problems, such as finances, inability to work or find a job, or the necessity of finding housekeeping help, were situations viewed by clients as problems with which the nurse could not assist. "What can she do? She can't get me a job." Increasingly, the client's medical problem became stabilized and assumed second place in relation to a more pressing new problem. When the PHNHVS continued to focus on the old problem, which the client felt was under control (and, in fact, it was), the PHNHVS was viewed as being routine and of little salience.

A man had been routinely followed for years as a tuberculosis patient. He had a "stroke" and was being cared for by his wife, who described the PHNHVS as just the nurse dropping by to remind her of his need for an x-ray. She felt this was not important, because "the nervous-like spells" of her husband constituted her present concern in caring for him. In another situation, a young woman discharged from the psychiatric unit of the county hospital said the public health nurse's concern for her children attending the child health conference would just have to wait. She first had to straighten out her marital problems.

Some clients expressed personal preference for an older nurse who knew the system and whose own experiences in living would supposedly render the nurse greater understanding of the clients' problems of marital discord and of the daily problems of living and rearing children, rather than a "book-oriented" young nurse whose advice had little applicability to the reality of the clients' needs.

When long-term illness occurred in young families who were engaged in the rearing of children and family planning, many other problems concerning family living were more likely to assume priority over the stabilized regimen of long-term illness. Surveillance for the condition of long-term illness thus was not relevant. Elderly clients with long-term illness whose family-rearing responsibilities were completed tended to view surveillance as unnecessary in terms of a kind of philosophical complacency. "What difference does it make? When you get to be my age you just expect things to happen to your health."

ACCEPTED BUT NOT HELPFUL

Clients who overtly expressed that the PHNHVS was not needed or who described the service as not being helpful constituted the category of accepted but not helpful. "There is no need for her to visit; she doesn't do anything, but she is a very nice lady" typified client response in this category.

The most characteristic feature of these clients is that they had been receiving PHNHVS for a long period of time, some to the extent of 3 years. The medical regimens and the clients' modes of obtaining medical care had long been established. Their illnesses could mainly be viewed as chronic and the nature of their regimens as routinized, consisting by and large of taking medications and carrying out general hygienic and precautionary measures for their conditions of illness. There were a few clients whose long-term illness was of more recent origin and who had previously experienced PHNHVS for another condition of illness in the family.

In general, care for patients in this category could be viewed as that of prolonged surveillance. The crucial factor that distinguished clients in this category from those in the ambivalent category, in relation to surveillance, was the fact that although these clients had received PHNHVS over a period of time and had accepted this service, they did not see it as needed or helpful. The legitimacy of this prolonged surveillance or the acceptance of it by clients was influenced by their perceptions of medical authority prescribed or imputed to the nurse as a routine agent of surveillance and by the behavior of the nurse. "It's her job; she has to check up; she doesn't do anything, but she has to make a report." The behavior of the nurse as a person, "a nice person," and her activity of "social chating" ("She just comes around and talks") made the routine function of asking "the same old questions all the time" tolerable and made prolonged surveillance more palatable.

Aspects of nurse authority and behavior and clients' conditions of illness combined to create various situations in which clients did not perceive PHNHVS as needed or helpful.

SUGGESTED QUESTIONS FOR DISCUSSION AND ANALYSIS

For undergraduate students

1. What major factors may account for an increased nurse-patient ratio in ambulatory versus inpatient settings?
2. What role changes may be experienced by patients with chronic respiratory or cardiac problems? How might you obtain this information?
3. When caring for a group of chronically ill patients, what baseline information is essential for establishing nursing care priorities?
4. What role conflicts might the nurse experience in this agency?
5. What kind of knowledge and clinical experience would facilitate your preparation to care for chronically ill patients and their families?

For graduate students and teachers of nursing

1. How might patient expectations of health professionals differ in ambulatory versus inpatient settings?
2. As part of a clinical course you are exploring the role of a clinical specialist in a public health agency. You observed that the public health nurses function very independently, and support between peers in almost nonexistent. What strategies can you use to increase colleagueship?
3. What does the nurse use to learn about the patient's perceptions of his illness?
4. Under what circumstances could a nurse assume primary responsibility for a group of patients? What issues and major factors must be considered?
5. What curriculum changes may be needed within your institution to facilitate student learning about chronic illness? Continuity of care?
6. What specific behavior promotes colleagueship between health professionals?
7. What positive outcomes may result from faculty involvement in the delivery of care?

16. The public health nurse: some aspects of work

Marcella Z. Davis, RN, DNSc

These field notes were collected over a 4-month period as part of research for a doctoral degree in nursing in the area of chronic illness. The sections selected for this book describe the quality of the day-to-day work situation of the public health nurse and the array of problems that she must cope with "on the spot" in her inner-city district. We follow the nurse along city streets through such work environments as roach-infested buildings, the city jail, and dreary boarding houses, some of which have been condemned. The field notes are of particular interest because they illustrate what some nurses do when confronted with a patient population whose cultural values, living conditions, and life-styles differ from their own and when the patient's problems are not of a purely medical nature and frequently are embedded in conditions that existed long before these nurses ever came on the scene.

In the past week I have gone out with two public health nurses, each taking me into a different section of the city. The first district to be described was in an impoverished area. I had no knowledge of this section except that it was a location for many warehouses, and I wondered whom we could possibly be going to see there. Much to my surprise, there were small, rather run-down, two-family wooden dwellings occupied by very poor people. The public health nurse I went out with today was a young woman in her late 20's. She and I took the bus from the public health office to her district. While we were on the bus, she made several comments about her district, such as, "There's very little point in out going there at this hour because most of the people there don't get up until 11 AM." She explained that they stay up all night and don't get up until late morning or noon. Most of her

223

clients were blacks; some were Chicano, and all were very poor. As it happened, we did visit several homes where people were awake and about. This was 9:30 AM.

ARTHRITIC PATIENT WHO LIVES ALONE

The first stop was at the home of an unmarried middle-aged black woman with a diagnosis of chronic arthritis. As we rang the bell, I asked the nurse if Miss Ryan was expecting her. She answered, "Oh, we don't make appointments in this area. It's absolutely useless." She added, "I just drop in, and anyway she is always home." After a few minutes' wait Miss Ryan came to the door and let us in. I was introduced as a nurse who was interested in seeing how the public health nurse worked. Miss Ryan led us in through a narrow, dingy hallway. We entered what appeared to be a living room–bedroom; however, all the furniture and accoutrements in there were clearly for a bedroom. The room was piled nearly to the ceiling with clothing, folded sheets, rags, boxes, and so on. In the corner was a small window with a torn curtain. It was closed and covered with condensed moisture, which prevented one from seeing out. Her bed in the corner was a pile of two or three very lumpy mattresses. Piled up at the head of the bed were several large lumpy pillows. There were any number of blankets of all different sizes and degrees of wear thrown over the bed. The dresser was piled high with medications and bottles (some filled, some unfilled), and unwashed teaspoons.

A chair was cleared so that I could sit down while the nurse made her visit. The nurse stood at the bedside talking with the patient who sat on the edge of the bed. Earlier the nurse had told me she had been "carrying" Miss Ryan for over a year. During this time she had been visiting her two to three times a week because Miss Ryan had been depressed and lonely and wouldn't eat. The patient was going "downhill" according to the nurse. However, at this point in her illness Miss Ryan looked very chipper and seemed quite well. The nurse explained that during the spiral downward she (the nurse) had contacted the homemaker service. A woman was sent out to the patient's home three times a week. The patient enjoyed this homemaker, who apparently was from Louisiana and who, according to the patient, "talks just like me and knows what I need." Between the nurse and the homemaker insisting that the patient eat because she was failing in health and strength, the patient had resumed her eating patterns and had improved physically.

Strategies and other tactics

The nurse told me later that she had to use "fear" with Miss Ryan as a way of getting her to do what the nurse wanted her to do. The nurse explained, "I told her if she wasn't going to do what I say, I was just not going to go there anymore." And too, when the patient complained of being lonely, the nurse, knowing her to be a religious woman, suggested that she read her Bible at those times.

Nurse-patient interaction

On this visit the patient happily told the nurse, "I washed my hair on Sunday." Both the patient and the nurse seemed to be quite delighted with this

224

accomplishment. Miss Ryan told the nurse about all the other things she had done since the nurse had visited last, "I managed to get to the back porch and water the flowers this morning. . . . I cleaned the mirror over there; see it." The nurse complimented the patient on the fact that she was wearing a dress. The dress was quite torn and was held together by large safety pins.

Through the social service the nurse got Miss Ryan a very sturdy large commode to keep by her bedside. Prior to this the patient had been using an old tin can that was inefficient.

Patient's social network

Miss Ryan had a sister-in-law who came in once a week to cook her one meal. Other than the sister-in law, the homemaker, who continued to come three times a week, and the public health nurse, who came about once a week, no one else came to visit.

Social worker's visit

Miss Ryan told me that once the social worker had come to visit (she never does, as a rule) and had begun to tidy up her place, which had upset the patient very much. Miss Ryan explained, "I told her I need everything out so I can reach it with my cane. I can't go looking for things and pushing drawers and closets open. If I need anything, I have to be able to pull it to me with this handle of my cane."

Miss Ryan was cared for through Medi-Cal. The public health nurse was in touch with her physician but said she communicated with him about her very infrequently.

Nurse-patient relationship

The nurse was very pleased with Miss Ryan during this visit and seemed equally pleased in demonstrating some of her accomplishments to me. The nurse told me, "This patient likes me. I think she thinks of me as a granddaughter. She bought me a small flashlight so that when I have to go home at night, I'll be able to see my door and keys."

POVERTY, SUPERSTITION, AND NURSING STRATEGY

We walked another few blocks to an old four-story wooden building. As we walked through the narrow, dingy, almost dark corridors, the nurse instructed me, "Take a deep breath; you're going to need it when we come into this house." In answer to the nurse's knock, the door opened slowly, revealing a very tiny girl. Within seconds, a bunch of little kids rushed to the door. The mother came, recognized the nurse, and fully opened the door by removing the chain. I was introduced. We came into a practically barren room; I guess one could designate it as a living room. On one side was a huge and completely broken couch. In the other corner was a single bed. There were two windows at one part of the room with torn shades and no curtains; the windows were shut tight. There was no covering on the floor; it was wooden and bare. On one wall was a woven picture of President

Kennedy tacked up near the ceiling. Across from it, also tacked up near the ceiling, was a picture of horses grazing in the fields. In the corner was a large TV that was turned on. There were no toys visible. There were five preschool-aged children here. All the kids had on torn, soiled undershirts, no other clothing, and no shoes. One child had begun kindergarten (this was the child who had opened the door). She went to the afternoon session and therefore was home that morning.

On a bed in another room, but visible from where we were standing, was an infant lying on top of the bed with a shirt and diaper on. The mother was a young woman, neatly dressed in pink slacks; a blouse loosely hung about her waist, and on her feet were sandles in good condition. She hadn't said one word to us; the nurse did all the talking. The mother shook her head "yes" or "no" in very small movements. From my observer's point of view I began to wonder if she understood what the nurse was saying, until at one point she yelled out to the children, "Stop making so much noise." The nurse asked to see the baby. When the mother brought the baby to the nurse, the nurse asked her about the baby's diet and if he was eating well. The baby looked very well and alert.

The nurse instructed the mother to take the baby to the well-baby clinic on Thursday for a checkup. The mother shook her head "yes."

When we left, I asked the nurse how she knew the mother would take the baby to the clinic. She answered, "Those kids look dirty, and they don't look like any kids we know, but I know this mother takes care of her kids." She went on to explain, "I told this mother to feed her baby on rice, and I know she is eating rice." I asked how she knew this. She explained that one day while she was out on the street, she happened to observe the mother (unknown to the mother) walking into the grocery store. She waited for the mother to come out, and sticking out the bag was a box of rice. The nurse was very pleased to see this, because it meant that the mother was following through with her suggestions.

Nursing strategy

This same mother used to put a penny over the baby's umbilicus. The nurse tried to get the mother to stop this practice and explained that the umbilicus would get infected. Each time the nurse visited, she took the penny off and gave the explanation. But on each return visit the penny was on the umbilicus. When the nurse realized that she couldn't get the mother to stop putting the penny on, she told the mother to be sure to put alcohol on the penny before putting it on the umbilicus and to wrap it clean. This seemed to work okay.

According to the nurse, at one time this home had an almost unbearable stench of urine, making it almost unbearable to stay in there. However, there was no strong smell of urine when we were there; I would describe it more like stale cooking odors. It was bearable at least for the 20 minutes we were there.

When the mother went out to the grocery store, as she did the morning the nurse observed her, she left her children unattended by a sitter and in the care of the 5-year-old child.

COPING WITH OUTSIDE ENVIRONMENTS

We walked a few blocks into another neighborhood with some trees, grass, benches, and swings in a small park area. The nurse told me that blacks lived on one side of this green area and Filipinos on the other. The nurse visited the homes of the blacks. As we walked up the street, I noticed a group of men standing idly against a parked car and others against a building, all watching us. I wondered if they were going to say anything to us and mentioned this to the nurse. She said at one time this had been a problem for her. She had received verbal abuse from the men and had been challenged with questions like "What the hell do you want here?" or "What are you doing in this neighborhood?" She told the men that she was there to give nursing care to some people in the neighborhood. Sometimes the comments to her were of a flirtatious nature, such as "Can I carry your bag; isn't it too heavy for you?" She said she was not frightened as she once had been, because she had never been harmed and felt she could handle the verbal comments. However, there were times when she would go out of her way to avoid certain streets when trying to reach her car. At times she would walk in the street so as not to pass too closely to these groups of men.

PATIENT WITH CANCER

We walked up to the second floor in the apartment house of a middle-aged black woman with terminal cancer. The patient was dressed in a pair of slacks and a blouse with worn slippers on her feet, and she was up and about. The cancer had metastasized and was now causing her to have difficulties in breathing. She was seen periodically at a clinic to get her lungs tapped. The nurse had been seeing her for slightly over a year, and she visited every few weeks. Since the nurse didn't make appointments with these clients, the patient was surprised but pleased to see her.

Public health nurse completes what others leave undone

The patient brought out a stack of pills she had recently been given and wasn't sure she understood how to take them. As it happened, the woman had not been taking the medication correctly. The nurse instructed the patient to eat something, such as some bread, before she took the pills. The patient complained that she was having diarrhea very badly. The nurse explained that this was because she was not taking any food before she took the pills, and her intestines were irritated. The patient happily reported to the nurse, "I went to the doctor a few days ago, and he listened to my lung and said I have only a little bit of fluid on it; that's a good sign, isn't it?" The patient continued in what sounded like a pleased tone, "I think I'm going to live until Christmas (this was October), maybe even past then, because I ain't in diapers yet, like Mr. . . . "(I didn't catch the name.) Apparently this woman knew a friend who also had cancer and in the terminal stages was so incontinent that he had to wear padding (diapers) in bed.

The nurse questioned the patient further, "Did the doctor tell you to restrict fluids and salt?" The woman said, "Nobody told me that." The nurse explained to   227 the patient that if she watched her diet and fluid intake, this would keep the fluid down in her lungs, and she could breath more easily. She instructed her to breathe deeply five times periodically through the day and stretch out her chest as much as possible, saying that this too would keep the fluid from forming too quickly. The patient was very visibly happy with these little bits of information and looked at me and said, "She's the best nurse I ever had; she's been wonderful to me."

While we were in the kitchen, the patient lifted her blouse, saying, "Look, look, I have a rash here," pointing to her midriff. Again the nurse questioned her about pills and discovered that the patient was taking Librium four times a day, Darvon, and a sedative at night. Each one of these medications had been prescribed at a different time in the patient's illness career for a different reason. No one had ever checked on the patient to see if her symptoms had subsided. The nurse explained, "If you're not feeling so nervous anymore, stop taking the Darvon and don't take the sedative, because the Librium should be enough to keep you relaxed and should put you to sleep at night."

POSTPARTUM VISIT

We left and walked along the street to another rather dilapidated building. We were to make a postpartum visit. The client was a 21-year-old white woman with three children, and all were living in a small, cramped dark apartment. The client was in the process of a divorce. Questions were asked about contraceptive pills. The nurse answered them, making it seem like a very complicated procedure. As the nurse was explaining, two little boys (under 3 years) were tugging at the mother and whining. To me it looked impossible for the mother to listen, let alone comprehend these very complicated instructions. The nurse was holding the infant in her lap as she talked to the mother. At one point one of the boys took some food from the kitchen. There was an altercation between the mother and the child. The nurse said to the mother, "You have to show them who's boss. Don't worry, you won't crush them, but you have to be firm. You have to be as stubborn as they are."

The client told the nurse she needed more money from welfare but the nurse either didn't hear (I failed to check this out) or else ignored the statement. As we walked away from this home the nurse explained to me how she tried to find ways for these people to save money. For example, if the baby was having problems with teething she didn't tell them to go out and buy "gummies" or toys for the baby to chew on, but since she was certain they all had whiskey in the house, she told them of a folk remedy. Apparently, one mixed some whiskey and sugar with warm water and gave this to the baby. She said that what she told them wasn't always scientifically correct, but it was adequate and appropriate.

CREATIVE NURSING

The nurse told me about a mother's group she had started for postnatal instruction. She had started it because she felt too lazy (those were her words) to

228

carry around all the equipment to each house. She had found that the mothers were willing to meet in each other's home for this instruction. The nurse continued to get referrals to the group from the mothers. At first the mothers had talked about the children and the problems of caring for them, but now the conversation had shifted to themselves. The mothers were pleased to have the time away from the children and to talk about things of interest to them. The group told the nurse that the level of instruction and information on physiology was better than anything they had ever had in high school. According to the nurse, this mothers' class had caught on in one of the other apartment houses and one of the mothers was acting as group leader. (This sounded like a creative idea of the nurse; I would have to ask her more about it.)

NONCOMPLIANCE AND THE NURSE

I indicated to the nurse that we had seen patients that morning who were very happy to see her and that I wondered if she had shown me her success cases. I asked if she had anyone who didn't want to see her, and she said she had. If she had a patient who didn't want to do what she thought the patient should do regarding clinic visits, taking medications, or anything else involving neglect of health, she would let the social worker know The social worker from the welfare department was the one who controlled the checks, so in this way the nurse used the social worker as leverage. However, she said the situation had to be pretty bad before she brought in the social worker. Another tactic of this nurse was as follows: if a patient was very sick and wouldn't do what she asked she let him get sicker until he "got his fill of it"; then, she commented, "I move in, and then he'll listen."

Another comment on the use of fear: this nurse said she did use fear quite frequently to get clients to do what she wanted them to do. However, she remembered she was told in nursing school never to use fear to move a patient. "I use it because it works," she observed. Fear, as she was using it, would seem to mean withholding some attention or service to get compliance.

FROM THE SOCIAL WORKER'S PERSPECTIVE

The nurse was talking about the kinds of difficulties she occasionally had with social workers. For example, a social worker phoned her one day and insisted that the nurse go into a particular home to see that the mother took her children to the clinic because it was thought that they were suffering from malnutrition. Apparently the social worker saw sores on the childrens' legs and assumed this to be a sign of malnutrition. The nurse went into the home and found the mother to be very angry with both the nurse and the social worker and was reluctant to let the nurse look at the children. However, the nurse did get a look at the childrens' legs and said they were flea bites that had become infected from scratching. The nurse did not insist that the mother go to the clinic. The incident raised a row between the nurse and the social worker. The nurse claimed that the social worker made a home visit about once a year, was very biased, and furthermore, had no background   229 in medicine; yet she went about diagnosing. The nurse accused the social worker of seeing everything as a case of malnutrition and the patients as all trying to get something out of the system for nothing.

THE ROACH

Several days later we were walking, and the nurse asked me if I had noticed the roaches in the houses we went to. I had not and was surprised, since I'm very wary about roaches. She then told me the story of how she had known she was at last a public health nurse. That was when she had seen a roach on her coat sleeve and had merely flicked him off. Prior to this "benchmark" she had responded with revulsion. However, on the next day's rounds I did notice roaches in one home. They were crawling up and down the walls like flies. According to the nurse, this was the home of a "hippie family."

HIPPIE FAMILY

As we walked to the door I heard very loud classical music playing in the background, and a pretty young woman answered the door. The woman and the nurse seemed to be very friendly. We walked into the kitchen, and lying on an old quilt on the floor was a 6-month-old baby boy fully dressed in bright blue corduroy overalls and a white polo shirt. (My thoughts harked back momentarily to the meagerly clad children we had seen a few days ago.) There were toys strewn about him. There was a huge turkey (about 15 pounds) sitting on the side table waiting to be put in the oven. Over the sink was a sign that read, "The best roach is a dead roach." The mother was neatly dressed in a blouse and slacks with cotton booties on her feet. Her hair was in a bun. The house, a tiny shack, was in utter shambles. Each room was piled high to the ceiling with clothing, equipment, and lots of boxes of all sizes. Nothing seemed to have a place except on top of the next item. This was to be a postpartum visit; however, it had all the overtones of a social call. The nurse and the client became involved in a long discussion on the Zen diet, its merits, and so on. The nurse shifted the conversation at some point to the baby's diet and suggested the mother start using table food for him. This family was on the highest level of welfare income one could have. Neither husband nor wife were working. While we were there, the husband answered a call about a friend who had just tried to commit suicide. The nurse suggested they take the friend to the city hospital, where there was a new psychiatric program for suicide cases. The young mother answered in a shocked voice, "We wouldn't do that to our friends; we're going to keep him here until he cools off."

COUNTY JAIL

After we left this house, we went to the county jail to give some prenatal instruction to a young mother who was there on a count of prostitution. When we got to the seventh floor, we had to show all kinds of identification that we were nurses. The nurse's bag, which was the official bag of the Public Health Service apparently wasn't enough for the police. We were led into the jail proper, where we met a woman police lieutenant. She filled all the stereotypes of a female cop; she was short, tough, and mannish. We went into her office, and on one side of the wall was a window looking out into a huge room. I was struck sharply by the similarity between what I saw in this jail room and a state psychiatric hospital. The room was filled with young women sitting on long benches; a couple of them were sitting at a table. No one was doing anything, and everyone had a very bored, lethargic, sluggish look on her face, with her body in a slumped position. They turned their heads very slowly and looked at us. Their faces were expressionless. Some stared at us the entire time we talked with the lieutenant, which was about 5 minutes, and others dropped their eyes and looked away.

As it happened, the woman we went to see was not there. She had delivered her baby, and as the lieutenant said, "We modified her." I later learned that this meant, "We let her go." They did not know where she went to live, so the nurse had to go to another section of the jail, to the probation officer, to find out for her records. If the woman were in the district, the nurse had to go visit her. If the woman were in another area of the city, the nurse had to officially indicate this on her records. We couldn't find the probation officer (they were not in their offices), and the nurse didn't pursue this any further. She closed the case.

FINANCIAL DISTRICT

On another occasion I went to the financial district of the city. The nurse I went with told me she had the smallest case load in the city because the area was primarily a business one. However, there were small hotels and some dilapidated houses that I had never noticed before, scattered among the business section.

The day we went out it was raining, and we walked to every visit we had to make. The first visit was to a hotel that housed only Filipino men. The visit was to check up on a man who had symptoms of TB. The man was on his way out when we saw him, and the nurse asked him to please come back to his room so that we could talk with him. He agreed, and we entered his tiny room with two walls filled with neatly hung up clothing. He sat down and pulled out some recent photographs of his family in the Philippines. We all looked at new and old photographs as the nurse asked him some questions. When we left, the nurse told me the story of the time she had come to visit this man, and on not finding him in had left her professional calling card. The very next day he had come to the clinic and wanted to know what he had done wrong. Since the nurse had left her card and he was now responding, the nurse had to reassure him that she had just been making a routine call.

We left this hotel, walked a few blocks, and arrived at a dilapidated apartment house. The door was locked, but the nurse pulled out a key from her bag. I expressed surprise. She said that the little old man she visited here had had the key made for her so that she could enter without his having to come down a long flight of stairs. The call was to check on his arrested TB.

We then made several other calls at hotels to see clients. One was an alcoholic with a fractured ankle; he was supposed to be on crutches. None of these people were in. It is of interest to note that this was something like 9:30 AM, and these people were already checked out of their hotel rooms for the day. The day was wet and rainy; where were they? One of the hotel managers said to the nurse about the client who was an alcoholic with the fractured ankle, "That guy don't need you; if he can manage a broken ankle and crutches in the rain, he don't need you."

MISSING LINKS IN COMMUNICATION

The next stop was the health center where we were to meet with a psychiatrist who had been called into consultation for this nurse's client, a man of 20 years weighing 350 pounds and standing 5 feet, 5 inches tall. According to the nurse, people from the hotel were complaining about his most recent behavior of inappropriate laughter, giggling, belligerency, and at times, actually fighting. During the discussion at the health center, another nurse overheard our conversation about the client and interjected some comments that she had known the young man when he had been a patient at the city hospital in the psychiatric division. The psychiatrist then asked her for more information. The nurse said the man she remembered was an awfully nice, bright kid and that he loved baseball. He lost his temper easily, though he did, on the other hand, get lots of teasing from other patients. Other than this, there seemed to be a scarcity of information about the young man.

After talking a bit more about this lad, we all picked up and the three of us—psychiatrist, public health nurse, and myself—walked some 15 blocks to the boy's hotel. We were let in by the landlord, who informed us the fellow had just stepped out. He had not known we were coming, so it wasn't as though he was trying to avoid us. We sat in the lobby for a few minutes waiting, at which point the landlady came over and offered some information. She said that he was being evicted this Friday and wasn't sure where he was going, but that some social worker was getting him placed somewhere else. We had no idea where that somewhere else was.

There seemed to be a very loose connection between and among the people who were involved with this boy. He was obviously a kid who needed help, was in trouble, and was rapidly getting into more trouble. The official people who were involved with his case had not communicated effectively with each other. The nurse left a note for the young man saying that we had stopped by and that she would be by again this coming Friday. Now here again, she could well miss him. Then what?

"CLOSING THE CASE OUT"

Some further comments on the use of the term "closing the case out": By this term, most public health nurses I talked with seemed to mean that they ceased going into that particular home or hotel to visit that patient. However, the three nurses I talked to most recently seemed to differ with respect to when they decided to close a case out. One nurse said she could not close a case out and kept everyone hanging on. Consequently, she had the biggest case load of all the nurses. She said, "I just can't seem to let any of my patients go." On the other hand, some other nurses said that if a patient did not comply with their orders and so on, they threatened the patient with closing the case out. However, they added that they didn't really do it. One nurse observed that it was the patient who kept the case open; that is, she closed the case out, but the patient called her when he needed her. Then another nurse said, "Once you lose a case they [patients] won't call you in anymore." Such conflicting information. There probably were some guidlines as to when to close a case out, but they got reshaped in the everyday work situation. I would have to get more information.

SUGGESTED QUESTIONS FOR DISCUSSION AND ANALYSIS

For undergraduate students
1. What do you think about this nurse's pragmatic approach to problems? ("I use it because it works," she observed.)
2. Did the nurse's perception of her clients influence what she did or did not do for them? Please explain.
3. What approaches did the nurse use that helped patients to learn about themselves and their condition?
4. Do you see similarities between the work of the public health nurse and that of the visiting nurse as described in Fagerhaugh's piece?
5. Should nurses be required to go into neighborhoods, buildings, and so on, where they feel their personal safety is jeopardized? If so, how should they manage this? If not, what are the alternatives?

For graduate students and teachers of nursing
1. Where in your curriculum do you offer preparation for nurses to learn to deal with the multiproblem situation faced by the sick poor and other groups marginal to our society? At what point in the nurse's education is this offered?
2. Referring to question one above, can this be done by offering a course of two? Or is some major shift required in perhaps the reorganization of curriculum, deemphasis of one perspective over another, as for example, medical versus social and psychological?
3. What relevance does the ongoing argument about the medical versus social and psychological orientation have for the work of nurses? For their education?
4. Is the work of the public health nurse and the visiting nurse so different as to require two separate organizational systems? Are these differences purely ideological?
5. The nurse as patient advocate is increasingly being asserted as the legitimate activity of the nurse. How do you see this fitting in with the work of the public health nurse, for example?

17. Dying at home

Barney Glaser, PhD, and Anselm L. Strauss, PhD

Because modern industrial societies place a high priority on productivity, youthfulness, and health, it has frequently been observed that those phases in the life cycle (the process of dying and death), that are seen to conflict with those values, are put out of sight and hence out of mind. Even those institutions whose functions encompass all the major life phases have been shown to be remiss when it comes to handling the process of dying. Glaser and Strauss, two professors of sociology who have done extensive research on the subject of death and dying in the hospital, offer us some observations about what nurses do who work with patients dying in their homes in the presence of family members. In reading this material, one might take note of where professional ideology and social and cultural norms and values come into play to influence what the nurse does for the patient, his family, and for herself as well.

Some light can be shed on lingering trajectories in the hospital by first considering briefly what dying at home is like—whether or not the family finally yields its kinsman, or he yields himself to the hospital during his last hours or days. Our data are drawn from interviews with nurses assigned by a public health agency to visit the homes of lower-income patients. Each nurse visited a number of patients; most were not regarded as "terminal cases," but typically had the degenerative diseases of old age.

Since most of these patients die at home rather than in a hospital or nursing home, a salient feature is their own or their family's wish to manage the dying for themselves. They do this, of course, with the help of the physician, who prescribes treatment and orders regimens, and with the additional good offices of the visiting

Reprinted from Barney Glaser and Anselm Strauss: *Time for Dying* (Chicago: Aldine Publishing Company, 1968); copyright © 1968 by Barney G. Glaser and Anselm L. Strauss. Reprinted by permission of the authors and Aldine Publishing Company.

nurse (or nurses) assigned from the public health agency. The most obvious problems of management—of caring for the patient—involve his physical needs. The closer he comes to death, usually the less he can do for himself. He must be bathed, shaved, have his pajamas changed, given the proper diet, and perhaps fed, given enemas, or watched for bedsores. Some of these operations are natural to ordinary family life, but some are not. Patients in great pain have to be bathed in special ways, for instance, and catheters have to be properly handled.

> His wife really needed somebody; she was almost at her wit's end. He had so many bedsores. The day I went in was the first he hadn't been able to be helped to the bathroom. In just two days she and I had developed good teamwork. I'd lift, she'd put the bedpan under, and so on. He had two tubes that had to be drained (he had cancer of the bladder), and she was already doing that, but I taught her about other things, especially bedsore care, and gave her help on his diet, told her of things very sick people are most apt to eat—custard instead of oatmeal.

Since the nurse visits only occasionally, and the family supplies the steady workers, the nurse's teaching arms both to increase the patient's comfort and to ease the family's work. It also tries to ease family anxiety about the work. ("I like to stay long enough to really *explain* the care. If you just tell them what to do, sometimes you come back and find the patient in worse condition than you left him.") The nurse tends to coach family members about psychological matters. She may remind a wife not to whisper about her husband's condition when in his room, for he may still be capable of hearing. ("The wife whispered right around him, thinking he didn't hear. Even people who didn't have cancer would think they did with her around!") Or she may caution relatives not to treat the patient "like a baby."

When the nurse is first assigned to the patient, she may not even know that he is considered terminal; his physician may not have signified this. But if she knows, or becomes aware, then she is in a better position to anticipate what the patient and his family are up against as he nears death. The lay images of what will transpire are likely to be far less accurate than hers. If the family does not realize their kinsman is dying, then "you work it so they know it's terminal by the end . . . sort of drop hints on the way," or persuade the physician to tell the family.

The sooner the family members know something of what to expect, the better they can carry on between the nurse's intermittent visits. As one nurse complained:

> So often we don't get in on terminal cases until close to the end. It would be much better to start when they are still in the hospital. . . . It's so much better if, before the family faces the pressure and emotion of the patient home from the hospital, I can tell them about the disease, and what they will be able to do to work with us.

She concluded her remarks with, "They need more preparation when they know it's going to be a long thing, chronic or terminal." So, to some extent, the nurse coaches responsible family members about what to expect in the way of bodily deterioration and worsening symptoms, and the change of work that probably will be entailed by the patient's decline: "We talk to them about the nature of the disease and what to expect and how to take care of it. You fear things   235 when you don't know about them, so knowledge of what to expect in a disease helps lower their anxiety." It is important also that they know something of what to expect because "sometimes a difficult thing is for us to get the person who is caring for the patient to do everything they ought to. They find it offensive, I guess." As the end draws near, the nurse may even step in and "question wives as to whether their husbands have drawn a will. . . . I've gotten the conversation along those lines, and then said I thought *everybody* should have a will—did her husband?" Whether or not she provides the family members with clear images of the anticipated trajectory, the nurse stands ready to signal them or answer their questions about what is happening right now, during the present phase of dying.

Several obstacles can frustrate the nurse in her efforts to coach family members in giving proper care to their patient. Sometimes they just do not understand the procedures, and she has to demonstrate them repeatedly. Sometimes kinfolk are recalcitrant—they know perfectly well how to care for the patient, and no outsider is going to show them. ("There's a problem in home nursing. In the hospital you are the boss. But at home you aren't the real voice of authority. Relatives will have ideas about diet, and they are on top, not you. Or home remedies.") The nurse may have to ask the physician to speak with more effective authority, though he will not always do so. Sometimes, as suggested earlier, The relative cannot face "offensive" aspects of the care (bad odors, for instance) and so cannot give proper nursing. The nurse may then attempt to counter possible guilt feelings: "Let them talk it out and reassure them there is reason for these feelings and that they are not alone in them."

There are also interpersonal relationships within families that decrease the efficiency of care. Perhaps the families serviced by the nurses we interviewed were even more prone to interpersonal difficulties than most, because many were only segments (or remnants) of families: an aged couple with no children; two sisters; a male patient and his two sisters-in-law who had come four years earlier to nurse him, and so on. ("The sister-in-law who took care of the housekeeping hated him and he knew it. . . . She said if only she had enough money she would leave. . . . She refused to help him; when he got very ill she wouldn't help with the bedpan, so we had to arrange things around him so he could help himself the best he could. . . . I always felt sorry for him, dying amid all that hostility.") Interpersonal family relations are extremely important to good comfort care, and nurses tend quickly to assess the prevailing temper of the household. They will judge a patient to be good, but his wife to be "difficult," or say that the attending husband is compassionate, thoughtful, and responsible, but that his wife is not at all a nice person. In this calculus of judgement, a cooperative family becomes increasingly necessary as the patient becomes less able to care for himself.

In the typical lingering death at home, the closer to the end, the more difficult the care becomes for the family members. The amount of deterioration and the work it entails are not easy for them to imagine unless they have experienced such deaths previously. Consequently, the nurse almost inevitably finds herself stepping up the number of her visits during this phase of dying: "Toward the end you generally have to start going in more frequently, and this gives you an idea the end is near." The nurse not only gives more physical care, but is likely to move in more on the family—sending them upstairs to rest, listening to their grieving, reassuring them about guilt over wishing the ordeal was over.

It is during precisely this period that some families get frightened, and cannot stand the pressure. (As one nurse said, "In general, if they die at home, it is very traumatic—they need 24-hour care and families can't do it. There are exceptions, of course.") Some families give in to the advice of the nurse or physician and let the patient go to the hospital or a nursing home. (Occasionally a patient has already been in a nursing home, but has been brought home because conditions there were distressing to him.) In general, however, the particular population visited by these agency nurses preferred to have its relatives die at home possibly because of cost but also possibly, as one nurse suggested, because this older generation, holding older attitudes, still considers that hospitals are not good places in which to die.

Usually the visiting nurse is not present when the lingering patient dies at home. She may not know about the death until informed by phone. (One nurse remarked that she had once arrived at a house, on a "routine" visit, during the funeral.) But, by chance, the nurse sometimes plays some role in the painful last moments.

> Just once I was there when a patient died. She was my own age, and I was very attached to her. Her mother called me at home early in the morning and asked if I could come out. I told her I'd rearrange my schedule and visit them first. When I got there I saw that she was dying, so I called her mother in to hold her hand and then phoned the doctor. You must handle it as naturally as possible. I let her stay holding her hand until the doctor got there; it seemed to help her.

Nurses report that they visit the survivors during the postmortem period, partly because their own personal careers have become "involved" and partly because, as nurses, they wish to help further. The family member may even request the nurse to return: "She asked me when we were on the phone at the time of her mother's death—she'd died the afternoon I went and found her failing—to please come back and see her—had made me promise. So I went and she told me all about the death." Or the nurse may casually visit once again just to see how things are: "I was in the neighborhood on a call about a week after the funeral and had a little spare time so I went to see her. And believe it or not, she was just as perky as could be! . . . She talked very calmly, wept a little, but not breaking down at all. Her children had asked her to sell her house and live with first one and then the other, but she said she wasn't going to do it." And the nurse's personal interest may be so great that she picks up news about the survivors much later; the nurse quoted directly above closed her narrative: "According to the RN in that neighborhood, who saw her recently, she has gained weight and looks well. . . . She must be 88 years old!"

Thus far we have emphasized three salient features in our account of lingering dying at home: first, the desire of the family and/or patient to shape the dying trajectory; second, the interrelationships of the experiential careers of nurse and responsible kin, and how together they handle the care of the dying; and third, the importance of the mode of dying in determining whether the family can sustain the drama until its very end. The intersection of the personal careers of the nurse and the family members can also be an important feature of dying at home. If the nurse arrives early enough in the trajectory and visits frequently enough, she can become "personally involved." Since some patients are visited over as long a period as two or three years, involvement is quite understandable; but even much shorter periods can bring considerable emotional engagement. Nurse and patient get to like and trust one another. The nurse also may be drawn into family feuds, or find herself balancing carefully to stay "neutral."

While the engagement of visiting agency nurses with families is probably not as great as that of private duty nurses, it is possible that the visiting nurse's involvement more directly affects the patient care, for since she must delegate most nursing care to the family members, their trust and their capacity to learn and follow through on instructions depends to a considerable degree on "personal" relationships with her. Some hazards of these involvements are suggested by these remarks:

> I think you've got to try very hard to keep objective because you're going to get a little emotionally involved anyway. The RN-patient relationship is better if you're not too close. They may get too dependent on one person and then another may have to take over. It shows even on the level of getting very upset if you don't come until two. You have to remind them that they have to be flexible—have to keep it on a professional level. . . .I know one nurse . . . she's in some sort of trouble with her supervisor because they started calling her instead of the department.

This nurse's most important point is the first: A nurse must balance her relationships among the various members of the family and keep her eye on the main job—care of the patient. The linkage between getting "drawn in" and giving good nursing care is underlined, again, by the comment of another nurse that she makes "a conscious effort to stay somewhat aloof" because being too empathetic takes its toll on her. But "of course, you have to get somewhat involved—or else you seem a cold fish to the family. They have to feel you're interested, not just a do-gooder. It's a strange paradox." Another nurse confessed that "there's a tendency to become too involved. If you sense this, you just have to tell yourself: now's the time to watch out. . . . You can get so involved that you forget what you're basically there for." Her supervisor repeatedly tells her "not to get so involved."

Although the intersection of a nurse's personal career with those of the family entails hazards, deep satisfactions sometimes accrue to her. Those satisfactions include enhancement of self as well as pride in jobs well done. Presumably the family's chief satisfactions in managing to care for their relative while he dies at home turn around maintenance of family solidarity and fulfillment of proper obligations to the dying person. Whether family members are able to endure until the very end, it must be emphasized, is closely linked with mode of dying. The point is dramatically underscored by a story told us, ten years after the event, by a

238   hospital nurse: Late at night her hospital received a frantic call from a family who

had been taking care of a relative without any assistance from a nurse. Their patient obviously was dying, was "turning black," and they had been unable to reach a doctor. The hospital quickly assigned this nurse to visit the family. On her arrival, she found them all so distraught that she "had five patients on my hands." The experience convinced her that no patient should die outside a hospital. Under ordinary circumstances, when the family faces such an impossible emergency, the patient is sent to the hospital rather than the hospital to the patient.

SUGGESTED QUESTIONS FOR DISCUSSION AND ANALYSIS

For undergraduate students
1. How would you assess the tactics and techniques of the nurses described in "Dying at Home"? Do they give what you consider good terminal nursing care? How might it be improved?
2. Discuss the problem of overinvolvement and underinvolvement when nurses give terminal care to patients in their homes.
3. Toward "the end" the nurse's work changes somewhat. In what ways and why?

For graduate students and teachers of nursing
1. If you have had experience in public health nursing, has it been comparable with what was described in the foregoing pages? If it has been different, how would you account for the difference?
2. How would you train public health nurses so that they might better be prepared for handling terminal patients and their families, and yet give good nursing care? Also, what alterations might have to be made in the structure of public health agencies in order to give better terminal care?
3. In hospitals, we nurse the patients; at home, sometimes we nurse the whole family. Should we sometimes be giving nursing care in hospitals to the families also? How would this be done for the families of terminal patients, or at least done better than is generally done now?
4. What changes in the health care system might be necessary for the nurse and physician to work more closely together in giving better terminal care?

18. The work of the visiting nurse

Shizuko Yoshimura Fagerhaugh, RN, DNSc

These field notes are from an interview with a former supervisor of a voluntary health agency. Fagerhaugh, while working on her doctoral degree in nursing, did the interview especially for this book. Not only do we learn in detail about some of the highly resistant problems the visiting nurse confronts, but we have an opportunity to see the strategies some nurses use to make their work day workable. These observations of the supervisor, distilled from years of experience, are of value in and of themselves. However, their worth is immeasurably enhanced because of the confirmation some of her observations receive from research material in this same collection.

These notes are an edited version of a 2-hour interview. The original field notes were rearranged into larger categories for readability and continuity. The fact that the interviewee was a psychosocially knowledgeable nurse enabled us to engage in a great deal of analysis during the interview process.

The supervisor

Miss Jean Davis is a nurse in her late 40's who has had a variety of professional work experiences. She is a graduate of a hospital nursing school, has an MA, and has completed some post-master's work. Her work experiences include many years of work as a staff nurse and supervisor in medical-surgical nursing and many years of teaching medical-surgical nursing, both in the United States and abroad. Jean worked at the visiting nurse agency, both as a staff nurse and as a supervisor. The staff nurse period was for approximately 4 years during the 1950's. The supervisor period was in the 1960's. In both periods of work Jean was considered a skilled nurse.

240

The visiting nurse agency

The agency is an old private one providing home nursing care services. Top administration is composed largely of old timers with many many years with the agency. The reason for this situation will be evident later.

Jean notes that the types of patients at this agency changed between the first and second work periods. In the second work period, reflecting the general trend throughout the country, there was a noticeable increase of patients with chronic diseases and of geriatric patients; there was a high number of patients with heart diseases, strokes, cancer, diabetes, emphysema, multiple sclerosis, and Parkinson's disease. There was a noticeable decrease in maternal and child health cases. Jean thinks the changes in cases are related to changes in the city's population, to the fact that hospitals and clinics are apparently doing a better job with maternal and infant care follow-up and teaching, and of course, to the passage of the Medicare program.

Clients come to the agency from referrals of private physicians, agencies such as social welfare, and the like. Occasionally there are self-referrals—persons who hear about the agency from friends and relatives who have had previous agency services. All self-referrals must first be authorized by a physician. Clients are evenly distributed among various socioeconomic classes. However, since the Medicare program came into being, there has been an increase in middle- and upper-middle-class patients. In general, Jean finds that middle-class patients tend to use the agency services more effectively. This situation seems to be explained in part by the fact that middle-class patients are more knowledgeable about disease and treatment and therefore are more capable of getting the doctors on their side than are lower-class patients. In addition to Medicare and insurance funds covering the service costs, the agency relies heavily on United Crusade Funds.

Over the years the agency has developed a special Home Care Program, a joint endeavor with many agencies, especially private general hospitals. Many private hospitals in the city have a nurse coordinator from the nursing agency who is located in the hospital. Her main focus is coordinating a variety of services for the patient discharged from the hospital to the home or another facility. The Home Care Program has teams of occupational therapists, physical therapists, speech therapists, home health aides, and professional and vocational nurses. The nurse coordinator assesses patient needs, coordinates other agency services and work of the health team members, and arranges for special equipment. Jean's involvement in this program was primarily working with staff nurses assigned to these patients.

The city is divided into districts according to population density and potential patients. These districts were established by the agreement of private health agencies of the city. How these districts compare with the official agency, Jean does not know.

Each staff nurse has a case load of about 150 to 160 patients. The number of nurses assigned to each district varies with the patient population serviced. Jean guesses that nurses care for about six to ten patients a day, depending on the complexity of the patient problem. Licensed vocational nurses care for the less complicated patients.

What visiting nurse work involves

The work is quite varied. It includes giving specific treatments as prescribed by private physicians, such as changing dressings, irrigating wounds, and giving injections (often of a diuretic drug) two or three times a week. These kinds of specific treatments most often involve patients who had been hospitalized.

Other tasks include bathing patients and taking general hygiene measures. Giving enemas is also common. Jean states that bowel problems seem to be a constant problem with older patients with chronic disease.

Health teaching and supervision is another large category. This includes teaching prenatal, postnatal, and infant care (bathing and formula preparation). There is a large group of diabetic patients who need a great deal of help, not only with specific things, such as learning to give injections, but with all the factors involved such as diet control, reading symptoms, and so on. For many diabetics, the nurse must prepare injections for a couple of days, using an automatic syringe, which is prepared for injection and stored in the refrigerator. Placement of all the equipment is worked out in accordance with the patient's life pattern. A constant problem among diabetics is lack of funds to afford the expensive high-protein, low-carbohydrate diets. In these cases the nurse negotiates for special increases in aid. Jean states that a visiting nurse has constant hassles in order to obtain financial aid for many of the patients, and this hassle is over the minimum level of food and shelter; never mind the clothing.

Checking patients' drugs is terribly important. A patient may have five different drugs—the red pill twice a day, the green one three times a day, the oblong one every 2 days, the orange one once a week, and so on. Not infrequently the patient becomes thoroughly confused, so the nurse must relabel the drugs in understandable terms. Jean states that a smart nurse checks out with the doctor all the drugs the patient is taking so that she isn't caught "flat footed" in the home. This is especially important because the prescriptions may not have the name of the drug on the bottle.

Jean states that with the increase in chronic diseases it is becoming increasingly important for nurses to know a great deal about diseases, such as the various stages of disease, signs and symptoms accompanying these stages, signs and symptoms of drug side effects, and so on. This is essential because the nurse is out there all by herself and cannot readily rely on others for immediate answers. Some crucial symptoms may be missed by plain ignorance. Then, of course, with all the gadgetry required in some diseases, such as emphysema, it is becoming more important for nurses to be knowledgeable about technical hospital care. Also, this knowledge is important to have to be able to negotiate effectively with doctors and agencies for such things as rehospitalization, getting immediate medical attention, getting orders changed, and so on.

242   **Improvising care.** Providing care in the home is vastly different from providing

care in a clinic or hospital setting. Carrying out nursing procedures and treatments in the home requires a great deal of ingenuity of the nurse. The agency does have an extensive orientation period in this respect. However, it is impossible to note all the contingencies and problems in the home that might modify the procedures. In general, Jean feels that the agency has developed ingenious ways of performing procedures in the home and of sterilizing and storing supplies with equipment available in the home.

Problems of living. A great part of visiting nurse work is concerned with the patient's problems of living, such as mobility, shopping, cooking (some patients may have only a two-burner stove and no refrigeration), laundry, sociability, and getting to the doctor. Thus, the nurse must mobilize relatives, home health aides, services of other agencies, managers of hotels, neighbors, and the corner grocer.

Negotiating for and coordinating services. Jean states that a variety of services from a variety of agencies must be mobilized for the patient's behalf. She estimates there are easily some 100 agencies the nurse needs to know about. To do a good job, the nurse must know the extent and limit of each agency's services. This knowledge includes not only the official pronouncements, but all the details, such as how much services can be stretched from the agency, its limits, and who in the agency to avoid. These are learned by word of mouth. For example, some agencies that commonly provide transportation for medical appointments are prohibited from chauffering persons who need assistance getting in and out of the vehicle (such as blind persons). This restriction comes from some feature of insurance coverage.

Because the home situation is so different from a hospital and because of the large number of agencies and services the nurse must learn, the agency has an extended orientation period. The orientation is for 2 months, and the hiring policy is that the nurse agrees to stay with the agency for 2 years. In general, Jean thinks that a new nurse cannot function effectively without 4 to 5 months of extensive orientation and supervision, but because of work pressures the nurse is given full patient load after 2 months.

In most nurse work, because of the doctor-nurse status relationship, the legal restraints placed on the nurse, and the constraints imposed by the institution, the nurse faces difficulty negotiating for the patient's behalf. She must learn to manipulate situations so that the delicate doctor-nurse status balance is not upset. In visiting nurse work, because of the large numbers of agencies and other health workers she must deal with, she becomes an expert in manipulating agencies and health professionals. Quite often patients are carefully coached to emphasize certain symptoms and aspects of their situations when talking with a social worker, doctor, and so on.

Patient-nurse and doctor-nurse relationships

Patient-nurse relationships. In visiting nurse work, the professional enters the home on the patient's terms. Thus, the professional perrogatives typical of hospital and clinic settings aren't workable. For example, to sterilize equipment and the   **243**

like, the nurse works with equipment in the patient's home. Visiting times are arranged in cooperation with the patient. The nurse doesn't ask family members to "leave the room" when working with patients. In fact, involving the patient and the family in the care, such as teaching patients and the family to be alert about specific signs and symptoms, is very important. Jean finds it interesting that patients are often poor judges of "what is good care." The patient's evaluation of the nurse's skill is frequently based on how the patient was previously managed by another nurse, either in the hospital or by another agency nurse. In performing nursing procedures and treatments, the nurse must ascertain from the patient how these procedures were previously done, his understanding of the treatment, and the like. The nurse must accept the patient's view of his priority needs, even though she might feel other priorities are more important.

Sometimes the agency policy may not allow what the patient wants, such as having the nurse sit with a patient for 2 hours while the wife does her errands. Generally, in the initial patient contract, the nurse informs the patient of the service limits of the agency.

Telephone as major source of communication. Aside from face-to-face contact among the agency nurses, practically all communications and negotiations between the nurse and other agencies and health professionals are done by telephone. For example, the doctor refers a patient to the agency by telephone, giving a brief description of the patient and specific prescriptions of treatment (a written authorized order to the agency). The nurse makes a visit to the patient. If she notes changes in the patient that require new orders, she telephones the doctor. Depending on the doctor, she can be very open about suggestions, or she might have to word the suggestions in such a manner that they may not be interpreted as "telling doctor what to do." The nurse forwards the new written orders to the doctor for his authorization of the verbal order. Jean has never seen most of the professionals she deals with. She tells a funny story about a black nurse on the staff who, after months and months of telephone conversations with other professionals, would accidentally meet a doctor or a social worker with whom she had had these phone conversations, and they would be shocked to discover that she was black.

Doctor-nurse relationships. In the main, doctors are willing to accept suggestions and judgments of the agency nurses. Jean has found that while the patient is still recovering from an acute stage of illness (after hospitalization), doctors are more directive about patient management. Once the chronic "not much more can be done" phase sets in, the doctors generally go along with the nurses' suggestions. Jean's main bone of contention is that doctors have to authorize the services of other agencies, all of which seems to be unnecessary back and forth negotiations for nonmedical matters. On rare occasions a doctor does not want services of other agencies that the nurse feels are essential, such as, the need for home health aides that the doctor feels make the patient "dependent." In these cases the nurse waits if there is no immediate ill effect. If the nurse estimates that the service is urgent, she coaches the patient on how to talk to the doctor, and she seeks the support of the nurse supervisor. It must be noted that all services from other agencies can only be rendered if the patient agrees.

In a sense, the doctors probably cooperate with the nurse because she relieves the doctor from having to make a house call.

What a typical work day is like

The agency services extend over weekends. All staff nurses and supervisors rotate weekend work. The work day starts at 8 AM at the agency office. The nurse lines up work for the day; she makes telephone calls to affirm visits with patients, and telephones doctors and other agencies about specific problems related to patients. The nurse must be aware of such contingencies as the weather (on nice sunny days a patient may decide to use the day for running neglected errands) or the doctor's work schedule (that Doctor so-and-so can usually be reached at such-and-such hospital between 8 and 9 AM because he is making patient rounds).

She usually plans the work so that complicated, time-consuming patients are cared for in the morning. She usually plans about 1 hour for each patient. Patients are cared for in the morning because patients demand it (to some extent patients are conditioned by a previous hospital schedule) and families demand it (it allows families to have time in the afternoon for their own life demands). Some patient visits, such as those for injections or dressing changes, may be only 15 to 20 minutes. These visits are called "short calls." Depending on the work load of the nurse, other nurses with less demanding patients assist in these "short calls." Work must be planned not only in terms of time with each patient, but also in terms of time requires for travel. Nurses with automobiles have less of a problem, but nurses on foot and dependent on public transportation may require considerable planning of travel time. The nurse supervisor often helps in decisions about equitable distribution of work among the staff, the licensed vocational nurse's role in the overall work, and special patient problems. Nurses go into the field sometime after 8:30. Some nurses go into the field later, but Jean made it a point to get into the field early by rearranging her work; more about this later. At about 1 to 2 PM the nurse calls the agency for new calls, cancellations, and the like. She is back in the office at about 4 PM to complete paper work, contact doctors and agencies, and so on. The afternoon hours are generally spent in such work as health supervision of patients and evaluation and assessment of new patients.

Problems of work and time

In any work situation there are problems of time, such as having time to complete all the necessary work tasks, scheduling work time, and making time with the patient count. Also, time is money; time and cost restraints imposed by the agency and the various funding agencies may pose problems for the nurse. Below are examples of various work problems the visiting nurse has that are related to time. These include problems of work timing, time stretching, hoarding, and balancing.

Work timing. A constant demand patients make of visiting nurses is that visiting times fit into the patient's life routine. In the hospital the patient's time belongs to the professionals; the patient fits into the schedule of the professionals and the hospital. In the home the patient's "sick time" is only a small portion of the daily time routine. The visiting nurse is caught in the problem of matching work time among a large number of distantly located patients who have all varieties of daily time routines. To complicate matters, the nurse must also contend with the patient's family times as well. Jean also points out that in the hospital patients see other patients and become aware that other patients require more or less of the nurses' time. In the home the patients could care less about the time demands of other patients. As a supervisor, the most common patient complaints Jean received were related to visiting time. There were very few complaints about the quality of patient care. Not infrequently the nurse is caught between two patients who are adamant that the nurse visit both patients at the same time. In these cases she works out a system of appeasing Mrs. A. on Monday and Mrs. B. on Tuesday. On occasion the nurse supervisor's assistance may be required to explain to the patient that the nurse is attempting to resolve the problem as well as she can. Sometimes a patient may rope in the doctor to support the timing of visits. More often than not, a doctor will understand the problem if it is explained, because he, too, is caught in the same timing problem.

Time stretching, hoarding, and balancing. Making time available for patient care is a constant problem for visiting nurses. Jean found that the paper work took up a great deal of time. She often took paper work home, which made more time to spend with patients. Thus, she was able to go into the field early. Taking work home is not required by the agency, but the more conscientious nurses tend to do this to make more time for the patients.

Although nurses help each other in work sharing, and it is important to be a good sport about work sharing, it is also important that one not get identified as a "speedy nurse." A reputation of a "speedy nurse" might mean getting assigned more and more "short calls," which thereby decreases time with one's own patient load—time that the nurse so carefully made.

Time is money, and the cost of care is not cheap. Over the years the cost of professional services has steadily risen, as have all costs of health services. The professional nursing service cost, at the time of Jean's employment, was approximately $8.00 for the first hour, and 50 cents for each half hour thereafter. Fees for Licensed Vocational Nurse services and Home Health Aid were less. Under these conditions the nurse is under constraints to make her patient contact time count. Frequently the patient engages in a variety of maneuvers to get more and more of the nurse's precious time. Jean notes that some patients who lead isolated lives just want someone to talk to them. Yet the nurse is under constraints to use the nurse's time in "essential nursing." Jean often felt frustrated because she was aware that extended chatting was necessary to discover areas of patient needs beyond the more superficial ones.

246

Many doctors are opposed to the idea that nurses charge for services. Now that part of the services are covered by Medicare, doctors complain less about the cost for nursing service.

Example of a case revolving around time. An elderly patient dying of cancer did not want to die in a hospital. The patient's wife also felt strongly about this. As the patient became more and more "terminal," the wife was getting more and more exhausted. There were no other family members or relatives to relieve the wife's work. Of course, the nursing time increased as the patient's condition worsened. Also, naturally, the wife wanted more of the nurse's time, not only for someone to pour out her problems to, but it was also a chance to get out of the house. In addition to professional nursing time, licensed vocational nurses and home health aides were assigned for longer and longer periods. The wife herself had health problems and required some assistance. Medicare finally placed limits on the hours of services. In general, Medicare does not approve of service time extending beyond 8-hour periods. Finally the licensed vocational nurse time was altered to shorter daily periods. The wife finally realized she could not handle the patient at home, but this took time for the wife to work through with the help of a nurse. Because the whole situation was terribly depressing for the staff, Jean finally had to work out a system of assigning a professional nurse and a licensed vocational nurse to take turns in sharing the work and to give each other emotional support. Jean states that "death work" is terribly trying both for the supervisor and for the staff nurse. As supervisor she was constantly used by the staff as a "shoulder to cry on." Also, in contrast to hospital "death work," the nurse must get involved in supporting the family. Quite often the nurse allows herself to be used by the family as for hospitalizing the patient instead of allowing him to die at home, thereby reducing the family's sense of guilt. Terminal patients are especially a problem, since so many patients have depleted their resources, and families dread the thought of family members dying at the city and county hospitals.

Control of work

A significant feature of visiting nurse work is that the staff nurse has more control of her daily work situation. She can also control work against the scrutiny of higher authorities. Because her work is not visible to those in authority, work can be controlled primarily by how and what the nurse reports to the supervisor. For example, Jean worked under a supervisor who tended to be judgmental about poor "down and out" patients from the depressed areas of the city; the supervisor thought that they deserved their plight, were morally weak, and so on. At the same time, this supervisor tended to favor the middle- and upper-middle-class patients, stretching more and more services for these patients, even though many of them had other resources they could have used. To complicate matters, the supervisor was favored by the higher authorities, since she knew how to "butter up" to those in authority. Jean would not report information of increases in a patient's income (fees were based on a sliding scale according to income), such as a patient with a   247 daughter who sent a small amount of money. If the supervisor knew this, she would see that the patient would be charged for higher fees, thus raising the charge higher than what the patient could afford. The presence of a common-law marriage or other similar information that the supervisor might use as moral judgment against the patient were "not reported." This supervisor was a stickler about "always having a doctor's order." She did not want the staff to give even a bath without a doctor's order, even if the patient were lying in filth. The staff soon learned what to report and what not to report. A kind of alliance developed among some of the staff about what were "reportable" and "nonreportable" items.

Because the staff nurse's work cannot be readily checked as would be the case of hospital work, the extent of the nurse's involvement with a patient is shaped to a great degree by the individual nurse's inclination to get involved or not to get involved. A nurse can be concerned with the patient's immediate superficial needs, or the doctor's immediate orders, and let it go at that. For example, a patient may have symptoms that require a visit with a physician. A nurse can merely tell the patient to see a doctor. A nurse willing to get involved may concern herself with ways of helping the patient get to the doctor, such as helping a mother with several preschool children who may not be able to locate a baby sitter and who may not have money to cart all the children along with her by public transportation. The nurse might also coach patients about what to say to the doctor.

Problems of young nurses. Jean has found that younger nurses often have difficulties with visiting nurse work because so many of the patients have multiple physical and psychosocial problems for which there is no immediate relief. The work is often depressing because of the many chronic disease conditions—most patients don't get better; they slowly deteriorate. This situation, together with the constant need to improve care for which she is not trained, makes the young nurse feel inadequate. Jean has found that all young graduates, from a hospital school, university, or otherwise, suffer the same painful breaking-in problem. A great deal of common sense, ingenuity, and patient commitment is required—but how do you develop common sense and commitment?

Backbreaking aspect of visiting nurse work. As the number of chronic disease patients increases, the work is becoming more and more backbreaking (caring for patients in low double beds, helping patients in and out of bathtubs, and the like). With the large number of patients who had strokes, work is often dirty. Planning for such a common thing as bathing may require the nurse to have the manager or the family to have clean linen available before the nurse visits the patient.

The irony of visiting nurse work is that the older the nurse is, the more valuable she becomes, because through experience she knows all the "ins" and "outs" of agencies and all the tricks of improvising care in the home. Yet the older she gets, the more the back gives out. (In fact, Jean could no longer do staff work because of back problems.) Jean stated that some of the old timer supervisors were walking encyclopedias on how to improvise care in all kinds of home situations, "ins" and "outs" of agencies, peculiarities of various doctors, and so on. The fact that so

248

many old timers are in supervisory positions is precisely because of this valuable asset. In general, Jean has found that supervisors are always willing to share information with staff members.

The fine line between nurse work and problems of living. Because problems of living are intrinsically a part of chronic illness, the nurse must learn the fine line of distinction between nursing and non-nursing actions related to problems of living. In other words, the nurse must learn to translate problems of living into medical and nursing problems. Because of this, a well-meaning, eager nurse can become involved in situations considered to be against the rules, by the agency such as picking up medicines for a patient or driving patients to the clinic in her own car (the agency does not cover accidents that might occur). Also, since the nurse may often play arbiter in family disputes and tensions, she must be careful not to get involved in touchy legal and financial matters that might implicate the agency. Visiting nurse work requires a mature person to understand the consequences and ramifications of rule stretching and rule breaking.

Assessing patient needs. Jean thinks that patient assessment requires a mature person because she not only must make an accurate physical assessment, but she must be aware of all the social contingencies, such as patients living alone, not living alone, reliability of family members, family relationships, residence location and facilities. Also conditions are constantly changing. Since time is so costly, the nurse must be able to make quick and accurate assessments. She is faced with the problem of matching priorities between the patient, family, doctor, and agency; at the same time she must deal with constraints placed on her by the patient, family, and others.

Numbers game. Since the agency is funded through community fund raising, justification of the number of staff members with the patients serviced is required. Staff members are placed in a position of playing the "numbers game" to make it appear that they are indeed seeing more patients. If a particular nurse's patient visit count is low because of patients requiring a great deal of time, she is asked by the supervisor to "make a few more check visits." Check visits usually refer to health supervision visits. If a patient has a family, that is all the better because by inquiring about the children's health, the count goes up.

Paper work. The large amount of paper work is, to Jean, "for the birds." This work includes recording patient visits, recording doctor's orders for authorization, filling out insurance and Medicare forms, making periodic summary reports to physicians and other agencies, and so on. The addition of secretarial help would greatly help the nurse and supervisor.

Supervisor's work. As supervisor, Jean was spending a good amount of time shuffling papers, a task she hated. Often she took home much of the paper work in order to make time available for helping the staff. In addition, the office had to be covered for telephone calls and for troubleshooting complaints from patients, doctors, and so on. Not infrequently, she felt like a taxicab dispatcher. As supervisor, she was constantly frustrated by the administrative demands that left   **249**

her little time for helping the staff. Situations such as the addition of several new young staff nurses requiring assistance and emotional support can be extremely frustrating. An inexperienced young supervisor can become quite flustered in these situations.

The most enjoyable aspects of supervision for Jean were patient contact through field visits with the staff and helping the staff with patient problems. She tried all methods of squeezing time to spend with the staff, such as bag lunching for staff chats, scheduling after-work conferences, and so on. In general, Jean, like many other supervisors, always tried to be honest with the staff about rule stretching, limits of rules, and the like. Because of her teaching orientation, Jean tended to see staff-supervisor encounters more in terms of teaching-learning situations rather than "checking on the nurse." According to Jean, staff-supervisor relations were the "least of the problems."

Satisfaction. In spite of the many constraints in visiting nurse work, Jean found staff nursing the most satisfying of all her many work experiences. If her back were better and if old age were not "creeping up" on her, she would have remained in this work. The independence of planning with families and patients is very satisfying. The nurse is forced to be more observant and has opportunities to use all her ingenuity and skills. Even though the nurse is accountable to the agency, she is primarily accountable to the patient, and this she likes.

Official public health agencies

Both Jean and I wondered what official public health agency nurses were doing about chronic illness in this city. For instance, if any treatment or nursing procedures were involved in patient care, the patient was referred to the visiting nurse agency—even patients with tuberculosis being given streptomycin injections twice a week, and tuberculosis is certainly a public health problem. Many of the visiting nurses spoke of official public health nurses in somewhat sneering terms as "talking nurses."

In general, Jean has found that hotel managers and families react warmly toward the visiting nurses. This is partly because older patients with chronic disease are neglected by just about everyone, and a sympathetic nurse is helpful, even if only as someone to listen to problems.

SUGGESTED QUESTIONS FOR DISCUSSION AND ANALYSIS

For undergraduate students

1. How might the nursing curriculum be altered to help you cope with some of the problems described above? How much can be reasonable accomplished through the curriculum, and what is the agency's responsibility?
2. What are some of the problems in making accurate nursing assessments in the home? Since time and money are of the essence, what form should the assessment interview take?
3. The supervisor in the interview refers to the nurse as requiring "common sense" in dealing with the complex problems she encounters. How would you describe "common sense" and the way that it fits in with the nurse's work?

For graduate students and teachers of nursing

1. The visiting nurse is obviously caught in a dilemma of playing negotiator, arbitrator, coordinator, and deliverer of care on behalf of the patient, while at the same time she is limited in power. If the nurse is committed and accountable to the patient, the dilemma reduces the nurse to be constantly engaging in subterfuge (or to put it another way, to becoming a great "con artist."). Identify the areas of dilemma that nurses face in fulfilling these various roles—social structural, interprofessional, legal. What should be the nurse's prerogative within the health team?

2. Since much of home care is related to problems of living, what aspects of care can reasonably be the domain of the nurse? What roles should nurses play in the varieties of support agencies?

3. With the emergence of primary nurses and the expanding roles for nurses, how will public health nursing, both private and official, probably change?

4. How might experienced older nurses be utilized other than in the supervisory capacity illustrated above, which tends to dissipate their real abilities and skills?

5. All health agencies have a "numbers game" problem. What kinds of evaluation methods would provide a truer assessment of quality and volume control? Keep in mind that visibility of work is a problem.

section H

Where is the nurse?

The title to this section should alert the reader that this section may be different from the previous ones. It is different—primarily in the striking absence of the nurse. The basic assumption underlying both Davis's and Reif's chapters is that nurses and health workers in general are not fully aware of, nor is there sufficient understanding of, the issues of (1) social isolation and (2) the intricate relationship between symptoms and life style. Their chapters are offered as an attempt to further the nurse's understanding and to maximize her performance with respect to these areas.

Davis's chapter on social isolation is excerpted from her doctoral dissertation on patients with multiple sclerosis. She attempts to analyze social isolation as a process, exploring how and why it occurs. The findings from the overall research show that while many patients are resourceful in their efforts to live with their progressively worsening chronic illness, they all become involved in the drift toward social isolation. Therefore, the important questions remaining for nurses and health workers are whether social isolation in long-term illness is inevitable and whether the process is inexorable. If not, then the question becomes, "How can nurses and other health workers involve themselves with patients to intervene in the process?"

19. Social isolation as a process in chronic illness

Marcella Z. Davis, RN, DNSc

The process of social isolation is analyzed in this chapter according to three main variables: (1) reciprocal nature of relationships, (2) stage in life career, and (3) rate of illness progression.

Generally, most persons are sustained in their image of themselves through their relationships with family and friends. When these relationships are severely disrupted through prolonged and worsening illness, such as multiple sclerosis, social isolation for the patient, and in some instances for his family, is not an uncommon consequence.

In this discussion the focus is on social isolation as a process, and attention is paid to its sources and consequences for patients with progressively debilitating chronic illness. As it is used here, social isolation is defined as the process whereby the individual increasingly becomes socially and psychologically separated from his former relationships and social activities, with decreasing opportunities for adequate replacement with new relationships and social activities.

One does not generally become socially isolated from others suddenly or even with much awareness. Rather, from the descriptions of those who now experience social isolation, the process seems to be vague, erratic, and imperceptible. As one young patient remarked on her repeated experiences of unreturned phone calls, with no response to phone messages left for friends, "At first, when they tell you that she's [friend] not in, you accept this, but then it starts to hit you, and it sinks in that you're being shut out." She believes that, "Anyone who is sick for longer than 6 months won't be remembered except for birthdays and holidays."

A longer version of this chapter appears in Davis, Marcella Z.: *Living with Multiple Sclerosis: A Social Psychological Analysis,* Springfield, Ill., 1973, Charles C Thomas, Publisher.

Still another patient, whose isolation from his family and former friends is now so severe that he has had to resort to hiring the attention of a neighbor to look in "now and then" just "to see if I'm dead or alive," made the observation that the isolation "is really getting to me. . . . Sometimes I think I'm going out of my mind."

The next patient, a married upper-middle-class woman was very active in social and political events prior to having multiple sclerosis. Over the 4-year period that she has had multiple sclerosis, her time spent at home has increased to where she now is home continually. She observed that she has more in common with a couple who recently moved into their neighborhood, because the husband is in a wheelchair, than she does with old friends. To be sure, this woman is not as socially isolated as the two previous patients, but she is removed from the mainstream of life as she once knew it. Because of the changes and alterations in all aspects of her day-to-day life, she finds that she has less in common with people who are old friends than with relative strangers who might be in similar circumstances.

CHANGES IN THE RECIPROCAL NATURE OF RELATIONSHIPS

Underlying the general process of social isolation is the change in the patient's relationships with others. In most instances, it is the patient who is unable to sustain reciprocities in the relationship sufficiently to maintain a viable undertaking. In some instances, when others redefine the relationship with the focus placed on the patient's illness and disability to the exclusion of all other characteristics, it is not uncommon for the patient to reject the relationship.

The following examples illustrate the nature of the difficulties patients have in sustaining reciprocities in their relationships. These are divided into two categories: (1) decline in shared experiences and (2) mutually unfulfilled expectations.

Decline in shared experiences

Miss Marks, an unmarried, 26-year-old woman has had multiple sclerosis since her senior year in high school. She continues to live with her parents and younger sister. After graduation from high school she did not take a job or continue with further schooling but remained at home and did some volunteer work in her local church. During this period she maintained a relationship with two friends. All her former high school friends other than these two had left the neighborhood to take jobs elsewhere. Her relationship with one remaining friend, a young man, has drifted apart since he learned of her suicide attempt.

With her married girl friend there seemed to be more opportunities to sustain a closer relationship for a longer period. Interestingly, it was Miss Marks who took the initiative in the relationship and visited the friend. However, the relationship continued to drift apart as her friend's family grew and home responsibilities increased. Miss Marks tried, as a way of reinforcing their relationship, to help in the care of the children, but was unable to sustain this physically. With the decline in shared experiences, the basis for friendship between the patient and the friend not only diminished, but their respective daily lives and interests became too disparate

for a mutually satisfying relationship to continue.

We see from this and other data that the patient's relationships with others are not repaired, rebuilt, or sustained easily, and in some cases, not at all.

Unfulfilled expectations

Mrs. Bond, a young mother who has been in a wheelchair for the past year, complained about the behavior of her friends since her shift to the wheelchair. She noted that she and her husband are no longer invited to their friend's homes, and if she is to see her friends at all, it is she who must invite them. While Mrs. Bond wants the sociability of her friends, she at the same time resents the fact that she and her husband are left "with cleaning up after them." When she pressed her friends for answers as to why they don't invite her or phone more frequently, she reported that they told her, "We don't know what to do and don't want to hurt you."

The patient and her friends have not established alternate modes of relating, and their former styles have proved unsatisfying and awkward. The friends no longer know how to be friends with the patient under the changed circumstances, and the patient finds sustaining friendship within the former patterns more than she can cope with.

Unfulfilled expectations also include the more intimate aspects of a relationship, as for example, sexual intercourse between husband and wife. Men patients commonly report that they experience sexual impotence and feel profoundly guilty for not being able to sustain a sexual relationship with their wives. Women patients, on the other hand, are able to sustain a sexual relationship should this be so desired by both parties. However, some women claim to have been abandoned shortly after their diagnosis on the grounds that their husbands found them sexually unattractive. Consequently, divorce and desertion of the partner is not an uncommon occurrence.

VARIATIONS IN SOCIAL ISOLATION AMONG PATIENTS

Unsustained reciprocities between the patient and others have explained one aspect of the more general process of social isolation. It does not explain the important variations among patients with regard to how quickly a patient experiences social isolation and the degree to which he experiences it. To understand and account for these variations two variables are simultaneously focused on: (1) the stage in his life career that the patient is in when he gets multiple sclerosis, and (2) the rate at which the illness and disability progress. These two factors are chosen for their relevance to the general process and offer a way of comprehending a wide range of factors that impinge on the process of social isolation.

Stage in life career

The stage in one's life career does not refer specifically to chronological age as such, but to the kinds of life tasks that are generally linked with a specific age range rather than with a specific age. For example, we generally associate career and

255

family building with persons in a young age group, and with an older age group we associate activities that function to phase out career and family involvements.

Unmarried patients. The stage in the life career of the patient must be viewed with respect to his peers, who generally are involved in a similar stage of their life career. Thus, when an event such as getting a progressively worsening chronic illness occurs, the style of life the patient gradually comes to live becomes increasingly misaligned with that of his peers. The previous examples illustrate the increasing discrepancies between the patient's round of life and that of his few remaining friends. For example, Miss Marks, whom we met earlier, had symptoms that progressed at a very slow pace; yet she experienced social isolation at a rate more rapid than another young woman who was bound to a wheelchair. Briefly, Miss Marks was 17 years old when she was diagnosed as having multiple sclerosis. After graduation from high school she never moved socially or psychologically into the next stage of her life career (career building, marriage, and so on) but remained, and was treated as such by her parents, as an older adolescent. She did not seek a job or continue any further schooling. Her social network, shortly after graduation, diminished instead of expanding and becoming more complex, as it did for her age mates. Activities and relationships that were lost were never adequately replaced, and new relationships were not initiated at all. Young persons who were at the same stage of their life career as she were involved in starting careers at school, jobs, or marriage, so that even those who had relationships with her were drawn away by competing demands. These persons were eventually unavailable as a source for further social contact. Because she had no commitments other than her illness, there were no competing demands for her time or concerns from outside involvements. Consequently, all the physical demands of her illness, whether minor or not, received first priority. Her routines and general life style widened the gap between the commonality of experience for her and her age mates.

The next example stands in sharp contrast. Miss Adams, now in her late 20's, was 23 years old, unmarried, and in her third year of college when she became ill with multiple sclerosis. Unlike Miss Marks, she had moved into the stage of young adulthood and had begun career building. Within a year's time of her first symptoms, her disease had progressed to the point where she had moved from using a cane to being confined to a wheelchair. In spite of her decreased mobility, this patient continued with her studies at school and with the same student group she knew. Activities such as attending classes, eating in the cafeteria, and generally being in the same location as her friends and acquaintances offered the patient and her friends easy access to each other. Most of the time there was an available supply of persons familiar to her to assist in some way, but even more important, there were friends and other young persons to talk with about topics of common interest. Her total sense of identity did not derive from her illness or disability, nor did others relate only to the disability.

In another example, Mr. James, a young unmarried man whose symptoms progressed rapidly, had to leave his work as an elevator operator in less than a year's time from the beginning appearance of symptoms. He lives alone with his widowed mother, who returned to work when her son was unable to work and was confined to home. His former friends visited him infrequently when he was first confined to his home, and eventually not at all. Such remarks from his friends as, "Jesus, how can you stand it!" seem to suggest that his confinement to his home appeared so completely out of their realm of common, everyday experience as to make it difficult, if not impossible, for them to identify with him any longer. These friends handled their discomfort and uncertainty by withdrawing from the patient.

In summary, we see that social isolation is less problematic when persons continue in their careers or jobs. Continuing in the mainstream with other nondisabled persons offers some commonality of experience for them with others. This serves to link them to the mainstream of life rather than solely to the day-to-day experiences of chronically ill and disabled persons.

Married patients. The patients are divided into two categories, those with preschool and school age children and those with children who are grown and, in some instances, away from home.

Mrs. Homer is a patient with two school age children. Her family's social situation has markedly changed (now 5 years later) since her symptoms have worsened and she has become increasingly disabled. For example, their move to the suburbs to a house with no steps in order to accommodate her failing mobility has removed them from a network of friends in the city. For the first few years in the new neighborhood she was able to get about with the aid of a crutch. She did volunteer work for the Girl Scouts, as well as in her children's school. It was through these activities that she befriended other mothers. Because her hands have now become affected and she requires more assistance than that of a crutch, her volunteer work has stopped, and she is confined to her home most of the time. She maintains some phone contact with other mothers. However, these women visit infrequently because of the pressures of their own busy round of life with young children.

Even though there are natural opportunities for sociability built into the very structure of their everyday world (playground group, shopping, and so on), as patients who are mothers with preschool age children become more physically disabled, these opportunities are closed to them. Consequently these patients are automatically cut off from the more casual contacts with other mothers. This source for sociability and informal information exchange, so useful to most mothers in the early years of child raising, is not to be theirs.

Among these young families, moving to a new location is not uncommon, either for reasons of the husband's work (if the wife is the patient) or to move to accommodate a spouse's disability through more appropriate housing. Ties with former friends are easily lost through these kinds of shifts.

From the above examples we see that social isolation for persons at this stage in their life career is associated not only with how fast the physical mobility decreases but equally with the fact that their peers are similarly involved with the time-consuming tasks of career building and family raising.

The circumstances surrounding the social isolation for men, whether or not they   **257** are fathers with families or single men, are closely associated with their jobs. All the men in the study had had, at some time, jobs that took them out of the home and that served as one of their major sources of social contact. Once these men were out of work and confined to their homes, their routines and temporal arrangements were in direct conflict with those of their nondisabled male friends who had jobs. While children's activities provide an opportunity for sociability for some mothers with multiple sclerosis, is this not the case for fathers with the disease. Based on the small amount of data in the study on them, men tend whenever possible, to replicate their time-pattern arrangements as close as possible to the temporal arrangements they knew at work. That is, some men in the study went to the recreational center for the handicapped 2 full days and 1 evening each week.

Patients in later stages of the life career. Some patients, whose first symptoms of multiple sclerosis occur in their early and mid 40's, do not at first think they have an illness but that they are experiencing signs of aging. This is in sharp contrast to persons in their late teens, 20's, and early 30's who find progressively worsening symptoms to be, as a rule, out of character with the expectations they hold about their bodies and health. These older patients, as well as their friends and relatives, who are also in a later stage of their life career, are less likely to reject a relationship where the major focus is on the patient's illness and disability. These patients and their friends are less likely to be mutually rejected on the grounds that all they want to talk about is sickness.

The children of the patients studied in this category were grown; some were married and living away from home. Therefore, family obligations were less pressing than for those families with pre-school and school age children. A few patients found their older children to be of comfort and of some assisaance to them.

Equally important, the onset and progression of symptoms does not progress at the same rate as for those in the younger age category. Not one of these patients in the study was in a wheelchair within a year of the onset of symptoms. All these patients were ambulatory, but all required some assistance in walking. Even though the rate of progress of symptoms was slower than in the younger age group, among those patients who were employed outside the home, all these patients had to leave their jobs within a 5-year period from the onset of symptoms. This severance from their work meant a break in a vital social network.

Some patients in this stage of their lives have friends whom they have known over a 20-year span of time and with whom they have established patterns of activities that help sustain the relationship once they become ill. Unfortunately, not all patients at this stage in their life careers have social networks of such long standing that they can depend on.

STRATAGEM OF WITHDRAWAL

Very much a part of the process of social isolation is the stratagem of withdrawal as it is used by patients and others with respect to the patient. In this discussion withdrawal is examined with respect to its function for patients and others.

Some patients withdraw from social interaction to shield themselves from whatever experiences they perceive as threatening to and incompatible with their more valued conceptions of themselves. These patients feel themselves to be set apart from the world of normals. On the other hand, they do not see themselves as completely identifiedable with those who are disabled or severely ill. Withdrawal, in effect, temporarily relieves the patient of experiencing the ambiguity of his social location and allows him to maintain his imagined view of himself as he prefers to think of himself as being thought of by others.

Withdrawal, in most instances, is as much a way of coping for others in relation to the patient as it is for the patient. In these instances, withdrawal can be viewed as mutual: patient from others and others from patient. Withdrawal of others, which is seen by most patients as a rebuff, in effect says, "You are no longer that person we once knew; you have something we don't want to hear about, and you have changed into something we don't want to see."

One man, now in a wheelchair and very socially isolated, described why he thought others no longer came to see him. He said, "I think sometimes people don't come to see me, because I'm gruesome. It's not pleasant to feel you're gruesome." Other patients explain to themselves why friends no longer visit or even phone by telling themselves that "nobody wants to see their friends go downhill" or that people are "too busy with their own lives." Still other patients feel that people are frightened that it might happen to them and that staying away keeps the frightening possibility "out of mind."

Withdrawal on the part of the patient and others from the patient in most instances results in increased social isolation of the patient. Some patients find themselves inextricably caught in a world so diminished and so devoid of communication with others that the idea of commiting suicide emerges as the only viable solution.

Withdrawal as a stratagem is not necessarily confined to persons who have been ill for long periods of time. One patient described how she purposely cut herself off from all her friends, even before she knew her diagnosis, when she first experienced symptoms. She did not tell her frineds, and this is not uncommon among undiagnosed multiple sclerosis patients, because she was certain they would think "I was going out of my mind." In fact, she wondered, too, when her symptoms continued after a year's time and in spite of frequent visits to a doctor, if this was what it was like to be "going out of my mind." When she was finally diagnosed, she recalled, "I felt like I had been brought back into the human race; now I had something other people had."

SUGGESTED QUESTIONS FOR DISCUSSION AND ANALYSIS

For undergraduate students
1. What conditions, in society in general and in your work specifically, foster social isolation in chronically ill patients?
2. What does being socially isolated mean?
3. Do patients want to be helped by others to avoid social isolation, or would they prefer to work it out on their own?

4. Can nurses be of help to patients to alter the course or ameliorate the process of social isolation?
5. Do attitudes of the public about persons who are chronically ill, disabled, and so on, play a part in the process of social isolation? If so, what are these attitudes? How would you go about altering them?

For graduate students and teachers of nursing

1. Do you see intervention in the process of social isolation as a legitimate function for nurses?
2. What organizational arrangements other than what currently exists do you envision could draw on the community and on psychological resources to intervene in the process of social isolation?

20. Beyond medical intervention: strategies for managing life in the face of chronic illness

Laura Reif, RN, MA, MS

Reif's chapter differs from all other ones in the book in that she takes as her point of departure the patient and his illness and from that extrapolates what the work of the nurse must be. It is of interest to note that in Fagerhaugh's chapter on the interview with the supervisor, the supervisor tells us that nurses who work with chronically ill patients in their homes must know the patient and his living situation intimately. Reif directs attention in precisely this direction. She systematically explores and carefully documents (1) how symptoms and medical regimens impinge on daily routines and social activities valued by the patient and (2) equally important, how the patient manages to get along and make a life for himself in the face of these disruptive influences. Reif, a nurse, collected these data as part of her work toward a PhD in sociology.

For the majority of the time the individual who is chronically ill is, just like the rest of us, concerned with getting along as well as he can. In other words, his central aim is to manage his work, his family life, and his social and recreational activities to his satisfaction. Standing in the way of his doing this are the problems associated

I would like to acknowledge Anselm Strauss, Barney Glaser, Leonard Schatzman, and Marcella Davis for their comments, suggestions, and criticism on earlier drafts of this chapter. A shortened and modified version of this chapter appears in the *American Journal of Nursing,* February 1973.

with his chronic illness. Unlike the individual who faces an acute, transitory disease, the person who is chronically ill confronts a condition that is, almost by definition, unresolvable medically and that is likely to have a profound effect on many aspects of his daily living. Given the limitations of current medical approaches to long-term illness, the individual himself is left to cope with many of the physical as well as the social-psychological ramifications of his disease.

Social scientists have long been concerned with the ways in which individuals respond to illness. Much of the work in this area, however, has been confined to investigating how the symptoms of a disease are perceived and the manner in which help is sought to cope with the situation. Although sick persons are viewed as taking an active role in dealing with some of the problems posed by their disease, they are seldom given credit for assuming major responsibility for managing their illness. Unlike disabled or visibly handicapped persons, who are depicted as being centrally involved in coping with the physical and social-psycholgical consequences resulting from their impairments, the sick person is not usually assumed to marshal his resources so effectively. Most often, medical personnel, rather than the sick person, are considered the "prime movers" in the situation. They are usually credited with providing the action and impetus needed to return the individual to normal activity.

While the above description may not be far off the mark for many *acute* illnesses, it applies somewhat less than satisfactorily to the individual who has a *chronic* disease. In this chapter, which focuses on the chronically ill persons, I present a rather different perspective on the activities and circumstances of the sick person. In the case of most chronic illnesses, the following are key elements that characterize the situation.

1. *The sick person is the central figure in efforts to deal with chronic illness.* By this, I do not mean simply that the patient is at the center of the medical treatment program, although that, too, may be important. The activities of the sick person are essential to the management of the problem, and the sick person is in a key position to effect the changes that need to be made to cope with the multiple aspects of the situation.

2. *The individual who is chronically ill is, for the most part, concerned with managing his life.* The ramifications of chronic disease are so extensive and long lasting that sick persons do not, for long, remain exclusively focused on their symptoms and medical regimen. Chronically ill persons are concerned with the overall problem of managing an acceptable life for themselves and are therefore primarily concerned with the impact of illness on day-to-day activities.

3. *The individual with a long-term illness deals with his difficulties by redesigning his life style.* Persons who are chronically ill are likely to face significant constraints that arise from the symptoms of disease, or the treatment program, or both. While medical interventions assist the individual in coping with the situation, they do not handle many of the problems associated with illness and, therefore, cannot serve as the total management scheme. If the individual is to live with his

illness, much depends on his altering the conditions under which he functions and on revising his expectations of the amount and type of activity he can perform. Chronically ill persons accomplish these changes by modifying daily activities and routines, rearranging their environment, and revising their patterns of interaction with others. In essence, they redesign their lives and circumstances in such a way as to compensate for, minimize, or surmount the difficulties they face.

4. *Chronically ill individuals are not only active but often remarkably effective at accomplishing what they would like to do occupationally and socially*. Particular instances of successful adjustment are even more impressive because they illustrate the extent to which sick persons exceed expectations based on medical prognoses.

In this chapter I am using one particular chronic illness as an example of how sick persons ensure acceptable lives for themselves. The disease symptoms and the medical regimen are seen as generating problems that have a substantial impact on the individual's occupational and social activities. The specific difficulties faced by this group of chronically ill persons are identified, as are the strategies they employ to deal with their situation. The implications of the foregoing remarks for the nursing care of persons who are chronically ill are indicated at the conclusion of this chapter.

ULCERATIVE COLITIS AS A CASE IN POINT

The individuals in this discussion were chosen because their disease, ulcerative colitis, was thought to be strikingly illustrative of the problematic character of several general features of chronic illness: (1) the disease symptoms interfere with many normal activities and routines; (2) the medical regimen is limited in its effectiveness; and (3) treatment, although intended to mitigate the symptoms and long-range effects of disease, contributes substantially to the disruption of usual patterns of living.

Medical aspects of ulcerative colitis

The individual who has ulcerative colitis faces an illness that is exceedingly difficult to deal with. To a large extent, this can be attributed to the nature of the disease and, more particularly, to the symptoms with which the individual contends. Ulcerative colitis characteristically manifests itself in the form of severe diarrhea, which means that the sick person is faced with drastically different bowel patterns. Not only are his bowel movements more numerous than before, but they are frequently spaced at very short intervals. Diarrhea often comes on suddenly and erratically, at any time of day or night. To make matters worse, voluntary control of defecation is extremely difficult.

This situation persists for long periods of time, with the illness cycling unpredictably between exacerbations and remissions over the course of many years and, not infrequently, a lifetime. Consequently, in both the immediate present and for the duration of the disease, the individual confronts a condition with an impact **263** on daily activities that is observable, pervasive, and inescapable and with symptoms that often defy prediction and control.

The cause of ulcerative colitis is not known. Medical treatment is aimed at slowing the progress of the disease and preventing physiological crises and death. It does not produce a "cure" in the sense that it removes or directly intervenes with the cause of the illness. Moreover, the regimen varies in its effectiveness; it is often quite limited in the extent to which it can ameliorate symptoms. The medical program, once embarked upon and if pursued as recommended, continues for long periods of time and frequently for the person's lifetime.

For most persons who are chronically ill with ulcerative colitis, the disease stabilizes to the point where treatment can proceed largely on an outpatient basis. There may be acute episodes of illness that require hospitalization; but for the majority of the time, the burden of treatment rests on the daily medical regimen that is implemented by the patient himself in his home.

The specifics of the regimen for ulcerative colitis include a somewhat variable combination of medications, special diet, corticosteroid retention enemas, and lengthy periods of rest. The flexibility and intensity of the regimen *as prescribed* may vary, but in general, strict adherence to the medical program involves constraints of a decidedly nontrivial nature: (1) the regimen is time consuming to learn and to execute; (2) it requires a moderate amount of skill to implement; (3) it necessitates revising usual habits and routines to a significant extent; and (4) it entails requirements that are often physically or psychologically stressful (prescribed drugs may have dangerous or adverse physical effects; procedures may be uncomfortable, painful, or repugnant to perform).

Impact of illness on daily life

It is obvious from the above description that both the symptoms and the medical regimen for ulcerative colitis generate many problems of a technical and physical nature: the individual faces the task of coping with technically difficult procedures, physical discomfort, pain, fatigue, various sorts of physiological disfunction, and even life-threatening episodes. What should also be apparent, however, is that many of the ramifications of this illness are personal and social in character. For the majority of the time, these problems arising from the social-psychological consequences of the illness are the foremost concern of persons chronically ill with ulcerative colitis.

The two major concerns of the sick persons I spoke with were (1) the personal and social consequences of the odor and excrement associated with their illness and (2) the ways in which being chronically ill restricted their use of time. In other words, two features of chronic ulcerative colitis, the odor and excrement it produces and its time-preempting character, generate the major social and psychological problems experienced by those who have this disease.

Pollution problems. It is easy to document how the symptoms of ulcerative colitis and the medical regimen prescribed for this disease lead to these two major concerns. Persons who have ulcerative colitis do, in fact, spend a great deal of time dealing with odor and excrement. It is not overstating the case to say that persons who have this illness face a pollution problem of substantial proportions. A large part of the problem stems from the symptoms: bowel movements are frequent, erratic, unpredictable, and often uncontrollable. Pollution problems are not only associated with symptoms, however; they also accompany various aspects of treatment. The sigmoidoscopic examinations, barium enemas, premonitoring preparations, and especially the daily retention enemas all have a great potential for creating problems with odor and excrement.

Time problems. This illness causes such demands on the individual's time that usual activities and routines are often displaced or crowded out by illness-related concerns. Again, both symptoms and regimen contribute to this difficulty. The individual accords symptoms top priority attention, because the personal and social costs of unchecked pollution are generally so high that few other concerns take precedence.

Dealing with symptoms and executing the medical regimen take large amounts of time, even under the best of circumstances. In addition, diarrhea and regimen procedures often slow the pace of activity through interruption and interference with ongoing tasks and thereby consume even more of the individual's time.

Moreover, the unpredictable occurrence of symptoms and the specific timing required by regimen procedures cut across and into conventional schedules and hours. As a result, many of the sick person's normal routines and time-bound arrangements are disturbed or displaced by the temporal patterning demanded by activities related to the illness.

Specific consequences

Pollution and time are significant concerns for persons with chronic ulcerative colitis because both problems have a tremendous impact on life style; that is, both lead to personal and social consequences of considerable magnitude. The constraints that arise from these two core problems manifest themselves in a wide variety of activities.

Problems with mobility and stigma. Pollution is a problem because it makes getting around from place to place exceedingly difficult, and it creates a potentially stigmatizing situation for the sick person.

Where the individual goes, how he travels, and the amount of time he spends at a particular place are all contingent on the extent to which odor and excrement are problematic for him.

Any social situation is a potentially embarrassing one when there is a chance that odor and excrement might be noticed by others. Even when the individual is understood to be legitimately ill, there is considerable risk that his symptoms will be viewed as repugnant and that he himself will be considered socially unacceptable.

Shortage of time and scheduling problems. As pointed out above, the symptoms

265

and regimen associated with ulcerative colitis complicate the individual's management of time because they consume time, preempt time, and interfere with the structuring of time. The sick person faces constraints of considerable magnitude because time is a scarce commodity, is unpredictable and unreliably available, and is often available at irregular or unconventional hours. As a result, the sick person's time for usual activities is very limited, his schedules and planning are highly variable, and the hours he keeps are unconventional and often subject to last-minute changes.

This means that the sick person can easily be out of pace with his associates, out of phase with the temporal requirements of his work situation, and either unavailable or unreliably available for various time-bound arrangements. Time problems manifest themselves most markedly when the sick person attempts to coordinate his activities and plans with others, tries to meet the time requirements of a conventional job situation, attempts to follow through on tasks, personal commitments, or social occasions that have been scheduled in advance.

Managing the consequences of illness

Ordinarily the task of dealing with the above problems falls largely to the sick person and his lay associates. Medical personnel generally direct their major efforts toward preserving or restoring physical functioning, retarding the deleterious effects of the disease, and preventing or postponing crises and death. While medical intervention is an essential ingredient in the overall management of the illness, additional actions need to be taken if the individual is to function effectively in the social and occupational realms. For the majority of the time, it is the chronically ill person himself who steps in to ensure the effective management of the overall situation.

Redesigning life style to deal with the consequences of illness. Because the sick person is primarily concerned with the consequences the illness has for his life style, the character of his interventions is markedly different from the typical medical approaches to the problem. Strategies largely consist of varying sorts of social and environmental manipulations and self-management tactics. That is, the individual draws upon various resources—personal social, environmental, financial, as well as medical—in order to work out new ways of handling his daily activities. To be specific, sick persons restructure the physical environment, utilize the help of other persons, or purchase special equipment and services in order to maintain themselves socially and occupationally. In addition, they develop ways of managing themselves physically, socially, and psychologically in order to circumvent or overcome their disabilities. For example, medications, dietary restrictions, and special interactional ploys are variously employed in an effort to sustain a normal appearance on the job or in a social situation.

Utilizing medical regimen selectively. It is important to note that the sick person utilizes the medical regimen quite selectively. That is, far from "buying" the treatment package outright, he implements medical recommendations when they

266

are effective for facilitating daily activities. In addition to judging the regimen in terms of its efficacy for improving the illness itself, the sick person evaluates treatment procedures, medications, and other medical interventions according to their costs and benefits for enabling participation in valued activities and ensuring attention to high-priority goals.

Before I delineate the specific strategies utilized by ulcerative colitis patients, I should make a few qualifications. Not all individuals make out equally well in their efforts to cope with their circumstances and not all management strategies are equally viable for all persons. There is, in fact, a great deal of variation among chronically ill persons in the numbers and types of tactics they employ. Differences in life styles, social circumstances, and access to resources such as money, people, information, and time, account for much of this variation. In addition, there are significant differences in the benefits and costs that individuals assign to various modes of coping; cost-effectiveness criteria vary depending on the individual's assessment of what constitutes appropriate behavior, the types of activities he hopes to engage in, the social context within which he operates, and the stage and length of his illness.

The interventions utilized by the persons I interviewed were primarily aimed at intervening on the two core problems, pollution and temporal preemption.

Dealing with pollution problems

Pollution-control tactics employed by the persons I interviewed suggest that at least three approaches to the problem are tanable: (1) preventing diarrhea from occurring in the first place, (2) keeping odor and excrement from being noticed by others (protecting self and others from the disruptive effects of pollution), and (3) correcting damage or disruption resulting from pollution.

Preventive strategies. Individuals who have ulcerative colitis employ a number of different techniques to prevent diarrhea from occurring. The sick person can effect short-term control of symptoms by fasting, regulating his diet, timing when he eats, or in certain instances, using drugs that provide temporary symptomatic relief. Over a long duration of time, he may obtain control of odor and excrement by restricting himself to certain foods, taking medicated enemas regularly, and utilizing a combination of drugs, varied to accommodate for changes in his condition.

While medical interventions figure prominently in such preventive approaches to the problem, it is important to note that the sick person's main purpose in employing a particular aspect of his regimen is to halt or delay the appearance of odor and excrement. In an attempt to obtian this sort of result, some persons use opiates to the point of overdosing themselves, restrict their diets to solid foods when they want to reduce liquid bowel movements, eat very little in order to cut down on the amount of excrement they produce, or avoid medicated enemas or diagnostic procedures that are seen as instigating polution problems. Thus, sick persons do not always utilize the regimen as prescribed, nor do they necessarily employ it for the purposes for which it was intended by health personnel.

267

Protective strategies. Protective strategies allow the individual to keep the odor and excrement accompanying his illness from impinging on others or becoming visible in social situations. Such interventions give the sick person an alternative approach to pollution problems, enabling him to negotiate a large number of situations otherwise closed to him were he to rely solely on preventive measures. The individual lessens the disruptive effects of his illness by (1) separating pollution-control activities in time and space from other pursuits, and (2) concealing odor and excrement so that their presence cannot be detected by others. The specific techniques for accomplishing these measures are many; the essence of the strategy, however, is to create such conditions that odor and excrement can be taken care of while away from other persons.

Persons who have ulcerative colitis carefully map out routes and places according to the accessibility of bathrooms. By restricting movement in space to these "safe" routes, the sick person is able to accomplish pollution control unobtrusively. When activities are not confined to familiar environs or previously mapped territory, the individual employs strategies for casing his new surroundings for the location of toilets. In addition, some sick persons ensure that they will not expose others to pollution by basing activities at home or avoiding travel and social encounters altogether when the risk of pollution is high.

Most ulcerative colitis patients I interviewed utilized some means for concealing and containing odor and excrement so that it would not be apparent or offensive to others until it could be safely and conveniently dealt with. Frequent change of clothing, rubber pants, absorbent pads, and deodorants served this purpose. While the above strategies do not prevent pollution from occurring, they enable the individual to keep its adverse consequences, for both mobility and social interaction, within reasonable limits.

Some persons who have ulcerative colitis utilize the help of one or more friends or associates to help them sustain ongoing interaction or activities despite frequent or abrupt exits from social scene. These persons know about the individual's illness and can serve as "front men." They can be relied on to work in collusion with the sick person, to speak in his behalf to conceal his disability, to explain or justify his unconventional behavior, to ensure his "normal" identity with other people. Protective strategies are often considerably more effective when coupled with the "fronting" or covering performed by the sick person's allies.

Corrective strategies. Correcting the physical damage or social disruption occasioned by pollution is viewed by some individuals as less costly in terms of time and effort than interrupting on ongoing activity. On other occasions such an approach to pollution is unavoidable; preventive and protective measures are not always effective or timely. Moreover, some individuals would rather tolerate the embarrassment of their problems being exposed to others than live in partial or total isolation. In any event, most persons who have chronic colitis have tactics for managing circumstances in which their problem is visible to others.

268   The individual who regularly has recourse to this approach is adept at

minimizing the deleterious effects of pollution on himself and others. Such a person is a master of the art of fast change of dress. He uses washable clothing and easy-to-clean work areas to help him repair disguises and environs with dispatch. He can deftly negotiate his way through an embarassing social situation, helping others retain their composure while he keeps his own.

Many individuals rely on the services of "front men" to supplement or ensure the effectiveness of corrective tactics. In addition, post-factum strategies are frequently buttressed by advance preparations. For instance, the individual who realizes his control of pollution is tenuous may select or educate his "audience" beforehand so that if an incident occurs it will not be entirely unexpected by those who witness it.

Managing time

The individual who has ulcerative colitis also ensures his occupational and social functioning by managing his time effectively. The chief aims of persons I interviewed were to conserve a reasonable amount of time for normal activity and to schedule time, given unpredictable and highly variable circumstances.

Time-conserving tactics. The patients I interviewed budgeted their time in an effort to utilize it more effectively. Time was portioned out in terms of priorities. Generally this took the form of explicitly designating (1) how activities ranked with respect to each other along a temporal-priority scale, (2) what minimum or maximum amounts of time would be spent on specific types of activity, and (3) what activities could be left until last or cut out completely should the person run out of time. These considerations provided the sick person with guidelines for the use of time, when and if it was available.

Another prevalent time-saving technique employed by the patients I spoke with involved the routinization and streamlining of illness-related activities. Routines incorporated certain time- and labor-saving devices that allowed the individual to handle symptoms and regimen as expeditiously as feasible. Individuals simplified procedural techniques, modified room arrangements, improvised special equipment, and kept stocks of needed supplies in order to shorten the time spent on illness. On occasion, persons economized further by omitting aspects of their regimen altogether in order to conserve time for other activities.

In addition to reclaiming time for normal pursuits by spending less time on symptoms and regimen, the individuals I interviewed made the most of time by "piggy backing" normal activity onto disease-related activity. For example, many individuals set up the bathroom as an auxiliary work area and set aside certain "lap work" that could be done while they were seated on the toilet. In other instances, individuals arranged necessary items so they could read, dress, shave, or put on makeup while they were occupied with symptoms. The time-consuming postenema rest period was also used for various sorts of activity. One self-employed man routinely handled his billing and bookkeeping while he was indisposed in this way.

Many sick persons were able to increase the pace of work and in so doing   **269** telescoped activities into shorter periods of time. Other individuals organized themselves in such a way that they could fill available time on the spur of the moment by plugging in a standby activity.

Strategies for scheduling time. Individuals who have ulcerative colitis cannot rely on conventional patterns and routines to structure time; if they do, the interruptions that result from symptoms and regimen requirements are likely to upset many, if not most, of their plans. One way in which these persons schedule time is by monitoring their illness, then working out a temporal routing that tailors the timing of disease-related and social-occupational activities to one another. By observing how often bowel movements occur, how long they last, and the amount of leeway between warning and appearance of diarrhea, most sick persons can predict how much time is available, when it is most likely to be available, and what period of time can be spent in uninterrupted activity. These individuals are then able to exploit time most free from both symptoms and regimen requirements to do what they would like to do.

The success of this type of temporal routing, however, is contingent on the individual's remaining flexible in scheduling time for normal pursuits; that is, normal activities must be fitted to the constraints of the illness. The sick person's chief strategy is to create such conditions that he can exercise greater control over the scheduling of work and social activities. If he can carry out his daily routines at his own pace and on his own time, he can generally avoid their being vitiated by illness-related activity. In an effort to do this, the individuals I spoke with worked out temporal arrangements with employers, work associates, family members, and friends. Some individuals had accomplished this to a remarkable extent. As a result, they were able to work at their jobs at irregular hours, work by contract or on a piece-rate basis, and, in general, complete tasks at their own pace.

Most persons traded off tasks or work times with associates so that they could put in time when it was convenient to do so. Many individuals had elaborate backup systems, so that if they were unable to follow through on a scheduled activity, another person would substitute for them. On occasion, sick persons worked with other individuals in a "buddy" arrangement. The buddy (whether work associate, friend, or family member) accommodated himself to the unconventional schedule and pace of the ill person and so ensured coordination of activities.

In addition, persons who have colitis often made special arrangements with close friends and family so that they can deal flexibly with social occasions. These individuals are familiar with the sick person's unpredictable symptoms and could frequently make last-minute adjustments to accommodate for changes in his plans.

It is apparent from the above discussion how important the assistance of other persons is to the sick person as he attempts to schedule time effectively. In instances where an individual cannot ensure coverage and coordination through the buddying or backup activities of friends and associates, it is usually necessary for him to drastically modify, if not completely curtail, certain activities. Ultimately, this might involve switching jobs, quitting work, or cutting out social and recreational activities.

As an alternative to this, many individuals who have chronic colitis intervene by modifying the temporal dimensions of activities related to the illness. That is, they attempt to regulate or delay the time spent dealing with symptoms and regimen in an effort to work out a more conventional allocation of time. This is generally most easily accomplished with regimen requirements for which time and timing can usually be adjusted. Most individuals attempt to implement regimen procedures at times that do not conflict with their normal routines.

As might be anticipated, symptoms are more difficult to time. It will be recalled, however, that these individuals employ various strategies for dealing with pollution. These strategies serve equally well as tactics for timing symptoms. That is, pollution control strategies allow the individual to stretch time by staving off symptoms or putting off the time that odor and excrement are dealt with. For example, by delaying a meal or wearing absorbent clothing, the individual could ensure the time necessary to make it through a social occasion or to follow through on a previously made commitment.

Consequences of effective management

In the course of developing and employing various approaches to problems generated by the illness, the sick person substantially redesigns his life style. That is the individual, over time, refines his strategies until ultimately he works out a series of new routines that allow him to carry out most activities to his satisfaction. Activities, once conceived as strategies for managing the problems posed by illness, come to be viewed by the individual as part of his usual style of living. At this point, the individual no longer thinks of himself as dealing with a situation that is out of the ordinary; nor does he see himself as having to create special conditions in order to function effectively. He simply sees himself as getting along well. This is not to say that the individual's life is as it would have been had illness not intervened; nor is it to assert that he leads a "normal" existence "like everyone else." It means that he is able to minimize many of the constraints of his symptoms and regimen and that he feels he can live with his chronic illness.

Implications for nursing

The model explicated in this chapter is a departure from the traditional way of viewing the sick person and his circumstances. The conventional medical perspective defines the medical problems as central, the goal as managing illness, the central managers as the medical personnel, and the central activity as medical intervention. The model I have presented identifies as central the consequences of illness—social and occupational, as well as medical; the goal, managing life in the face of chronic illness; the central actor-manager, the sick person; and the central action, redesigning of life style coupled with medical intervention.

My major purpose in presenting specific material on one long-term disease was　**271** to illustrate the extent to which illness impinges on the daily life of the chronically ill person and how effective the chronically ill person can be at managing the social and occupational ramifications of his illness. I pointed out that chronic illnesses generate very specific social-psychological problems for the sick person and that medical treatment and the regimen, as well as the disease itself, contribute to these difficulties.

The foregoing remarks have a number of implications for nursing. Nurses could help improve the situation of chronically ill persons if they were to give systematic attention to the social, personal, and occupational consequences of chronic illness and assist the sick person by facilitating the medical management of his chronic disease. Nurses do currently attend to these activities, but clinicians could be more effective if they had systematic guidelines for both the social-psychological and medical counseling of chronically ill persons.

The following concrete suggestions indicate the variety of ways in which nurses might specifically address these two areas. Nurses can help patients cope more effectively with the social and occupational impact of chronic illness by (1) inquiring about the specific social and occupational problems the patient has and counseling him in strategies for dealing with these difficulties; (2) directing the patient to professional resource persons who might assist him with problems outside nursing expertise (the social worker, dietitian, rehabilitation therapist, or vocational counselor could serve in this capacity); (3) helping the patient to develop lay support systems by educating family, friends, and employers to be aware of the sick person's specific limitations and needs for help; and (4) utilizing chronically ill persons as resources; the perspectives and experiences of persons with chronic diseases could be shared with other patients directly or via a nurse.

Nurses can also assist the patient to manage the medical aspects of his care and lessen the impact of the regimen on day-to-day activities. This might be accomplished by (1) obtaining information from the patient on the ways in which the regimen impinges on his activities and assisting him to tailor medical interventions so that they fit into his usual routines more readily; (2) showing the patient how to streamline medical management, teaching him ways of overcoming the technical difficulties involved in executing the regimen; and (3) providing counseling on the cost effectiveness of various aspects of the regimen, indicating priorities for investment of time in medically relevant intervention.

There is a great need for research designed to identify the specific ways in which various chronic diseases impinge on the lives of patients. The information obtained from such research, if put into readily accessible form, could immeasurably assist nurses in their efforts to counsel chronically ill persons. Until the time when more information of this kind is available, nurses should be encouraged to look beyond purely medical intervention to alternative strategies that would help chronically ill persons to manage their lives.

SUGGESTED QUESTIONS FOR DISCUSSION AND ANALYSIS

For undergraduate students

1. What activities would you anticipate might be problematic for an individual who has been disabled by a myocardial infarction, stroke, emphysema, multiple sclerosis, diabetes, or arthritis?

2. A chronically ill adult being seen regularly in the outpatient clinic reveals to you that he is not carrying out some aspects of his medical regimen. How might you find out why this is occurring? What might you do about it?

   a. What aspects of the medical regimen would you anticipate would be problematic for a person with heart disease, emphysema, diabetes, tuberculosis, or ulcerative colitis?

   b. How might the medical procedures prescribed for a patient with one of the above illnesses be viewed as problematic by members of his household or by his employer? In what ways might the patient's regimen impinge on these persons or their activities?

   c. How might the nurse lessen the impact of the regimen on the patient and his associates? Give specific examples of how this might be accomplished, using a patient with one of the diseases mentioned above.

3. How might a nurse go about providing social-psychological and medical counseling to chronically ill persons (a) in a hospital setting, (b) in an extended-care facility such as a nursing home or a residential treatment center, (c) in an outpatient facility, (d) in a private doctor's office, or (e) at home? In what ways might her orientation and activities differ depending on the setting in which she and the sick person interact?

4. What services *outside* the medical system might be useful to persons who are chronically ill? How might the nurse facilitate access to these resources?

5. How can nurses employ the information gained from persons who are chronically ill to help other patients faced with the same sorts of difficulties?

For graduate students and teachers of nursing

1. What knowledge and skills would enable the nurse to be more effective in her work with chronically ill persons and their families? What clinical assignments might provide her the necessary experience?

2. How would you go about incorporating the function of a social-psychological counselor into the job of a nurse currently working as (a) a clinical specialist, (b) a primary care agent for a group of chronically ill persons coming to an outpatient facility, (c) a discharge planner for a hospital unit designed for the care of acute phases of chronic diseases, or (d) a nurse in charge of a residential treatment center housing chronically ill and aged persons?

3. What changes would you make in medical settings (such as a hospital, an outpatient clinic, or an extended-care facility) to improve the variety and quality of services provided for chronically ill persons?

4. How would you go about informing and encouraging other professionals about using service agencies and community groups?